The first book of its kind, this collection contains a variety of classic essays and seminal works by researchers from many disciplines, as well as policy statements and research guidelines from professional and governmental bodies. Among the issues considered are: the norms of ethical conduct in science and their origins; scientific honesty, skepticism, and self-deception; the ethical standards of laboratory practice; the use of human and animal subjects; the qualifications for authorship and publication; the ethics of learning and teaching; and the relationships of science, industry, and society.

This anthology is intended for a general audience of students and professionals in the biological sciences whose education has included both theoretical and laboratory work. It is especially useful for graduate students and postdoctoral fellows, and is ideal for faculty responsible for teaching ethics in science as required by federal training grants. Introductory essays, questions for discussion, and references for additional reading that accompany each section not only provide a helpful framework in which to consider the readings, but also stimulate readers to reflect on broader contexts and their own personal experience.

The Ethical Dimensions of the Biological Sciences

The Ethical Dimensions of the Biological Sciences

Edited by

RUTH ELLEN BULGER
Institute of Medicine, National Academy of Sciences

ELIZABETH HEITMAN
University of Texas Health Science Center at Houston

STANLEY JOEL REISER
University of Texas Health Science Center at Houston

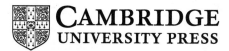

CAMBRIDGE
UNIVERSITY PRESS

Published by the Press Syndicate of the University of Cambridge
The Pitt Building, Trumpington Street, Cambridge CB2 1RP
40 West 20th Street, New York, NY 10011-4211, USA
10 Stamford Road, Oakleigh, Victoria 3166, Australia

© Cambridge University Press 1993

First published 1993

Printed in Canada

Library of Congress Cataloging-in-Publication Data
The Ethical dimensions of the biological sciences / edited by Ruth
Ellen Bulger, Elizabeth Heitman, and Stanley Joel Reiser.
p. cm.
Includes bibliographical references.
ISBN 0-521-43463-7 (hardback). – ISBN 0-521-43599-4 – (pbk.)
1. Bioethics. I. Bulger, Ruth Ellen. II. Heitman, Elizabeth.
III. Reiser, Stanley Joel.
QH332.E73 1993
174'.9574 – dc20   92-26258

A catalog record for this book is available from the British Library.

ISBN: 0–521–43463–7 hardback
ISBN: 0–521–43599–4 paperback

Contents

Preface

Biological science has become a public enterprise. While biologic discovery continues to be a product of private and group work in laboratory and research centers, the social and economic effects of these discoveries have drawn the attention of powerful public constituencies – government, industry, legislatures, and the population at large – whose support is crucial to maintaining the scientific endeavor.

This new position of biomedical science is epitomized by a recent cover story from *Time* magazine, which portrayed science as "under a microscope" and "under siege." The review outlined a "crisis" brought on by "a budget squeeze and bureaucratic demands, internal squabbling, harassment by activists, embarrassing cases of fraud and failure, and the growing alienation of Congress and the public."[1] The fact that the topic could generate sufficient public interest to warrant an eight-page feature in an international magazine is itself a large part of the story.

As the discoveries of bioscience foster profound changes in our view of ourselves and our ability to overcome threats to human health, and create enormous investment opportunities for entrepreneurs, bioscience is increasingly perceived as an essential social enterprise that requires both the support and decision-making involvement of those outside of the scientific community. For students and professional researchers to live in this new environment successfully, they need the knowledge necessary to understand it.

Researchers' difficulties over the past decade in sorting out the ethical questions involved in their work make a strong case for explicit teaching about these problems in the course of professional training. The scientific community's experience in dealing with fraud in research has demonstrated that faculty and students need a forum in which to discuss the ethical issues that may arise in a scientist's career. Ethics enters into basic questions that scientists face continuously, from their responsibilities to the human and animal subjects of their research to the social consequences of their discoveries.

Until recently, many scientists have seemed content to leave such education in ethics to the role-model format: older scientists transmitting standards to younger ones by their demeanor and through random conversations and actions. But as has been well demonstrated in clinical medicine, role models, though important, are not sufficient to educate students in the complex ethical problems of modern science.

A crucial feature of disciplines that call themselves professions is systematic reflection about the ethical traditions that govern them and their relationship with society. Such reflection is critical to fostering the public trust that sustains the professions' right of self-regulation and claims of authenticity. The consideration of the ethical dimensions of science as part of the curriculum of scientific learning and research can be tangible evidence that the scientific community warrants public trust, and can serve as a major underpinning for ethical behavior in science.

Although the scientific community is developing ways to respond to unprofessional behavior, too little attention has been given to the place of education in preventing it. The time has arrived, as public and scientific concern about fraud has demonstrated, for scientists to consider formally, through scholarship and classroom teaching, the ethical context of their work.

In 1985, prompted by an ethical conflict involving a student, and encouraged by R. W. Butcher, the dean of our graduate school of biomedical sciences, we developed a course to provide such instruction; the course has since been required of all entering graduate students in the biomedical sciences. We believed then, and believe more strongly after eight years of experience, that the lack of systematic teaching about the nature of scientific discovery and the scientist's life in the context of ethics, leads to ambiguity about the moral aspects of gathering, interpreting, and reporting evidence; the social responsibilities of science; and the personal obligations of scientists to their colleagues, their discipline, and themselves.

The course that we designed does not enumerate standards that students must adopt or commit to memory; rather, it attempts to stimulate students' interest and to provoke them to further reading and consideration of the issues and their implications. Although honesty, integrity, truth, and professional responsibility are all key elements of the course, they are complemented by considerations of creativity, the process of discovery, and the implications of Pasteur's dictum that "In the field of experimentation, chance favors only the prepared mind."[2] The very existence of the course, and the fact that entering graduate students in biomedical sciences are required to attend it, demonstrates to students the commitment of the institution to examining ethical values within the scientific process.

A similar educational requirement has now been accepted as part of the administrative guidelines for the National Research Service Award institutional training grant applications submitted to the Alcohol, Drug Abuse, and Mental Health Administration and the National Institutes of Health (NIH). As stated in the NIH *Guide for Grants and Contracts,* a program concerned with the understanding of the concepts of scientific integrity must be a part of any proposed research training effort.[3] The guidelines, however, make no concrete recommendations for either the format or the content of such a program, leaving many directors puzzled about compliance.

To share the benefits of our experience with such a program, we developed this volume of readings, commentaries, and questions. The book attempts to do two things. First, it presents in one place a variety of readings organized according to several fundamental topics of ethics in science. Second, the introductory essays and discussion questions in each section provide a focus on aspects that we believe warrant particular consideration.

The book introduces students to the norms of ethical conduct in science as established by the profession and by legislative bodies; scientific honesty and its relationship to objectivity and self-deception; professional policies of coauthorship and plagiarism; the use of human beings and animals in research; the relationship between science, scientists, and society; and the ethics of teaching and learning. The readings also provide an opportunity to discuss other issues basic to research but often not formally considered in graduate science education, such as: methods of scientific investigation (and scientists' difficulty thinking outside the paradigm upon which their own work is based); the creative process; and the problem of describing reality.

The three faculty members who selected the readings and prepared the introductory essays, and who have been responsible for the course from which they come, include a bench scientist now working in health sciences policy, an ethicist in medicine and the professions, and a physician/historian of science. The material is intended to be accessible to students and faculty from a wide variety of backgrounds and expertise.

We have used a number of formats in teaching this material. For some subjects we used predominantly lecture, while other sessions were led in a Socratic style; however, time has always been reserved for group discussion, and the readings provide many issues for debate. In class we have also supplemented these readings with material from our own academic environment. For example, to consider using animals in research, the students served as an Animal Care and Use Committee, reviewing a fictitious application on the forms used by our institution. Since all our students have worked in a laboratory, their actual experiences have also been a focus for discussion. We recommend that the general material in this book be tailored similarly to the specific needs and situations of the students and institutions that will use it.

Our anthology would not have been possible without the support and assistance of a number of people. We would like to thank, in particular, R. W. Butcher, Kristin Heitman, James M. Berry, Kara McArthur, and Janice Glover for their efforts on behalf of this project.

R.E.B., E.H., and S.J.R.

Notes

1. Nash, J. Madeleine, & Thompson, Dick, "Crisis in the Labs," *Time,* Vol. 138, No. 8, August 26, 1991, p. 44.
2. Pasteur, Louis, quoted in Hilaire Cuny, *Louis Pasteur: A Man and His Theories,* Patrick Evans (trans.), New York: Fawcett World Library, 1963, p. 149.
3. NIH Guide for Grants and Contracts, Vol. 18, No. 45, December 22, 1989.

Overview

The ethics movement in the biological sciences: A new voyage of discovery

Stanley Joel Reiser

The modern voyage to chart the ethical bases of the biological sciences is an important episode in its history and also in the annals of society. Its purpose has been to identify, for biological scientists from different disciplines who probe human function and for the surrounding society, principles for setting the goals of this research, creating the resultant knowledge, and influencing its subsequent use. This essay traces seminal events of this journey, which began near the midpoint of the twentieth century, and seeks to identify directions the journey may take as it continues on a course into the future. This passage has occurred in four phases, in each of which biological scientists have altered a fundamental relationship: in the first phase with the individual research subject, in the second with society, in the third with their research procedures, and in the fourth with their institutions of learning.

Phase I   1945–1966: Fathoming the human subject

Revelations emerging from the Nuremberg War Crimes Trials at the end of World War II disclosed the forced induction of prisoners of war and civilians into experiments that injured and killed many. These activities were officially sanctioned and promoted by government authorities of the Nazi regime, and conducted by scientists and physicians. To prevent future harm to subjects of human studies, instruct investigators about the ethical precepts needed to protect subjects, and delineate the responsibilities of investigators to carry out these goals, a set of ten principles was developed by the war crimes staff. It came to be called the Nuremberg Code.

The code focused on giving the potential subject of an experiment the opportunity to decide whether to participate. It enumerated the conditions necessary to assure the freedom and capacity of individuals to make this choice. This included the absence of a coercive environment that would hinder choice, the presence of a mental capability and adequate data about harms and benefits that would facilitate choice, and the freedom of the subject to withdraw at any time from the experiment. The code made investigators responsible for assuring the adequacy of the consent process, the scientific credibility and safety of the experiment, the qualifications of those conducting the experiment, and the ending of an experiment when the likelihood of injury or death to subjects emerged.[1]

With the code in hand, and the consequences of moral insensitivity to the possibilities of harm in human studies so starkly taught, biological scientists believed that major ethical problems now could be avoided or adequately handled if they occurred. As they entered the 1950s they also were caught up in the excitement of a period of unsurpassed growth in biomedical research. This was a time when the public accepted scientists as benevolent

1

experts, whom they trusted to select the projects and determine the goals of science. Biological science was a good of which the public wanted more, and they were willing to give considerable sums of money for this purpose. The National Institutes of Health (NIH) became a major scientific funder in the postwar period, its grants rising from $75 million in 1948 to $150 million in 1954.[2] Understandably, the research community wished to focus on scientific questions. Hence the 1950s produced little commentary about the ethical issues of human studies or the relation of the biological sciences to society.

However, in the 1950s a small group of lawyers was interested in strengthening legal protections for human subjects. They attempted to encourage research organizations in the United States to build on the ideas in the Nuremberg Code. They urged scientists to seek ways to refine scientific practices used in human studies, and to develop innovative principles to guide the research. But as one of these lawyers, William Curran, now Professor Emeritus of Legal Medicine at Harvard, writes of his efforts in the 1950s to gain attention to research ethics: "We had only very limited success in this ambitious undertaking. We were working at a time somewhat before the researchers were ready to believe such action was necessary."[3]

Attitudes changed in the 1960s. The catalysts were the discovery of particular cases in which investigators disregarded the canons of the Nuremberg Code, the burgeoning civil rights movement that heightened social sensitivity to the needs of vulnerable groups, and legislative and regulatory actions that changed the procedure of research on human subjects.

A case that drew wide attention occurred in 1963, when three physicians experimentally injected live cancer cells into twenty-two elderly and debilitated in-patients at the Jewish Chronic Disease Hospital in Brooklyn to determine whether such patients would reject such cells. Several physicians opposing this experiment and particularly concerned that the subjects never consented to participate brought the matter to the hospital's board of trustees. One of these physicians took the hospital to court to see the records of involved patients. In the complicated proceedings that followed, several of the study's investigators contended that a doctor could rightfully withhold data that patients might find threatening. This position was not upheld when the Board of Regents of the State University of New York reviewed the case. It asserted the investigators had an experimental, not a thera-peutic, relationship with subjects. Thus no basis existed for the exercise of the "usual professional judgment applicable to patient care."[4] As the story unfolded in the media, however, there was public and professional surprise and consternation that existing ethical principles of scientific research had not prevented the occurrence of such an experiment.

Federal interest in this subject had emerged a year earlier in 1962. A group of U.S. senators devoted to civil rights issues and led by New York Senator Jacob Javits added a requirement to the Food, Drug, and Cosmetic Act being amended that year. It mandated investigators of experimental drugs to obtain a formal consent from subjects in their trials. In 1965, more pressure for reform was introduced. In March of that year Harvard anes-thesiologist Henry Beecher delivered a paper at a conference in which he cited cases in the published literature showing disregard of the consent process in human experiments. This speech, published in 1966 as an essay, received widespread coverage in the public media. In December 1965 The National Advisory Council to the NIH added its weight to the issue, and went much further than had the food and drug legislation. It announced that guidelines would be developed requiring prior review of all research protocols on human subjects before a study could begin. A February 1966 memorandum from the

U.S. Surgeon General spelled out what these guidelines would mean. Scientists now would be required to obtain an informed consent from all research subjects and provide an assessment of the possible harms and benefits of the studies they proposed. Evaluation of this material would be given to a group of peers within the investigator's institution. In a July 1966 revision these institutions were made responsible for assuring that all research funded in them by the NIH met its review requirements.[3] The panels became known as Institutional Review Boards, or IRBs.

With the IRBs in place, the private world of the individual investigator was opened not only to peers but to social others, as the membership on IRBs became enlarged to include community participants who were not scientists. The IRB requirement made investigators consider and discuss explicitly with subjects ethical questions connected with their research. This discourse, involving issues of consent and the risks and benefits of medical interventions, dovetailed with and further stimulated consideration of these matters in clinical medicine. Indeed the scientists whom such regulations involved often worked in the milieu of hospitals where human subjects could be recruited from among patients. Accordingly these events influenced investigators doing basic and applied research in the clinical community more than it did those working on biologic questions in laboratories removed from patient care.

This 1945–1966 period began as the era of the individual in the biological sciences. In the 1940s and 1950s social authority was used to free both the individual scientist and the research subject. The NIH increasingly freed scientists from monetary constraints to pursue their research projects; the Nuremberg Code liberated research subjects from the authority of scientists to decide their own welfare. However, in the 1960s, the introduction of the IRB diminished the scientist's authority to determine the content of research procedures used on the human subject, while it further enhanced the self-determination of the subject.

Phase II 1966–1974: The social engagement of biological scientists

While the first part of this ethics movement focused on the danger of the scientist's work to particular individuals, the second part emphasized its threat to society at large. In the context of exploring potential social threats, a searching examination was conducted concerning the respective roles of the public, government, and investigators in deciding the course of scientific work that posed a possible threat to populations. This phase began in the mid-1960s and lasted about a decade.

The proximal antecedents of this phase were calls of alarm in the early 1960s by a number of prominent intellectuals such as Lewis Mumford, Jacques Ellul, and Raymond Aron. They and others were concerned about the growing hegemony of science in determining the course of civilization. Through innovations in transportation, communication, and warfare science was altering basic patterns of life, and scientists were becoming the quintessential experts of society. As the power over the way society lived flowed to the experts upon whose scientific knowledge social change was based, anxiety arose about the ability of the laity to question their authority. Raymond Aron wondered whether democracy could function in this situation. How, he asked, could legislators, politicians, or the electorate evaluate the complex facets of social problems when the most basic knowledge about them increasingly fell into the domain of the scientific expert? He worried that democratic institutions were threatened by the emerging dominance of a scientific elite.[5]

Ironically, this problem stemmed in part from the retreat of scientists from political dialogue and not their entrance into it. Scientists, including those in the sphere of biology, generated these transforming innovations without a clear view of the changes their work produced. They largely were unprepared to discuss the social consequences of their innovations when called into public forums for this purpose. Scientists held the knowledge to create transforming social change, but lacked the understanding or will to evaluate its influence on social institutions or values. They exercised power, but seemed unwilling and unable to take responsibility for its effects.

The main exceptions in this period were found in the community of atomic scientists. During the late 1940s and 1950s J. Robert Oppenheimer, Leo Szilard, and other leading physicists urged scientists to participate in discussing the use of their innovations. But the example of the physicists was not widely followed in other scientific disciplines. Scientists for the most part stayed out of social controversies for several important reasons. Too much involvement would take time away from the reading, reflection, and experimental work that made them "expert" in the first place: an excessive public profile threatened their scientific status. Public discourse required oversimplification of complex issues, and too much public exposure could turn scientists into celebrities. These effects could taint their image as detached analysts. Further, their training did not prepare them intellectually or emotionally for the social and political forums of public debate. Some worried, rightly, that when they entered into social debate, they descended from the platform of the expert to the ground of the layperson.[6]

However, by the mid-1960s a small number of biologists and medical scientists began actively to embark on an involvement in social issues. They were joined by a public grown increasingly interested in and perturbed about the power of the biological sciences to alter human life. The trust that the public had imposed on the scientist to decide alone what research to pursue was fading. In no aspect of biology and medicine was this concern deeper than in genetics.

The modern scientific transformation of this field had occurred in 1953 when James D. Watson and Francis H. C. Crick described the structure of DNA. This development made possible dramatic advances in understanding the architecture and function of human genes. During the 1960s, particularly the latter half of the decade, discussions were held in growing numbers on the ethical, social, and medical consequences of this research. Concerns grew that a second eugenics movement would emerge as more was learned more about genetic functions. Worry began to compete with exhilaration about what the knowledge might bring. One of the earliest efforts to study these issues began in 1966. A small research group at the newly created Harvard Program on Technology and Society was formed to explore the social implications of advances in the biomedical sciences. The group convened conferences that brought together scientists, humanists, and policy experts. A book describing its early work noted that the issues being addressed had "to do specifically with the social control of the new biomedical technologies. . . . They relate to how science and technology can be used to social advantage. . . . It is evident that what were once considered exclusively professional decisions are increasingly coming to be regarded as decisions that need to be made by the larger society."[7]

As the 1960s came to an end, popular books began to appear that portrayed the threatening sides of the emerging understanding of biological function. A typical one, by the journalist Gordon Rattay Taylor was called, ominously, *The Biological Time Bomb*. The titles of its eight chapters tell its story: "Where Are Biologists Taking Us?" (a chapter describing how biological knowledge is outpacing society's ability to control it), "Is Sex Necessary?" (a view of test-tube babies), "The Modified Man" (a look at transplantation), "Is Death Necessary?" (prolonging life through hibernation and freezing), "New Minds for Old" (manipulating emotions, memory, and intelligence), "The Genetic Engineers" (the possibilities of genetic surgery and eugenics), "Can We Create Life?" (making cells and viruses), "The Future, If Any" (social discord as the above innovations mature). In this and in similar publications, analogies were made between the possible destructive force of biological discoveries and the problems caused by the knowledge of atomic energy. The book's cover included a quote from Arthur Koestler from which its title apparently was taken: "Biology is just reaching the critical point of sudden acceleration which physics reached a generation ago . . . the biological time bomb is about to explode in our face."[8]

These concerns extended into the 1970s. In 1971, ethicist Joseph Fletcher made a comment about genetic research that mirrored an emerging social fear that biological knowledge could be used to harm or control society: "Even though its medical aim were only to gain control over the basic "stuff" of our human constitution it could no doubt also be turned into an instrument of political power."[9]

It was against this background of rising anxiety that in 1971, a member of the research staff of the Cold Spring Harbor Laboratory, Robert Pollack, telephoned Stanford biochemist Paul Berg. He called to discuss his concern with Berg's research to determine if the simian virus 40 could be used to transfer a foreign gene into bacteria. Because it had been shown that this virus produced tumors in hamsters, Pollack worried about the consequences of placing it into a strain of bacteria that grew in the human intestine, such as the widely used *Escherichia coli,* the one that Berg had intended to employ. Given the possibility that the virus could cause tumors in the human population, Pollack asked whether more knowledge was needed before conducting such an experiment. After much consultation Berg decided two things: He would postpone the experiment, and he would seek to convene a conference on the hazards of using tumor viruses. The conference was held in January 1973, at Asilomar, California, with about 100 scientists attending and Berg as chair. The meeting concluded that firm evidence of hazards of laboratory viruses inducing cancer was not available, but that caution should be used in work with these viruses.

Later in 1973, the ability to splice and recombine different DNAs became possible. On first learning of this possibility at a Gordon research conference in New Hampshire, several scientists became alarmed. As Donald Frederickson writes, they reacted "to this hint that biology was approaching something akin to the nuclear physicists' chilling arrival at 'critical mass.' " Maxine Singer of the NIH and Dieter Söll of Yale drafted a letter, with the backing of others attending the meeting, to the National Academy of Sciences. It asked the academy to convene a committee to study the consequences of making biological alterations such as joining DNA from animal viruses with DNA from bacteria. "In this way," they wrote, "new kinds of hybrid plasmids or viruses, with biological activity of unpredictable nature, may eventually be created."[10]

The letter, and a general societal concern that this work posed a potential threat, produced a second Asilomar Conference held in September 1974, chaired again by Paul Berg. Its explicitly announced purposes were threefold: to review progress on research on recombinant DNA molecules; to discuss whether what were called "the biohazards of the work" still required a "pause" in certain of its aspects; and to decide how to conduct this research with minimal risk to laboratory workers, the public, and plants and animals.[11]

The conferees produced a set of guidelines for recombinant DNA research. It specified that the research should proceed, but that biological and physical safeguards were to be used to contain the new organisms it generated. The biological barriers were bacterial hosts that could not survive in the material environment, and vectors able to grow only in specified hosts. The physical barriers were containment technologies – for instance, gloves, hoods, and filters – applied in a strategy that matched the level of containment to the risk of the experiment. However, experiments involving highly pathogenic organisms were to be deferred until more knowledge was gained. These guidelines were to be implemented by codes of practice in different countries. But until such codes were developed, scientists as individuals were to decide on how to comply. A clear statement also was made about the ethical duties of principal investigators to their staff: they were to inform the staff fully about the hazards of experiments before initiating them, assure they were properly trained in containment procedures, and monitor their health.

Like the events that led to the creation of the IRBs, Asilomar reflected a growing public need for a voice in shaping the research agenda of biological science. In this sense, as Dorothy Nelkin argues, Asilomar was a challenge to the autonomy of biological science.[12] But Asilomar also stood for the recognition by a small vanguard of biological scientists that consideration of effects of their work on society should be a factor in developing the scientific agenda. Perhaps most fundamental, concern over the social harms and benefits of biological science became appreciated more widely in the 1970s as a shared responsibility of scientists and the public. However, this phase is marked more by the public's growing interest in biological science than by scientists' concern with public issues. The large majority of scientists still were focused on performing their basic work in the laboratory.

Phase III   1975–1989: Challenges to the process of creating knowledge

The third part of the ethics movement, which directed attention to the procedures within the biological sciences used to generate and transmit knowledge, had four distinct components. It began in 1975 with the publication of Peter Singer's book *Animal Liberation;* continued with the highly publicized events of 1981 when John Darsee, a scientist at Harvard Medical School, admitted to falsifying scientific data; kept on into mid-decade with the growth of large project grants for the biological sciences made possible by its new relation with industry, and the development of social interest in the human genome project; and concluded in 1989 when the NIH and the Alcohol, Drug Abuse, and Mental Health Administration (ADAMHA) published a requirement that a program on principles of scientific integrity be given to students by institutions receiving their grants. The growing density of events perceived as ethical issues by the biological sciences community marks this phase as one of greater openness of that community toward ethical discourse and reflection. By the end of Phase III the stage was set for the development of a collective self-consciousness among biological scientists about the moral dimensions of their work, and a greater understanding of why public accountability should be important to them.

In 1975, with a number of worldwide movements for human rights as background, Peter Singer published his book *Animal Liberation*. In it he disputed commonly held views about animals, such as the belief that they lack the capacity to suffer. He argued that the human claim to a right to life should be extended to animals, whom society should not cause to suffer regardless of particular characteristics (or lack of them) they might have. He urged us to "bring non-human animals within our sphere of moral concern and cease to treat their lives as expendable."[13]

This book, and the rights-conscious social environment fostered by the civil rights and medical ethics movements, were important catalysts of a re-examination of the ethical issues concerning animals in experimental work that occurred in the 1980s. Groups emerged such as the Animal Legal Defense Fund, The International Society for Animal Rights, and the Coalition to End Animal Suffering in Experiments. By 1986, eighty bills dealing with the use of animals in research had been introduced in state legislatures around the United States.[14] By the decade's end, federal legislation had extended to animals protections similar to those given human subjects in the mid–1960s. Institutional review boards to examine all experiments involving animals from the viewpoint of humane treatment now were required. However, the controversy over their appropriate use continued, marked by heated discussions and even violent entries by activists into laboratories to free animals being used in scientific experiments.

The second component of this phase arose at the turn of the 1980s, as big business became interested in the biological sciences. Up to then, apart from the funding of drug research by pharmaceutical companies, main sources of revenue for the biological sciences were from the federal government, mainly through the NIH, private foundations, and universities. However, the possibilities to develop profitable innovations led industrial corporations to make significant investments in biological research. For example, in the 1980s the Massachusetts General Hospital received two major industrial grants: one of almost $50 million was from a German drug and chemical company for molecular biology research, and a second of $85 million was from a Japanese cosmetics company to study the skin. In this period, the founding of the Biogen Company by Nobel Laureate Walter Gilbert and colleagues marked another milestone – the emerging viewpoint among biological scientists that work in a business corporation is an appropriate extension of their lives in science. During that decade many scientists developed relationships with industry to produce commercial products. By 1984 industrial funds accounted for almost a quarter of the external support of university research in biotechnology, which included projects on genetically engineered drugs and genetically altered bacteria, cell and tissue cultures, DNA technology, monoclonal antibodies, and fermentation.[15,16]

The growing relationship between biological scientists and industry posed ethical issues for investigators, universities, science, and the public. With new interests in profit-making activities, would the scientific agenda of research shift from seeking basic knowledge to seeking profitable knowledge? Would openness of communication be damaged by the introduction of competition among scientists working under grants from different companies? Would industrial relationships undermine the obligations and allegiance of scientists to the universities in which they held appointments? What obligations did universities have to ensure timely dissemination of inventions developed within them that might significantly further the public's health? How could universities avoid compromising the education of students and fellows employed by faculty supervisors to work on industry-sponsored research? Studies indicated the existence of such problems.[16,17]

In addition to large grants from industry, a major effort that led government to invest, over time, several billion dollars in a single biological research project emerged in the second half of the 1980s, when proposals appeared to delineate the human genome. In 1984 Robert Sinsheimer and colleagues at the University of California at San Diego attempted to create a genome sequencing institute. "They likened the effort to the exploration of the moon, arguing it would provide insights into who we were, and serve as an integrative focus of all DNA cloning techniques," wrote R. M. Cook-Deegan.[18] The proposal failed to attract private or federal funding. But in 1984 the parallel efforts of Charles DeLise and David Smith at the U.S. Department of Energy to begin a human genome project did garner governmental and scientific support, ultimately with the NIH jointly sponsoring the project with the Department of Energy. In 1987 the NIH made an initial appropriation of $17 million, and in 1990 Congress allocated $87 million for human genome research.

The organizers of the genome program recognized the ethical implications of gaining a genetic portrait of human beings, particularly James Watson, named as head of the NIH genome office created in 1988 and then as director of the National Center for Human Genome Research initiated in 1989. As a result of this recognition, a working group was created and funds dedicated for social, ethical, and legal research as part of the project. This research brought up issues such as: How will knowledge of human propensity for genetically determined illness influence employment and insurance coverage? Will it lead to wholesale discrimination in both? What right to such information does government have? Can the confidentiality of genetic data be assured? This new project has promised to make biological scientists more sensitive to the social significance of their work. As Paul Berg put it, "Judging the ethical value of basic research prospectively and preemptively would be a considerable departure from current practice."[19]

While scientists in the 1980s debated aspects of discovery that affect society, another set of events pointed to problems within the biological sciences themselves. In 1981 John Darsee, a medical scientist working in clinical and experimental cardiology, admitted to falsifying data in one of his papers. Darsee had published 18 research papers in major biomedical journals and about 100 abstracts, book chapters, and other works. Investigations at institutions where he worked – Emory and Harvard Universities and the NIH, which funded some of his studies – revealed that his fabrication was more widespread.

What troubled many was not only that Darsee had been dishonest, but that his coauthors had not detected the flaws in his work before it was published. This led to concern about whether the responsibilities of authorship are sufficiently clear to members of the scientific community. It cast doubt on what Walter E. Steward and Ned Feder, NIH scientists at the forefront of this discussion, called "the integrity of the scientific literature." In a 1987 article in *Nature* that produced much comment and controversy, they claimed that Darsee's coauthors had not been adequately vigilant, that in some cases the contributions of coauthors were minimal and not entitling authorship. For instance, one coauthor's role had been to encourage Darsee and provide grant support.[20]

Sensitized by the Darsee case, the scientific and lay press publicized several other instances of alleged improper conduct in research during the decade. One of the most prominent of these cases involved a Nobel laureate, David Baltimore. In 1986 he was one of the authors of a published article concerning genetic influences on the immune system; the main investigator was a colleague, Thereza Imanishi-Kari of Tufts University. Baltimore's role was that of a senior advisor who reviewed the paper's data and research but did not personally participate in the laboratory work on it. Following publication of the article, Dr. Margot O'Toole, a junior researcher in molecular biology at Tufts who questioned the validity of some of its experimental data, lost her job. The ensuing controversy about the facts and meaning of these events brought the case to the NIH and to the U.S. Congress. As a result, Baltimore was called to testify before a congressional committee about the issue, and the laboratory notebooks of the experiment were even subpoenaed by the Secret Service.[21] Responding to this case, *The New York Times* published a lead editorial headlined, "A Scientific Watergate?" The newspaper criticized the fact that Baltimore, who was never accused of fabrication, and several committees of scientists had investigated the affair and found no basic problems, yet a draft report by the federal investigators involved in the case did find problems. The *Times* faulted the scientific community's mechanisms for investigating such controversies.[22]

These events led, as had revelations of problems in human experiments in the 1960s, to a review of procedures of research used in the biological sciences. One of the earliest outcomes of this examination was a careful look at the duties of scientific authorship. While the subject had been discussed before, it had never received the focused attention of investigators that it did in the mid–1980s. For example, in a 1986 article Edward J. Huth, editor of the *Annals of Internal Medicine,* defined what he called "unjustifiable authorship," a situation in which authors cited in a paper lack basic involvement in its generation: that is, the gaining and analysis of the evidence, and the writing and revision of the findings.[23] Such action appeared to be a leading cause of the burgeoning number of papers cited on the vitae of scientists. Some scientists and, more emphatically, members of the public believed that this behavior, like the highly publicized cases of fraud, represented a breakdown in the fidelity of scientists to truth in the oversight and reporting of their investigations, and that it thus damaged the scientific community as a whole.

But within the scientific community these discussions were received with mixed feelings. Many believed that it remained appropriate, for instance, for the persons who obtained the funds for a project to be named as authors. They pointed out that the stream of help and obligations that flows through a laboratory and touches many of its staff in the course of a study, makes rigid criteria for defining authorship too difficult to devise or implement. Many preferred to determine themselves, on an ad hoc basis and with less rigidity, who should be given the credit of assistance that the title of author conveys.

These events and discussions prompted a number of private and public institutions such as Harvard University, the University of Texas Health Science Center at Houston, and the NIH, and professional societies and journals to publish corrective guidelines delineating the responsibilities of authorship.[24] They led also to two developments in 1989, which demonstrated a social and governmental interest in areas that before were the private preserve of the biological scientist: the oversight of scientific misconduct, and the teaching of students.

An announcement in the *Federal Register* of March 16, 1989, told of the establishment at the NIH of an Office of Scientific Integrity. Its task was to delineate for investigators the responsibilities of handling and reporting possible scientific misconduct, and of investigating it. The office defined such misconduct "as fabrications, falsification, plagiarism, or other practices that seriously deviate from those that are commonly accepted within the scientific community for proposing, conducting, or reporting research."[25]

While some welcomed the introduction of a formal mechanism to deal with misconduct, others were concerned that because it came from government it was intimidating. An article by Bernard Davis, an emeritus professor at Harvard Medical School, titled "How Far Should Big Brother's Hand Reach?" seemed to express a widely held viewpoint within the scientific community. Davis was concerned that the office reached too deeply into the interstices of research, and threatened its freedom. He thought that inadequate distinctions were being made between fraud and normal error, and that the investigation of science by government authority could foster a repressive atmosphere that would cast a shadow over the environment of openness needed for creativity to thrive.[26]

Following this article, in December of 1989, a new administrative rule concerning teaching was placed in the NIH Guide for Contracts and Grants.[27] The rule stated that all institutions seeking National Research Service Award training grants from the NIH and ADAMHA were required to have "a program in the principles of scientific integrity" as an integral part of their efforts in researcher training. The subject matter of this program, it was suggested, could include material on conflict of interest, professional standards and codes of conduct, responsible authorship, issues of human and animal experimentation, and the recording and retention of data. It expressed a concern about integrity in the conduct of research, and the hope that these efforts to train scientists in research ethics early in their career would be meliorative.

This phase of development uncovered ethical problems in the major procedural aspects of the work of the biological sciences, from its use of animal subjects to its authorship claims. Still, it seemed that many biological scientists and students had not yet integrated the ideas generated in the controversies of this period into the way they thought and ran institutions. But with the suggestion by the NIH and ADAMHA that a formal examination of the ethical meanings of scientific work was important, a new pedagogic element in the development of the biological sciences had been introduced. It would mean that faculties and students would have to decide what material and what ethical issues should become part of scientific training. The possibilities for new thinking about these issues within the biological sciences seemed at hand.

Phase IV   1990–?: Turning inward and institutionalizing ethical discourse

The ethics movement in the biological sciences is entering a fourth phase, one that promises to enhance ethical self-awareness about research issues among scientists as education in ethics enters their institutions of learning. Evaluation of what has happened can help to determine where best to go from here. This process was started by challenges to the view that the biological sciences can be managed and directed essentially by the professional community of scientists. The creation of the Institutional Review Boards in 1966 in Phase I of the ethics movement, the Asilomar Conference of 1974 in Phase II, and recently the Office of Scientific Integrity of 1989 in Phase III are witness to society's efforts to join scientists in evaluating standards and setting goals. The sharing of authority with society, the voyage of the biological sciences from a private to a public enterprise, has been a key theme and issue of controversy in the events discussed.

The debate of the biological scientists among themselves and with others in society about the values that should undergird key functional activities in scientific research also has been a recurring theme, particularly strong in Phase III. This is mirrored in the attention given to evaluating the procedures that govern the keeping and reporting of evidence and the awarding of authorship. At the heart of the public's concern about these activities was the significance it attached to the fidelity of scientists to honestly obtain, record, evaluate, and reveal their findings, and to seek to depict nature truthfully. Some members of the public thought that they could not trust scientists to properly use the funds given to them by society, or the conclusions generated by their work, if the rule of honesty seemed threatened.

While some scientists viewed this public concern as an intrusion and did not believe that significant problems existed, others became convinced that the issues were real and necessitated action. One result of this debate was the conclusion that informal attention to education in ethics is not enough. This conclusion led to the development of the 1989 federal guideline that required such education as a basic part of graduate studies.

Opposition to this requirement coalesces about the view that the informal system of ethics education – observing and learning from mentors – remains adequate for the biological sciences. The same argument was heard during the modern medical ethics movement, a search for ethical precepts to guide practice among clinicians from different disciplines, which has run in time alongside the ethics movement in the biological sciences. The mentor-based argument failed to carry the day in clinical medicine because the ethical issues of patient care had grown too complex even for mentors to fully understand. Many clinicians reached the conclusion that scholars who were knowledgeable about ethics needed to join those learned in medicine in order to deal with the ethical questions of practice. A similar association between investigators and ethicists is needed now in the biological sciences to produce innovative educational formats and materials, and to stimulate discourse on ethical issues arising in scientific work.

There are other parallels between the ethics movements in clinical medicine and in the biological sciences. In the medical ethics movement, the phase when medicine changed from a private calling to a public enterprise was followed by a period of self-reflection about the ethical bases of clinical practices and medicine's accountability to the public. As this self-reflection deepened, it stimulated the spread of course work and other institutional innovations in education such as ethics case rounds, which in turn caused this learning to be expressed in the research, policies, and goals of medicine.

The ethics movement in the biological sciences is evolving in this way.[28] The movement now is entering a period in which it should, and I think will, encourage a greater sense of public accountability and self-reflection among scientists concerning the ethical parameters of actions and goals, as well as institutional activities to further these developments. This activity should lead to efforts that clarify and increase the connections of the biological sciences with humanistic ideas and learning. It should produce more empirical and analytical research on the ethics of significant relationships in science such as those between students and teachers, researchers and funders, investigators and staff, and scientists and society. It should stir a closer examination of the institutions of the biological sciences – such as professional societies, research organizations, and schools – to clarify their goals and to assure that their policies do not create pressures that impede their constituents from meeting ethical responsibilities.[29] It should cause scientists to rethink the expectations and aims of their lives in science. It also should stimulate thought on how the scientific community should treat members involved in inappropriate ethical actions. No sound policy on these issues yet exists.

Conclusions

To realize the possibilities of Phase IV will require a decision by scientists to support change rather than to retain the status quo. Such a challenge is not new to science, which is perennially concerned with modification. A response to a shift in theory or technique that alters concepts and practices is continually demanded of scientists. But this situation can be difficult. Change can require new learning, disrupt research patterns, and shift institutional authority and social standing. The biological sciences now must consider whether a change of a kind they are not used to encountering is appropriate: to relinquish the view of biological science as a private professional enterprise to one that sees its activities as engaging the ideas and values of society and its institutions. Ideally, the research community will draw on its own experiences with scientific change so that it can wisely face these novel issues.

Some may find it tempting, comforting, and perhaps safer to argue that things should be left as they are. However, experiences from the medical ethics movement provide a perspective and encouragement for change. Like biological scientists now, clinicians felt highly uncomfortable when ethical issues arose in the 1960s concerning medical decisions such as whether to withdraw life support measures or perform abortions. Many doctors believed such decisions were personal matters, and not proper issues to consider with experts outside the field of medicine or with the public, both of whom lacked the doctor's experience and knowledge. Gradually, physicians recognized that the significant ways in which society is affected by medicine required collaboration with it in discussing and defining medical problems and goals. Physicians further saw that the new ethical questions raised by advances in their own technology and in their new social relationships demanded a different experience, which they did not have. This was an expert experience in the analysis of ethical questions; in the organization and financing of health care services; and in defining the needs, values, and preferences of social institutions with which they now collaborated. As medicine has accommodated these experts into its fabric, it has emerged stronger and more able to deal with the new reality that its innovations in part created. This experience and outcome for medicine, difficult but salutary, offers the biological sciences an important reassurance as it charts its future course.

If the community of biological scientists comes to agree that change is appropriate and beneficial, then the educational effort now required by the NIH and ADAMHA can be shaped to give students and faculty the capacity to meet prospective problems. The subjects of such an education span matters from the ethical aspects of the relationships of scientists with colleagues in the work of research, to the scientist's ethical obligations to society and the enterprise of science itself. Since ethics is the study of the right-making and wrong-making characteristics of action, significant features of this education involve discerning which ethical values can best serve as yardsticks to determine whether actions contemplated or taken in the biological sciences are right or wrong, and learning how best to resolve ethical dilemmas.

Some examples of ethical values particularly relevant to the biological sciences are truthfulness, trustworthiness, stewardship, autonomy, and doing no harm. Maintaining truthfulness as a characteristic of action is essential for the scientists themselves and the public to remain open to ideas and conclusions presented by investigators, and for the triumph of objectivity over bias and self-interest in science. Trust in the intentions, reliability, and honor of colleagues is necessary for the confidence it provides investigators to participate in the relationships essential for the interdependent enterprise that science is. Assuming a responsibility for safeguarding the beings, resources, and institutions used and influenced by science, embodied in the concept of stewardship, is relevant to issues that bear on how scientists should deal with the effects of their discoveries. Autonomy, or the ability to be free and self-governing, is a value that in science encourages inquiry and the creation of novel ideas. The value of avoiding harm to others is also important to an enterprise like science, which forges knowledge that produces significant power.

Ethical dilemmas arise when uncertainty exists about which ethical values are most cogent to the problem at hand, or when the relevant values are recognized but found to be in conflict with one another – for example, when pursuit of one value requires the others to be minimized or disregarded, and participants must decide on the appropriate weights to give the conflicting values. In these situations, ethical analysis has as its aim delineating the balances and compromises that will produce for participants the best available choice under the given circumstances.[30]

Formal courses on the ethical dimensions of the biological sciences and discussions of the ethical aspects of scientific cases are the basic structures within which this education should take place. The two are complementary for ethical learning. Courses provide students with the methodological and analytical capabilities needed for ethical inquiry. Cases provide the material to which this rational approach can be applied. While the development of courses is familiar to the biological sciences community, the concept and formatting of case discussions generally is not.

A key aspect of the development of clinical medicine has been to record the experiences of patient care as cases. These cases provide data not only to advance knowledge, but also to inform instruction.[31,32] In the medical ethics movement ethics case discussions have been a valuable means to learn precisely what ethical problems exist in the care of patients, through discussion to decide on a course of action, and through record keeping to preserve important experiences otherwise lost to learning. Such case discussions that reflect the daily experiences of work and thinking in the biological sciences community could serve its research, education, and policy needs equally well (See Appendix).

This next phase of development in the biological sciences will produce new discoveries, but some will be of a different sort than those to which biological scientists are accustomed. Until this time biological scientists have explored single-mindedly the environment of nature. They must now turn their attention to the environment of profession, and focus their vision inward, on themselves.

Appendix: The case discussion

Typically a case discussion lasts an hour. It begins with the brief presentation of a case that raises some ethical questions, ideally but not necessarily given by a person involved enough in the case to provide specific information. Details of the case should be modified where confidentiality or privacy is an issue.

An effective way for the moderator to begin the discussion is to ask the audience of students, faculty, and staff to identify the ethical questions that they discern in the case, and to write out the questions so that the audience can see them. This formulation of the issues is a very important aspect of the exercise. It reveals the presuppositions, convictions, and uncertainties of the audience, which must be addressed for the discussion to be successful.

The questions are discussed in the order in which they are posed, with attention to the values that underlie them. The group then makes an effort to draw conclusions and suggest specific actions to resolve the problems that the case involves.

The positive experience in medicine with the case discussion and formal courses in ethics indicates that they also can be helpful to the biological sciences in analyzing and coping with the challenges that lie ahead.[33]

References and Notes

1. Nuremberg Code, in *Trials of War Criminals Before the Nuremberg Military Tribunals Under Control Council Law*. No. 10, Vol. 2 (Washington, DC: U.S. Government Printing Office, 1949), pp. 181–182.
2. S. J. Reiser, Human Experimentation and the Convergence of Medical Research and Patient Care, *Annals of the American Academy of Political and Social Sciences,* May 1978, pp. 8–18.
3. W. J. Curran, Current Legal Issues in Clinical Investigation with Particular Attention to the Balance between the Rights of the Individual and the Needs of Society, in *Psychopharmacology: A Review of Progress, 1957–1967* (Washington, DC, U.S. Public Health Service Publication, No. 1836, 1968), pp. 337–343.
4. J. Katz, *Experimentation with Human Beings* (New York: Russell Sage Foundation, 1972), pp. 9–65.
5. R. Aron, The Education of the Citizen in Industrial Society. *Daedalus* Spring 1962, pp. 253–258.
6. S. J. Reiser, The Public and the Expert in Biomedical Controversies, in Institute of Medicine, *Biomedical Politics* (Washington, DC: National Academy Press, 1991), pp. 325–331.
7. E. Mendelsohn, J. P. Swazey, I. Taviss, eds., *Human Aspects of Biomedical Innovations* (Cambridge: Harvard University Press, 1971).
8. G. R. Taylor, *The Biological Time Bomb* (New York: The Wood Publishing Company, 1968).
9. J. Fletcher, Ethical Aspects of Genetic Controls: Designed Genetic Changes in Man, *New England Journal of Medicine* 285, 1971, pp. 776–783.
10. D. S. Frederickson, Asilomar and Recombinant DNA: The End of the Beginning, in Institute of Medicine, *Biomedical Politics* (Washington, DC: National Academy Press, 1991), pp. 258–298.
11. P. Berg, D. Baltimore, S. Brenner, R. Roblin III, and M. F. Singer, Asilomar Conference on Recombinant DNA Molecules. *Science* 188, 1975, pp. 791–794.
12. D. Nelkin, Commentary in Institute of Medicine, *Biomedical Politics* (Washington, DC: National Academy Press, 1991), pp. 299–301.
13. P. Singer, *Animal Liberation: A New Ethics for Our Treatment of Animals* (New York: Discus, 1977).
14. R. E. Bulger, Use of Animals in Experimental Research: A Scientist's Perspective. *The Anatomical Record* 219, 1987, pp. 215–220.
15. D. Blumenthal et al., Industrial Support of University Research in Biotechnology. *Science* 231, 1986, pp. 242–248.
16. D. Blumenthal et al., University–Industry Research Relationship in Biotechnology: Implications for the University. *Science* 232, 1986, pp. 1381–1386.
17. Association of Academic Health Centers, *Conflicts of Interest in Academic Health Centers* (Washington, DC: Association of Academic Health Centers, 1990).
18. R. M. Cook-Deegan, The Human Genome Project: The Formation of Federal Policies in the United States, 1986–1990, in Institute of Medicine, *Biomedical Politics* (Washington, DC: National Academy Press, 1991), pp. 99–168.

19. P. Berg, Commentary, in Institute of Medicine, *Biomedical Politics* (Washington, DC: National Academy Press, 1991), p. 171.
20. W. W. Steward and N. Feder, The Integrity of the Scientific Literature, *Nature* 325, 1987, pp. 207–214.
21. P. S. Hilts, Hero in Exposing Science Hoax Paid Dearly, *NY Times,* March 22, 1991, pp. A1, B6.
22. A Scientific Watergate? *NY Times,* March 26, 1991, p. A14.
23. E. J. Huth, Irresponsible Authorship and Wasteful Publication, *Annals of Internal Medicine* 104, 1986, pp. 257–259.
24. International Committee of Medical Editors, Guidelines on Authorship. *British Medical Journal* 291, 1985, p. 722.
25. J. V. Hollum and S. W. Hadley, OSI: Why, What, and How, *ASM News* 56, 1990, pp. 647–651.
26. B. D. Davis, How Far Should Big Brother's Hand Reach? *ASM News* 56, 1990, pp. 643–646.
27. National Institutes of Health Guide, Requirement for Programs on the Responsible Conduct of Research in National Research Service Award Institutional Training Grants, No. 30, Vol. 19, August 17, 1990, p. 1.
28. The common paths of development taken by these two ethics movements suggests the need for further study to determine if this pattern is typical of ethics movements in general.
29. R. E. Bulger and S. J. Reiser, eds., *Integrity in Health Care Institutions: Humane Environments for Teaching, Inquiry, and Healing* (Iowa City: University of Iowa Press, 1990).
30. Two useful texts on the basic elements of biomedical ethical analysis are T. L. Beauchamp and J. F. Childress, *Principles of Biomedical Ethics*, 3rd. ed. (New York: Oxford University Press, 1989), and R. M. Veatch, *Medical Ethics* (Boston: Jones and Bartlett Publishers, 1989).
31. S. J. Reiser, The Clinical Record in Medicine, Part 1: Learning from Cases, *Annals of Internal Medicine* 114, 1991, pp. 902–907.
32. S. J. Reiser, Administrative Case Rounds: Institutional Policies and Leaders Cast in a Different Light, *JAMA* 266, 1991, pp. 2127–2128.
33. The author gratefully acknowledges R. E. Bulger and E. Heitman for their review and comments on this paper.

PART I

The Conceptual and Social Foundations of Science

INTRODUCTION

Scientists seeking to understand the values that influence their actions should first inquire into the ways in which new ideas emerge. One of today's most prominent models of science, developed by Thomas Kuhn, describes the historical record of research as one of tension between tradition and innovation.[1] Generations of researchers work to develop a theoretical consensus, or *paradigm,* which has two primary characteristics: a breadth that attracts adherents from competing modes of scientific activity, and an open-endedness that offers new problems for researchers to solve. Kuhn calls this problem solving *normal science,* an activity based on scientists' assumption that they know how the world works.

Continued research eventually reveals anomalies and discrepancies in the paradigm, which, after a certain point, the conceptual views of normal science can no longer suppress. New investigations generate a revolutionary new theory that resolves these discrepancies, but only by rejecting the fundamental assumptions of the old paradigm. Kuhn thus claims that the canons of scientific knowledge inhibit the acceptance of findings that depart too radically from what the existing scientific practice anticipates.

Many scientists will spend their careers doing normal science. Yet developments in science depend on researchers' ability to see and interpret information in new ways. In exploring the creative process, Silvano Arieti shows how the recognition of anomalies leads to creative breakthroughs. Arieti recounts a variety of such discoveries from the personal histories of creative scientists, tracing how new data, random events and images, and even creative interpretations of *gaps* in knowledge may stimulate significant new understandings of old information.

Although meaningful research depends on careful planning and methodical execution, creative breakthroughs cannot be planned. Julius H. Comroe, Jr. and Robert D. Dripps illustrate this situation persuasively in their discussion of national research policy and the usefulness of applied versus basic research. Their chronology of the development of electrocardiography demonstrates that it is impossible to predict a conceptual breakthrough or to assess the potential uses of data from their immediate practical applicability. What appears to be essential applied research may prove fruitless, and broad conceptual work may yield insights vital to specific projects in widely disparate fields. Even where research policy aims for practical ends, science must always seek to generate new questions that promote ongoing creative work in the field.

Note

1. Thomas Kuhn, *The Structure of Scientific Revolutions,* Chicago, IL: University of Chicago Press, 1970.

1
Science

Silvano Arieti

At the present time the creative process is being studied more intensively in relation to science than to any other field. There are several reasons for this focus on science. The first is the twentieth century's bias in favor of scientific knowledge. A second reason is found in the belief held by many investigators that it is easier to study the creative process in scientists than in artists. Scientists seem to be more methodical in their observations and therefore seemingly should be more capable of reporting their inner experiences. A third reason is the assumption by many investigators that the process of scientific creativity consists of logical or mathematical steps that can easily be traced back.

As to the first reason, we must accept its historical validity. The second and third reasons, however, contain only grains of truth. The scientist's methodology is of little help in the attempt to recapture the inner experiences leading to a scientific innovation. Moreover, although the tracing back of logical steps is indeed important, it does not lead to insights into unconscious mechanisms or even into the overall modes of operation that are followed consciously.

Before examining the process of creativity in scientific discovery, we must clarify one point: discoveries are not always the result of scientific creativity. An explorer who discovers an unknown land is not necessarily endowed with creative ability. Inventions that require only the rearrangement or practical application of principles discovered by others are more properly considered as pertaining to technology than to creativity, no matter how important their practical effects are. On the other hand, some scientific principles that are among the highest products of creativity may not have practical applications for long periods of time.

The contributions of Poincaré and others

One of the aims of students of scientific creativity has been to recapture the different phases of thinking that lead to the creative act. Personal accounts given by great scientists are particularly valuable, but unfortunately only a small percentage of them have provided this information. One who did so was the physiologist Helmholtz (1896), who recognized three stages in his creative work: (1) an initial investigation carried on until it is impossible to go further; (2) a period of rest and recovery; and (3) the occurrence of a sudden and unexpected solution.

One of the best accounts of the creative process in science was given by the mathematician Poincaré (1913). In a report that has become a classic in the literature on creativity, Poincaré described the discovery of the theory of Fuchsian groups and Fuchsian functions that made him famous. He studied the problem for fifteen days, trying to reach a conclusion that later proved to be false: that no such functions existed. A sleepless night spent on this problem brought no apparent results. He had drunk black coffee and could not sleep, and he later wrote about that memorable night: ''Ideas rose in crowds; I felt them collide *until pairs interlocked,* so to speak, making a stable construction.'' The following day, on the way to a geological excursion, he got on a bus. At the moment he put his foot on the step, the idea came to him – apparently without any conscious effort and without his even thinking about this problem – that the transformations he ''had used to define the Fuchsian functions were identical with those of non-Euclidian geometry.'' This was the creative moment. Poincaré went on with the business of the day, but later he verified this sudden illumination. A few days later, in another sudden flash, he realized that the ''arithmetic transformations of indefinite ternary quadratic forms were identical with those of non-Euclidian geometry.'' These breakthroughs led to a great expansion in the field of mathematics.

Poincaré added another stage to those described by Helmholtz: a second period of conscious effort, after the illumination, to validate the insight obtained. Wallas (1926) named and described the stages already individualized by Poincaré. Hadamard (1945), in his interesting book on the psychology of invention in the field of mathematics, follows Poincaré's ideas for the most part.

Poincaré carefully considered the important topic of how some connections or combinations lead to the acquisition of new knowledge, to discovery, or to the experience of sudden illumination – the ''Eureka!'' of Archimedes. Combinations that will lead to new knowledge are a small minority; useless combinations are potentially endless in number. How is it that ''good combinations'' are made during the incubation period and reach consciousness in the subsequent stage of illumination? It seems impossible to attribute good combinations to mere chance, as some authors do. For how can chance explain the fact that many creative people make more than one discovery? Poincaré in fact believed that these combinations occur in the unconscious or subliminal self, and he offered the hypothesis that the subliminal self is in no way inferior to the conscious self. He wrote: ''Does it follow that the subliminal self, having divined by a delicate intuition that these combinations would be useful, has formed only these, or has it rather formed many others which were taking an interest and have remained unconscious?''

In trying to understand how the selection leading to the useful combination is made, Poincaré advanced two hypotheses. The first concerns the aesthetic quality of the combination: perhaps the mind, like a delicate sieve, lets pass through the threshold of consciousness only those combinations that are striking for their beauty and elegance. The second assumes that during the preparatory work the mind does not put into motion all possible ideas but only those that have something to do with the object of study. Poincaré says that if we think of these ideas as ''atoms'' hooked on the mind's walls, we can imagine the mind unhooking only those ingredients that are possible for the new ideas. The mobilized ''atoms'' are those from which we may reasonably expect the desired solution. Some of these ''atoms'' collide and enter into new combinations. A good combination is one in which at least one ''atom'' was freely chosen by the will.

The first hypothesis does not seem convincing. It is true that several useful mathematical formulas have the characteristics of beauty and elegance that Poincaré mentioned, but their being aesthetically attractive does not make them *valid*. Poincaré himself has stated that some false ideas can still gratify "a natural feeling for mathematical elegance." On first examination, Poincaré's second hypothesis seems more acceptable. Certainly in the preparatory stage the creative person consciously mobilizes only those ideas that have something to do with the object of his research. In many instances, however, the new combinations that emerge in the subsequent flash of illumination have been suggested by something completely unrelated to the object of inquiry. Often it is by the unpredictable application to one field of what is valid in another field that valuable new combinations have occurred. Now in the case of Poincaré, obviously he put only mathematical ideas into motion in his preparatory work, not – let us say – historical, geographical, and literary notions. This restriction, however, does not seem very important, because the field of mathematics was vast enough even in his time to permit infinite combinations.

The process of discovery

Let us reconsider the first important illumination that Poincaré experienced. "At the moment when I put my foot on the step the idea came to me . . . that the transformations I had used to define the Fuchsian functions were identical with those of non-Euclidian geometry." The act of illumination consisted of seeing an *identity* between two transformations previously reputed to be dissimilar: those that Poincaré had used to define the Fuchsian functions, and those of non-Euclidian geometry. A later illumination came when Poincaré had the idea "with just the same characteristics of brevity, suddenness, and immediate certainty, that the arithmetic transformations of indeterminate ternary quadratic forms were identical with those of non-Euclidian geometry." Again the moment of illumination was the moment when Poincaré saw an identity between two subjects reputed to be dissimilar.

Similar instances could be multiplied endlessly in which great discoveries were made by the act of perceiving an identity among two or more things that had been thought dissimilar or unrelated. In the classic example, Newton observed an apple falling from a tree and saw a common quality in the apple attracted by the earth and the attraction between heavenly bodies. He perceived the similarity between two forces: that which causes an apple to fall to the earth, and that which holds the moon in its orbit. He validated this insight by comparing the rate at which bodies fall to earth with the rate at which the moon deviates from the path it would follow if the earth did not exist.

We could say that many scientific discoveries are the result of individualizing a common characteristic or connection between things that were deemed dissimilar or unrelated before. But of course the observation of similarity is not enough. The transformations used by Poincaré are not identical in every respect with those of non-Euclidian geometry. And an apple is very dissimilar in size, origin, and chemical structure to the moon. Yet Newton saw a similarity. In what way, then, *are* the moon and the apple similar? What does their partial identity consist of? Of being members of a class of bodies subject to gravitation. That is, when Newton saw this similarity between the apple and the moon, *a new class was formed,* to which an indefinite number of members could be added thereafter. The new object for which he was searching, and which he found, was a class. The discovery of this class revealed a new way of looking at the universe, because each member of the class came to be recognized as having similar properties.

Is this new class a primary class . . . ? Obviously not. It differs on many counts. First, when Newton perceived the identical element, he did not respond to the stimulus but to the class. Had he been a regressed schizophrenic, after seeing a similarity between the moon and the apple, he could have paleologically identified the moon with the apple and thought that the moon could be eaten like an apple or sucked like the maternal breast – as Renée, a by-now-famous schizophrenic patient reported by Sechehaye, did during a stage of her illness (1951). Second, Newton's creativity consisted, after seeing a common property in the moon and the apple, not in identifying them but in seeing them as members of a new class. An increased ability to see similarities – a property of the primary process – is here connected with a concept; and the tertiary process emerges. The secondary class loses all its original connections with the primary process.

Is the new class discovered by Newton exclusively the result of secondary-process mechanisms – that is, what Reichenbach called "induction by enumeration" (1951)? (Induction by enumeration is the procedure by which a man, having observed that some sequences – say, the daily alternation of light and darkness – recur again and again, feels entitled to draw a general principle such as "night follows day".) Induction by enumeration is a simple procedure, even for the average man. Obviously this is not what Newton did. His is a case of what some authors have called "induction by intuition" and others "induction by imagination" or "induction by guessing" (Frank 1957). I shall call it *induction by creativity,* which creativity consists of (1) individualizing a common property (as, for instance, the property shared by the moon and the apple); (2) *not* identifying the objects (as, again, the moon and the apple) having some such common property by putting them into a primary class; and (3) recognizing that they belong to an unsuspected secondary class (such as gravitational bodies). In this type of induction, an increased ability to recognize similarities – a characteristic of the primary process – is connected with a concept; and the tertiary process emerges. *The concept of the new class is much more important than the recognition of the similarity; but the mental grasping of the similarity is necessary to evoke the concept of class at the level of consciousness.*

Once the concept of the new class is created, it will be easy to use thereafter in induction by enumeration; for instance, in recognizing that all bodies are subject to a gravitational force. It will also be easy to apply the concept in deductive procedures: since *A* is a body, it is subject to a gravitational force.

From this description it can be seen that the tertiary process in scientific creativity uses mechanisms that are different from those found in aesthetic creativity. Blake's poem "The Sick Rose" compares the sick woman to the sick rose and makes us aware of a class "beautiful life destroyed by illness." However, the rose and the woman, although not identical as they would be in schizophrenic thinking, are not clearly distinct either, the way the apple and the moon are. The members of a secondary class that emerges through the aesthetic process retain the tendency to fuse together, or to exchange non-essential predicates. Consequently, even the class "beautiful life destroyed by illness" is not as definite as the class of gravitational bodies is. The poet leaves things somewhat indistinct. It is part of our aesthetic appreciation first to experience the ambiguity of the unfinished statement, and then to attempt a clarification of that statement by finding psychological resonances in our feelings and ideas. The scientist instead tries to make the statement as clear as possible, leaving no room for doubts or exceptions. His new secondary class loses all its original connections with the primary process. Here, too, however, although the new class is very well defined, the search is not ended. The understanding of the Newtonian system is a prerequisite to the eventual discovery of the Einsteinian world of classes.

In many instances the process of creativity consists of discovering a similarity between one system or field of knowledge and another. One of the most important examples of this type is that of Darwin. In 1838 Darwin happened to read the book written by Malthus 40 years before, *Essay on the Principle of Population.* Malthus had advanced the idea that Rousseau's optimistic views about humanity are unsound because (1) the natural tendency of population is to increase faster than the means of subsistence; and (2) this fast increase results in a struggle for existence. Darwin, abstracting from all the observations that he had made in the Galapagos Islands, had the vision that reproductive competition between members of the same species is similar to the Malthusian competition found in human society. Thus principles formulated in relation to human society were applied by Darwin to organic life in general. According to Ghiselin (1973), he also initiated a radically new way of studying behavior.

The whole theory of evolution is based on the similarities between species, as well as on the differences interpreted as leading to greater complexity. The greatest evidence for the Darwinian theory rests on the similarities collected from anatomy, embryology, and paleontology. The more closely related the groups of animal and vegetal organisms the greater is the number of like structures and functions. The recognition of similarities often leads not only to the formation of a class, but of a class of classes, that is, to the formation of a system.

Typical is the example of the Russian chemist Dmitri Mendeleev, who in 1869 announced to the world his "Periodic Table of Elements." Prior classifications, made by Johann Döbereiner in 1829, by Jean B. Dumas in 1850, and by John Newland in 1865, had not been successful. Mendeleev had noticed that some groups of elements had common properties. His great discovery was that these common properties (or similarities) recurred periodically if the elements were arranged in order of increasing atomic weight. Thus, for instance, fluorine, chlorine, bromine, and iodine have common qualities. Their atomic weight is quite different: 18.99 for fluorine, 35.45 for chlorine, 79.90 for bromine, and 126.90 for iodine. However, if we arrange all the known elements according to their atomic weight, we find that the above-mentioned four elements fall into the same column and therefore are expected to have similar properties. The genius of Mendeleev appeared also in the fact that he was not deterred by serious obstacles. When he could not place any elements in available places in the table that he had put together, he left holes. In several cases the accepted atomic weight of some elements did not correspond to that anticipated by the periodic law. He challenged the correctness of those atomic weights and subsequent investigations proved that he was right.

. . .

Many discoveries that are not of the highest creative order reach the stage of invariable association without going through the stage of similarity. And of course, it can happen that their individual practical results are more consequential than those of discoveries of the highest type. For instance, an observer is struck by an unusual sequence, never noticed before: an unusual event *B* occurs after an unusual occurrence of *A,* and he jumps to the conclusion (which later he has to confirm with other experiments) that there is an invariable association between *A* and *B*. At other times the association is a negative one: *B* cannot be associated with *A*. A great deal of medical research is based on negative association (for instance, if penicillin *A* is present, a certain microorganism *B* will not multiply).

Many inventions and discoveries have occurred by this method of seeing an invariable association or by filling some gap between invariable associations.* When the invariable association is discovered without going through the stage of the mode of similarity, we have only a practical invention or at most an *empirical law*. The law is explained only by the empirical proof; it is not sustained by a new class or by a greater understanding of the world. It is doubtful that the tertiary process is used in discoveries made by empirical relation.

Some inventions seem to have occurred purely by accident. If Roentgen had not chanced to observe a glowing barium platinocyanide screen, X rays would not have been discovered. The creativity, if we can use that term, here consisted of not accepting the chance, the accident, the seeming anomaly, but of trying to understand the event as part of the order of the universe. In such incidents, what appears fortuitous or anomalous is recognized as an inevitable occurrence. The accidental result may immediately show itself to have great practical consequences or applications.

It is a curious fact about scientific discoveries that fortuitous incidents, such as that of Newton and the apple or that of Galileo and the lamp in the cathedral of Pisa, are frequently of importance. Many people doubt the historical validity of these episodes, which seem almost like myths that have grown up around the memory of great men. The stories have the flavor of parables, "artistic concretizations" that popular culture has created out of the ideas of these men. Early in life Galileo had neglected the study of mathematics because his father had convinced him to study medicine. In 1581, when he was seventeen, he was in the cathedral of his native city Pisa and watched the swinging of a lamp. He observed that whatever the range of the oscillations of the lamp, the time span for each remained the same. The subsequent verification of this fact led him to the discovery of the principle of the isochronism of the pendulum.

One of the most famous of these stories about creative men concerns the mathematician and inventor Archimedes, who was born at Syracuse, Sicily, in 287 B.C. Hieron, the King of Syracuse, had asked Archimedes to determine whether a crown given to him and supposed to be of gold, did not actually contain a quantity of less valuable silver. Archimedes did not know how to solve the problem. One day, however, while entering his bath, he noticed that he displaced a certain volume of water, and he had a sudden illumination. He realized that he would be able to solve the enigma if he put the crown and equal weights of gold and silver separately into a container of water and observed the difference in overflow. Struck by this sudden insight, he shouted "Eureka! Eureka!" an expression which throughout centuries has remained symbolic of scientific discovery.

At the risk of appearing gullible, I must say that I believe in many of these little episodes which led to great illuminations. That small, chance episodes are responsible for some inventions and discoveries is beyond doubt and has been verified by a number of observers. There is no reason why incidents such as those reported about Archimedes, Newton, and Galileo could not have occurred, thus offering a genius the opportunity to grasp a regularity he was searching for. The episode becomes a concretization of the idea, just as a work of art stands for an abstract concept. The falling apple concretizes the force of gravity. Here it is nature that does the concretizing, not man. Man's genius

---

*See J. Rossman, *The Psychology of the Inventor* (Washington, DC: Inventors Publishing, 1931).

lies in recognizing the concretization and unraveling it by finding the universal in the particular. The particular is not just a symbol of the universal, as in art; instead it belongs to the class of the universal. Both are parts of the same reality.

Imagery

However, it is true that many innovators have not needed some concrete episode to grasp the universal. Nor have they relied directly on seeing an identity among dissimilarities, as Poincaré did. These innovators have relied on other forms of primitive cognition, and especially on images.

In answer to a questionnaire prepared by the mathematician Hadamard (1945), Einstein wrote:

(A) The words or the language, as they are written or spoken, do not seem to play any role in my mechanism of thought. The psychical entities which seem to serve as elements in thought are signs and more or less clear images which can be 'voluntarily' reproduced and combined . . .
(B) The above elements are, in my case, of visual and some of muscular types . . .
(C) According to what has been said, the play with the mentioned elements is aimed to be analogous to certain logical connections one is searching for . . .

Hadamard himself reported that he thought creatively in visual pictures. Some authors have stressed the role of visualization in scientific creativity. For instance, Walkup (1967) writes that creative individuals, in the field of science at least, have intense visual imagery. They "almost hallucinate in the areas in which they are creative." He soon tempers his statement by adding that he uses the word "visualize" in its broadest sense to include the mental synthesizing of many sensory experiences, not just ocular experiences. He also writes that inventors with whom he talked reported "thinking visually about complex mechanisms. . . . So it appears that ideas which can be grasped when drawn on paper can be visualized without being put onto paper. . . . Also, the nature of the *seeing* or sensing is peculiar. It is almost a *feeling like* the object being visualized." (Italics in the original.) It seems to me that the "peculiar seeing" that Walkup describes is imagery.

In a very interesting article, Dreistadt (1974) examines the importance of the role of visualization in Einstein's creativity and in his discovery of the theory of relativity in particular. (Einstein was fully aware of this role. In a letter to his friend Janos Plesch (Clark 1971, p. 87), he wrote, "When I examine myself and my methods of thought, I come to the conclusion that the gift of fantasy has meant more to me than my talent for absorbing knowledge.") For instance, in one of his fantasies, Einstein visualized himself as a passenger who rode on a ray of light and held a mirror in front of him. Since the light and the mirror were traveling at the same velocity in the same direction and since the mirror was a little ahead, the light could never catch up to the mirror and reflect any image. Thus Einstein could not see himself in the mirror. In another instance, Einstein fantasied some physicists in an elevator that was falling freely in a high building. The physicists, unaware of what was happening, were performing some experiments. They took coins and keys out of their pockets and let go of them. The coins and keys remained in mid-air because they were falling at the same rate of speed with the elevator and the men. The physicists might have interpreted the strange phenomenon in unusual ways. For instance, they might have thought they had been transported outside the gravitational field of the earth and were in empty space, where every body follows Newton's law of inertia and continues in its state of rest or uniform straight line.

Dreistadt aptly describes how these imaginary events, and others reported in his article, were analogous to real events. We remember that Einstein himself, in point C of his answer to Hadamard, had said that these visual elements were "*analogous* to certain logical connections one is searching for."

I believe we can go a step further and state that these fantasies had the same value that some little episodes, reported in the previous section of this chapter, had for people like Galileo and Newton. The apple in the case of Newton, the moving lamp in the case of Galileo, did not need to be imagined. They were both analogous to the logical connections implied in the physical law. They were also a particular instance of a universal phenomenon, an actual embodiment of a notion of the highest generality. The particular became identical to a potentially infinite number of cases in which the same conditions apply.

Now the problem with people like Einstein is whether the fantasy comes first, or whether it is a concretization or perceptualization of mental processes that occurred previously. Galileo and Newton saw an identity. Einstein had to create a visual identity. Einstein may be in good faith when he says that the visual part of creativity comes first, because his antecedent mental work might have been unconscious. His situation may be similar to that of a person who examines a dream he has had, and who had not been previously aware of the antecedent mental processes that gave origin to that particular dream. The difference between a person like Poincaré and a person like Einstein may be that whereas Poincaré could proceed from an endoceptual to a preconceptual and finally a conceptual level, Einstein had to go from the endoceptual back to the image level before reaching the conceptual.

References

Arieti, S. I., 1967, *The Intrapsychic Self: Feeling, Cognition and Creativity in Health and Mental Illness*. New York: Basic Books.

Cassirer, E., 1953, 1955, 1957, *The Philosophy of Symbolic Forms*. Vols. 1, 2, 3. New Haven: Yale University Press.

Clark, R. W., 1971, *Einstein: The Life and Times*. New York: World.

Darwin, C., 1872, *The Expression of the Emotions in Man and Animals*. London: Murray. Quoted by Keith-Spiegel, 1972.

Dreistadt, R., 1974, "The Psychology of Creativity: How Einstein Discovered the Theory of Relativity." *Psychology*, 11:15–25.

Frank, P., 1957, *Philosophy of Science*. Englewood Cliffs, N.J.: Prentice-Hall.

Ghiselin, M. T., 1973, "Darwin and Evolutionary Psychology." *Science*, 179:964–968.

Hadamard, J., 1945, *The Psychology of Invention in the Mathematical Field*. Princeton, N.J.: Princeton University Press.

Helmholtz, H. von, 1896, *Vortrage und Reden*, 5th auff. Brammschweig: Vieweg und John.

Keith-Spiegel, P., 1972, "Early Conceptions of Humor: Varieties and Issues," In Goldstein and McGhee (eds.), *The Psychology of Humor*, pp. 3–39. New York: Academic Press.

Poincaré, H., 1913, "Mathematical Creation." In *The Foundation of Science*, Lancaster, PA.: The Science Press, 1946.

Reichenbach, H., 1951, *The Rise of Scientific Philosophy*. Berkeley: University of California Press.

Sechehaye, M. A., 1951, *Symbolic Realization*. New York: International Universities.

Walkup, L. E., 1967, "Creativity in Science through Visualization." *Journal of Creative Behavior*, 1: 283–290.

Wallas, G., 1926, *The Art of Thought*. New York: Harcourt, Brace.

2
Scientific basis for the support of biomedical science

Julius H. Comroe, Jr. and Robert D. Dripps

Our project had only one goal: to demonstrate that objective, scientific techniques – instead of the present anecdotal approach – can be used to design and justify a national biomedical research policy.

Our interest in this project began in 1966 when President Lyndon Johnson said, "Presidents . . . need to show more interest in what the specific results of research are – in their lifetime, and in their administration. A great deal of *basic* research has been done . . . but I think the time has come to zero in on the targets – by trying to get our knowledge fully applied. . . . *We must make sure that no lifesaving discovery is locked up in the laboratory* [italics ours]."

The position of the Johnson Administration on basic research was bolstered by a preliminary report of a study, "Project Hindsight," commissioned by the Department of Defense and published in 1966.[1] A team of scientists and engineers analyzed retrospectively how 20 important military weapons came to be developed. Among these were weapons such as Polaris and Minuteman missiles, nuclear warheads, C–141 aircraft, the Mark 46 torpedo, and the M 102 Howitzer.

Some of the conclusions of that study were as follows. (i) The contributions of university research were minimal. (ii) Scientists contributed most effectively when their effort was mission-oriented. (iii) The lag between initial discovery and final application was shortest when the scientist worked in areas targeted by his sponsor.

The President's words and the Department of Defense's report popularized a new set of terms such as research in the service of man, strategy for the cure of disease, targeted research, mission-oriented research, disease-oriented research, programmatic research, relevant research, commission-initiated research, contract-supported research, and payoff research. These phrases had a great impact on Congress and on the Office of Management and Budget and led to a sharp upsurge of contract research and commission-initiated research supported by the National Institutes of Health (NIH).

Medical and other scientists countered with carefully prepared case reports that illustrated the important contributions of basic, fundamental, undirected, non-targeted research to advances in medicine, social sciences, and physics.[2]

Since 1966 there has been a continuing debate whether the federal government would get more for its biomedical research dollars if they were used to support clinically oriented research or if they were used to support research that was not clinically oriented.

We believe that the Department of Defense's study suffered from two factors. (i) Only a preliminary report has been released (and that 9 years ago) and even it is not yet widely

From *Science*, 1976, 192, pp. 105–111. Copyright 1976 by the AAAS.

available. (ii) Some who have read it have transferred conclusions drawn from that study on development of military weapons directly to biomedical research. However, the reports of those who countered Project Hindsight also suffered from one or both of two problems. (i) Some presented single case reports and so were anecdotal or ''for instance'' arguments. (ii) The cases were selected by those who did the study and so were subject to their bias.

It is easy to select examples in which basic, undirected, nonclinical research led to dramatic advance in clinical medicine and equally easy to give examples in which either clinically oriented research or development was all-important. A classic example of the great importance of research completely unrelated to clinical medicine or surgery was that of Wilhelm Roentgen. While studying a basic problem in the physics of rays emitted from a Crookes' tube, he discovered x-rays that immediately became vital for precise diagnosis of many diseases and later for the treatment of some. A classic example of the importance of mission-oriented research was that of Louis Pasteur. Pasteur, originally trained as a chemist, was employed by the French government as an industrial trouble-shooter. Among the problems assigned to him were the practical ones of how to keep wine from turning to vinegar, how to cure ailing silkworms, and how to save sheep dying of anthrax and chickens dying of cholera. The solution of these practical problems led Pasteur to discover bacteria and become the founder of modern bacteriology and the father of the germ theory of disease. A classic example of the importance to medicine of development (as opposed to research) was the mass production of penicillin in the United States in the early 1940's when it was required immediately for England's war effort and later for our own.

The anecdotal or ''let me give you an example'' approach provides fascinating after-dinner conversation and even interesting testimony before congressional appropriations committees. However, we believe that the time has come for the nation's biomedical research policy to be based on something more substantial than a preliminary analysis of weapons development by the Department of Defense and informal let-me-give-you-an-example arguments by concerned scientists, and that Congress and the Administration should require more than for-instances from proponents or opponents of any policy for the support of medical research. We believe that the design and the broad scope of our study avoid the weaknesses of previous studies and provide an example to show how long-term policies on support of biomedical research can be developed on an objective basis.

Scope of our study

Because the heart of our thesis is that the support of research should not be based on selected examples or anecdotes, it was mandatory that we study all of a broad field. We selected the field of cardiovascular and pulmonary diseases because these are responsible for more than half of all deaths in the United States each year and because we have some competence in evaluating research on the heart, blood vessels, and lungs, or know where to go for advice. To ensure that our study was concerned directly with the health of the nation and not with esoteric scientific discoveries, we directed our attention only to clinical advances since the early 1940's that have been directly responsible for diagnosing, preventing, or curing cardiovascular or pulmonary disease; stopping its progression, decreasing suffering, or prolonging useful life.

To avoid our own bias, we asked 40 physicians to list the advances they considered

Table 1. *The top ten clinical advances in cardiovascular and pulmonary medicine and surgery in the last 30 years.*

Cardiac surgery (including open-heart repair of congenital defects and replacement of diseased valves)
Vascular surgery (including repair or bypass of obstructions or other lesions in aorta, coronary, cerebral, renal, and limb arteries)
Drug treatment of hypertension
Medical treatment of coronary insufficiency (myocardial ischemia)
Cardiac resuscitation, defibrillation, "cardioversion" and pacing in patients with cardiac arrest, slow hearts, or serious arrhythmias
Oral diuretics (in treatment of patients with congestive heart failure or hypertension)
Intensive cardiovascular and respiratory care units (including those for postoperative care, coronary care, respiratory failure, and disorders of newborn)
Chemotherapy and antibiotics (including prevention of acute rheumatic fever and treatment of tuberculosis, pneumonias, and cardiovascular syphilis)
New diagnostic methods (for earlier and more accurate diagnosis of disease of cardiovascular and pulmonary-respiratory systems)
Prevention of poliomyelitis (especially of respiratory paralysis due to polio)

to be the most important for their patients. We then divided their selections into a cardiovascular and a pulmonary list and sent the appropriate list to 40 to 50 specialists in each field, asking each to vote on the list and to add additional advances that they believed belonged on the list. Their votes selected the top ten advances (Table 1). With these as a starting point, we worked retrospectively to learn why and how they occurred.

With the help of 140 consultants,[3] including 46 interviewed personally, we identified the essential bodies of knowledge that had to be developed before each of the ten clinical advances could reach its current state of achievement. To make clear what we mean by this, let us consider cardiac surgery.

When general anesthesia was first put to use in 1846, the practice of surgery exploded in many directions, except for thoracic surgery. Cardiac surgery did not take off until almost 100 years later, and John Gibbon did not perform the first successful operation on an open heart with complete cardiopulmonary bypass apparatus until 108 years after the first use of ether anesthesia. What held back cardiac surgery? What had to be known before a surgeon could predictably and successfully repair cardiac defects? First of all, the surgeon required precise preoperative diagnosis in every patient whose heart needed repair. That required selective angiocardiography which, in turn, required the earlier discovery of cardiac catheterization, which required the still earlier discovery of x-rays. But the surgeon also needed an artificial heart-lung apparatus (pump-oxygenator) to take over the function of the patient's heart and lungs while he stopped the patient's heart in order to open and repair it. For pumps, this required a design that would not damage blood; for oxygenators, this required basic knowledge of the exchange of O_2 and CO_2 between gas and blood. However, even a perfect pump-oxygenator would be useless if the blood in it clotted. Thus, the cardiac surgeon had to await the discovery and purification of a potent, nontoxic anticoagulant – heparin.

These are just a few examples; obviously Gibbon needed many more essential bodies of knowledge. Table 2 lists 25 that we believe he needed in 1954 before he could perform

Table 2. *Essential bodies of knowledge required for successful open-heart surgery.*

Preoperative diagnosis of cardiac defects
Anatomic and clinical
Physiologic: electrocardiography, other noninvasive tests
Physiologic: cardiac catheterization
Radiologic: selective angiocardiography

Preoperative care and preparation
Blood groups and typing; blood preservation; blood banks
Nutrition
Assessment of cardiac, pulmonary, renal, hepatic, and brain function
Management of heart failure

Intraoperative management
Asepsis
Monitoring ECG, blood pressure, heart rate, EEG, and blood O_2, CO_2, and pH
Anesthesia and neuromuscular blocking agents
Hypothermia and survival of ischemic organs
Ventilation of open thorax
Anticoagulants
Pump-oxygenator
Elective cardiac arrest; defibrillation
Transfusions; fluid and electrolytes; acid-base balance
Surgical instruments and materials
Surgical techniques and operations

Postoperative care
Relief of pain
General principles of intensive care; recording and warning systems
Management of infection
Diagnosis and management of circulatory failure
Diagnosis and management of other postoperative complications
Wound healing

open-heart surgery with confidence in the result; we list all of these because some, such as antibiotics, are so commonplace in 1976 that we forget that even they once had to be discovered! For the ten advances, we identified 137 essential bodies of knowledge.

The knowledge essential for these advances has accumulated over decades or centuries from the lifetime work of many thousands of scientists. It was clearly impossible for us to read all of their publications to determine how and why the research of each was done. But, because we were determined to avoid the let-me-give-you-an-example approach, we did examine about 4000 published articles. Of these, we identified about 2500 specific scientific reports that were particularly important to the development of one or more of the 137 essential bodies of knowledge. We arranged these chronologically in 137 tables. From these, with the advice of consultants, we then selected more than 500 essential or key articles for careful study.

Why did we spend several years collecting and reading thousands of articles and arranging more than 2500 of these in 137 chronological tables before doing our final analysis? There were several reasons.

1) It was essential that we have tangible evidence that our selections came from painstaking, scholarly review and not from the imperfect memories of a group of scientists at a cocktail party.

2) The chronological lists facilitate analysis of lags between initial discovery and clinical application (to be reported elsewhere).

3) They emphasize to the reader that scientific advance requires far more work than that reported by the discoverer or by those who wrote key articles essential for his discovery. We believe that a major defect in education in science in high school and colleges is the perpetuation of the one person = one discovery myth (for example, Marconi = wireless; Edison = electric light) and that this is partly responsible for the anecdotal approach to national science policy. Without a long chronologic tabulation, such as the electrocardiography (ECG) list in Table 3, some might consider that Einthoven in 1903 invented the ECG in its 1976 form, without help from those who preceded or followed him. Chronological tables provide specific evidence for policy-makers that scientists earlier and later than the discoverer have always been essential to each discovery and its full development. A defect in tables is that they can convey only a bit of the message, because even a long list includes only a small fraction of the good, original research that helped to move us away from complete ignorance toward full knowledge.

Definition of a key article

1) It had an important effect on the direction of subsequent research and development, which, in turn, proved to be important for clinical advance in one or more of the ten clinical advances under study.

2) It reported new data, new ways of looking at old data, a new concept or hypothesis, a new method, new drug, new apparatus, or a new technique that either was essential for full development of one or more of the clinical advances (or necessary bodies of knowledge) or greatly accelerated it. The key article might report basic laboratory investigation, clinical investigation, development of apparatus or essential components, synthesis of data and ideas of others, or wholly theoretical work.

3) A study is not a key study (even if it won the Nobel Prize for its author) if it has not yet served directly or indirectly as a step toward solving one of the ten clinical advances.

4) An article is a key article if it described the final step in the clinical advance, even though it was an inevitable step requiring no unusual imagination, creativity, or special competence (for example, first person to report on a new drug in humans even though basic work on animals had been done and results in humans were largely predictable).[4]

Selection and analysis of key articles

Because these key articles formed the basis of our analysis, we devoted considerable thought to their selection. We realized that bias in selecting them could invalidate our study and that their careful review by consultants was essential. At the same time, experience with pilot studies showed us that scientists are rarely unanimous in voting that Jones's discovery is more important than Smith's. Sometimes this is because of justified differences in judgment; sometimes it is because there is no one article that can be singled out from many in a steady advance with many equal contributors. We solved this problem for the purposes of this study (though not for election of individual scientists

Table 3. *Chronological events in the development of electrocardiography. The scientists' names that are printed in boldface type indicate key articles.*

Year of discovery	Scientist	Event and publication
B.C.	Ancients	Early manifestations of electricity: electric fish, rubbed amber, lodestone, terrestrial lightning
1660	von Guericke	First electricity machine (friction of glass and hand) [*Experimenta Nova Magdeburgica* (Jansson, Amsterdam, 1672), book 4, p. 147]
1745	von Kleist	Charge from electricity machine stored in glass bottle and delivered as static electric shock [Letter to Dr. Lieberkühn, 4 November 1745; J. G. Krüger, *Geschichte der Erde* (Luderwaldischen, Halle, 1746)]
1745–1750	Musschenbroek	Electricity stored in Leyden jar; shocks killed small animals [*Introductio ad Philosophiam Naturalem* (Luchtmans, Leyden, 1762), pp. 477–1132]
1752	**Franklin**	Kite and key used to charge Leyden jar from lightning; identity of lightning and electricity proved [*Philos. Trans. R. Soc. London* **47**, 565 (1751–1752)]
1756–1757	Caldani	Nerve and muscle excited by discharge from Leyden jar [*Institutiones Physiologicae* (Pezzana, Venice, 1786)]
1780	**Galvani**	Stimulation of nerve by Leyden jar and "electricity machine" caused identical muscle contraction [*Bononiensi Scientiarum et Artium Instituto Atque Academia Commentarii* **7**, 363 (1791)]
1786	**Galvani**	Concept of animal electricity [*Bononiensi Scientiarum et Artium Instituto Atque Academia Commentarii* **7**, 363 (1791)]
1791	**Galvani**	Contraction of heart muscle produced by discharge from electric eel; contraction of muscle caused by injury current [*Dell'uso e dell'attività dell'arco conduttóre nelle contrazioni dei muscoli* (Tommaso d'Aquino, Bologna, 1794)]
1800	Volta	Electricity generated by dissimilar metals; voltaic pile or battery [*Philos. Trans. R. Soc. London Part 2* **90**, 403 (1800)]
1839	Purkinje	Purkinje's fibers in the cardiac ventricles [*De Musculari Cordis Structura* (Friedlaender, Bratislava, 1839)]
1842	**Matteucci**	Muscle contracts if its nerve is laid across another contracting muscle [see Dumas, *C. R. Acad. Sci.* **15**, 797 (1842)]
1843	DuBois-Reymond	Action current in nerve as well as muscle [*Untersuchungen über Thierische Elektricität* (Reimer, Berlin, 1848–49)]
1852	Stannius	Ligatures demonstrating specific conduction paths in heart [*Arch. Anat. Physiol. Wiss. Med.* p. 85 (1852)]
1856	Kölliker and Müller	Frog muscle contraction used as indicator of cardiac currents [*Verh. Phys.-Med. Ges. Würzberg* **6**, 428 (1856)]
1875	Lippmann	Use of capillary electrometer [*Ann. Chim. Phys. Ser. 5* **5**, 494 (1875)]

Table 3 (*cont.*)

Year of discovery	Scientist	Event and publication
1876	Marey	Refractory period in early cardiac systole [*Physiol. Exp. Trav. Lab. Marey* **2**, 63 (1876)]
1878	Engelmann	Studied electrical excitation of isolated frog heart [*Pflügers Arch.* **17**, 68 (1878)]
1879–1880	**Burdon-Sanderson and Page**	First ECG in intact animals (frogs) [*J. Physiol.* **2**, 384 (1879–1880)]
1883	Gaskell	Sequence of contraction from sinus venosus to atria to ventricles [*J. Physiol.* **4**, 43 (1883)]
1887	**Waller**	First human ECG using Lippmann's capillary electrometer [*J. Physiol.* **8**, 229 (1887)]
1887	McWilliam	Noted fibrillary contractions of heart [*J. Physiol.* **8**, 296 (1887)]
1893	**His**	Atrioventricular bundle [*Arbeit. Med. Klin. Leipzig.* **14**, 14 (1893)]
1893	Kent	Atrioventricular bundle [*J. Physiol.* **14**, 233 (1893)]
1897	Ader	Thread or string galvanometer [*C. R. Acad. Sci.* **124**, 1440 (1897)]
1903	**Einthoven**	Sensitive string galvanometer for measuring human ECG; telemetry of ECG signals [*Pflügers Arch.* **99**, 472 (1903)]
1906	Tawara	Atrioventricular node [*Das Reizleitungssystem des Säugethierherzens* (Fischer, Jena, 1906)]
1907	Keith and Flack	Sinoatrial node, mammals [*J. Anat. Physiol.* **41**, 172 (1907)]
1908	Mackenzie	Polygraph, venous pulse and arrhythmias [*Diseases of the Heart* (Frowde, London, 1908)]
1909–1920	**Lewis**	ECG and arrhythmias in man (numerous articles in *Heart*, a magazine he founded)
1913	Einthoven, Fahr, de Waart	Equilateral triangle theory of ECG [*Arch. Ges. Physiol.* **150**, 275 (1913)]
1914	Garrey	Mechanisms of flutter and fibrillation; "circus" movements [*Am. J. Physiol.* **33**, 397 (1914)]
1915	Lewis and Rothschild	Excitation wave in dog heart [*Philos. Trans. R. Soc. London Ser. B* **206**, 181 (1915)]
1918	Smith	ECG changes after ligating a branch of coronary artery in dogs [*Arch. Int. Med.* **22**, 8 (1918)]
1926	Rothberger	Arrhythmias in man [in *Handbuch der Normalen und Pathologischen Physiologie* (Springer, Berlin, 1926), vol. 7]
1927	Wenckebach and Winterberg	Arrhythmias in man [*Die Unregelmässige Herztätigkeit* (Engelmann, Leipzig, 1927)]
1930	**Wilson**	Laws of distribution of potential differences in solid conductors; modern theory of ECG [*Am. Heart J.* **5**, 599 (1930)]
1939	Hodgkin and Huxley	Transmembrane action potential recorded in giant axone of squid [*Nature (London)* **144**, 710 (1939)]
1946 1949	Graham and Gerard Ling and Gerard	First measurement of transmembrane potential in skeletal muscle with intracellular microelectrodes [*J. Cell. Comp. Physiol.* **28**, 99 (1946); *ibid.* **34**, 383 (1949)]

Table 3 (*cont.*)

Year of discovery	Scientist	Event and publication
1949	Coraboeuf and Weidmann	Intracellular electrode to record mammalian cardiac potentials [*C. R. Seances Soc. Biol. Paris* **143**, 1329 (1949)]
1951	**Draper and Weidmann**	Intracellular electrode used to measure transmembrane potentials of heart muscle cells [*J. Physiol.* **115,** 74 (1951)]
1958	Alanís, González, López	Electrical activity of bundle of His [*J. Physiol.* **142**, 127 (1958)]
1960	Giraud, Peuch, Latour	Electrical activity of bundle of His in man [*Bull. Acad. Natl. Med. Paris* **144**, 363 (1960)]
1967–1968	**Scherlag** *et al.*	Recording from bundle of His by cardiac catheter in man [*J. Appl. Physiol.* **22**, 584 (1967); *ibid.* **25**, 425 (1968)]
1967	Watson, Emslie-Smith, Lowe	Recording from bundle of His in patient undergoing cardiac catheterization [*Am. Heart J.* **74**, 66 (1967)]

to a "Hall of Fame") by first selecting key articles in 42 of our tables and then sending the same tables (with no clue to our choices) to reviewers for their independent selection. We then analyzed the articles that we had selected to determine the goal of the investigators and repeated the same process for the articles selected by our reviewers. Although there was not complete agreement on the selection of individual key articles, there was almost exact agreement on the type of articles selected. Thus the percentage of key articles reporting research that was not clinically oriented was almost identical in their selections and in ours (Table 4). Because our interest was in determining the type of research reported in key articles (for example, clinically oriented research or that which was not clinically oriented) rather than in identifying specific scientists and their reports, we believe that the agreement on type, based on a sample of more than 50 percent of our key articles, justifies our extending it to the whole group.[5]

Once the key articles were selected, we re-read and analyzed each article to determine

Table 4. *Goal of authors of key articles as selected by reviewers and by us from the same 42 tables.*

Key articles selected by	Number of articles	Goal was not clinically oriented	Goal was clinically oriented	Percent of total not clinically oriented
Reviewers	494*	189*	305*	38.3
Us	267	101	166	37.8

*Total number of key articles selected by reviewers is higher than number selected by us because (i) the reviewers on the average selected 8.4 key articles per table and we selected on the average only 6.7 for these 42 tables; and (ii) we sent some tables to more than one reviewer.

the answers to the following questions. (i) How many key studies were clinically oriented? How many were not directed toward the solution of a clinical problem? (ii) How many key articles reported basic research? Other kinds of research? Development or engineering?

Was the key research clinically oriented?

To eliminate uncertainty about our definitions, in this section we avoid classifying research as clinical investigation, basic research, fundamental studies, directed or undirected research, or targeted or nontargeted research. Instead, we use only two terms; (i) clinically oriented research, and (ii) research that was not clinically oriented.

We define research as clinically oriented, even if it was performed entirely on animals, tissues, cells, or subcellular particles, if the author mentions even briefly an interest in diagnosis, treatment, or prevention of a clinical disorder or in explaining the basic mechanisms of a sign or symptom of the disease itself. Thus the Nobel Prize–winning research of Enders, Weller, and Robbins on extraneural culture of poliovirus in vitro was classified as clinically oriented because the team expressed an interest in multiplication of poliovirus outside the nervous system (for example, in the patient's gastrointestinal tract).

We define research as not clinically oriented if the authors neither state nor suggest any direct or indirect bearing that their research might have on a clinical disorder of humans, even though their work later helped to clarify some aspect of it. An article can be classified as not clinically oriented even if the research is done on a human (for example, Oliver's administration of an adrenal extract, later known as epinephrine, to his son in 1895 to see whether it would narrow the diameter of his radial artery).

Each article was classified as one or the other without consideration of earlier or later work of the same investigator and without being influenced by later stories (written or verbal) of "Why I did my research." The results of classifying 529 key articles into these two categories are shown in Table 5.

These data strongly support our contention that those concerned with preserving or changing national biomedical science policy should disregard anecdotal "evidence" no matter how convincingly the case is presented. Table 5 shows that someone looking for evidence to defend any position on the support of research can get it by choosing the right clinical advance as his example, his for-instance. If one picks vascular surgery or antibiotics or poliomyelitis, one can "prove" that clinically oriented research deserves major support; if one selects hypertension or oral diuretics or new diagnostic tests, one can "prove" that research that is not clinically oriented deserves major support.

The most important figure in Table 5 is that, for cardiovascular and pulmonary advances as a whole, 41 percent of all work judged to be essential or crucial for later clinical advances was not clinically oriented at the time of the research; 41 percent of the investigators, when they did their work, expressed no interest in a clinical problem – their goal was knowledge for the sake of knowledge. These data indicate clearly that planning for future clinical advances must include generous support for innovative and imaginative research that bears no discernible relation to a clinical problem at the time of peer review. Because of many unknown factors (for example, ratio of clinical as compared to non-clinical scientists who do not produce key articles to those who do; relative costs of supporting one type of scientist versus the other), we cannot translate "generous support" into a percentage of NIH's budget for extramural programs. Nor can we transfer conclusions from a study of cardiovascular and pulmonary research to other research fields,

Table 5. *Goal of authors of 529 key articles that later were judged to be essential for a clinical advance.*

Clinical advance	Clinically oriented	Not clinically oriented	Total	Percent of total not clinically oriented
Cardiac surgery	53	35	88	39.8
Vascular surgery	40	8	48	16.7
Hypertension	35	44	79	55.7
Coronary insufficiency	44	21	65	32.3
Cardiac resuscitation	24	16	40	40.0
Oral diuretics	19	24	43	55.8
Intensive care	*	*	*	*
Antibiotics	40	13	53	24.5
New diagnostic methods	41	53	94	56.4
Poliomyelitis	16	3	19	15.8
Total	312	217	529	41.0

*A key article is assigned to only one advance even though it may have been essential to more than one. Because practically every key article in intensive care was also essential to other advances, these articles were assigned elsewhere (for example, to cardiac or vascular surgery, coronary insufficiency, resuscitation, or antibiotics).

such as cancer research. But the conclusion seems inescapable that programs to identify and then to provide long-term support for creative individuals or groups (judged more likely than others to produce key research) should be expanded.

Was the key research basic or not?

Earlier, we avoided using the term basic research. We must now use it and define what we mean by it. We classify research as basic when the investigator, in addition to observing, describing, or measuring, attempts to determine the mechanisms responsible for the observed effects; with our definition, basic research can be on healthy or sick people, on animals, tissues, cells, or subcellular components. Our definition differs from the layman's (and some scientists') concept that research is more and more basic when the unit investigated is smaller and smaller; further, it allows that work on small units, such as cells, need not be basic if it is purely descriptive. It steers clear of whether the research was initiated by the investigator or by a commission, whether it was undirected or directed, whether supported by grant or by contract, because who initiated, directed, or supported the research has nothing to do with whether it is basic.

We analyzed each key article to determine how each investigator carried out his research and put each article in one or more of six categories.

1) Basic research unrelated to the solution of a clinical problem.

2) Basic research related to the solution of a clinical problem.

The clinical relationship was obvious when the investigator studied basic mechanisms of disease in patients; when it was not obvious, we depended on the investigator's statement, no matter how brief, that he initiated his research to gain further insights to the diagnosis, treatment, or prevention of human disease.

Two examples will clarify the difference between categories 1 and 2. When Landsteiner discovered human blood groups in 1900 he was investigating a basic problem in immunology and had no thought of the importance of his discovery to the transfusion of blood; this was clearly basic research unrelated at the time to the solution of a clinical problem (category 1). When Landsteiner, in 1909, found that a nonbacterial material (a virus) caused poliomyelitis in monkeys, this again was basic research but, since it was clearly related to a clinical problem, it fits category 2.

3) Studies not concerned with basic biological, chemical, or physical mechanisms.

These include purely descriptive studies (for example, description of a new disease, such as Stokes-Adams disease, without an investigation of the mechanism); an important observation that initially required no research (inhalation of ether causes anesthesia); a new procedure that required no research (cardiac catheterization); a new operation on humans that first required only perfecting surgical techniques in animals; and clinical tests of a new diuretic, antibiotic, or antihypertensive drug in humans without measurements designed to determine its mechanism of action.

4) Review and critical analysis of published work and synthesis of new concepts (without new experimental data).

5) Developmental work or engineering to create, improve, or perfect apparatus or a technique for research use.

6) Developmental work or engineering to create, improve, or perfect apparatus or a technique for use in diagnosis or care of patients.

The difference between categories 5 and 6 can be clarified by an example. Bayliss and Müller developed a roller-pump in 1929 to solve a problem in basic cardiac physiology; we classify this under category 5 even though later, as the DeBakey pump, it had widespread clinical use. The Drinker respirator (iron lung), developed for clinical use, we classify under category 6.

The results of classifying 529 key articles into these six categories are shown in Table 6. Note that of 567 entries, 209 are in category 1 and 141 in category 2; the total of studies in basic research, either unrelated or related to a clinical problem, was 350, or 61.7 percent of the total number of entries. Other types of clinically oriented studies (some inevitable once the basic research was done)[4] accounted for 21.2 percent of the total; development and engineering (much of it inevitable once the basic research was done)[4] accounted for 15.3 percent; synthesis accounted for less than 2 percent. Basic research therefore was responsible for almost three times as many key articles as other types of research and almost twice as many as non-basic research and development combined.

Objectivity of our study

Research on the process of discovery is unusually difficult in that the data come from judgments and decisions and not from physical measurements. Further, no matter how many consultants participate in the judgments and no matter how distinguished each is, to be a consultant each must be an expert in his field of knowledge (we cannot ask clergy, lawyers, or ethicists to determine which were the key advances leading to the prevention of poliomyelitis), and as such, each is likely to have some bias.

In the case of our study, its objectivity is strengthened by the fact that, although the data and conclusions emphasize the importance of nonclinically oriented research and of

Table 6. *Types of research reported in 529 key articles.*

Type	Basic: not clinically oriented	Basic: clinically oriented	Not basic	Review and synthesis	Development: research	Development: clinical	Total
Cardiac surgery	34	23	19	0	3	11	90
Vascular surgery	9	7	14	3	0	21	54
Hypertension	42	16	21	2	0	0	81
Coronary insufficiency	21	20	22	1	1	3	68
Cardiac resuscitation	16	11	9	0	0	6	42
Oral diuretics	23	13	6	1	0	0	43
Intensive care	*	*	*	*	*	*	*
Antibiotics	12	18	21	1	0	2	54
New diagnostic methods	49	21	5	2	17	22	116
Poliomyelitis	3	12	3	0	1	0	19
Total	209	141	120	10	22	65	567[†]
Percent of total	36.8	24.9	21.2	1.8	3.9	11.4	

*Because practically every key article in intensive care was also essential to other advances, these articles were assigned elsewhere (for example, to cardiac or vascular surgery, coronary insufficiency, resuscitation, or antibiotics).

[†]The total number of entries in the six categories (567) exceeds the total in Table 5 (529) by 38 entries. This is because some key articles fit into more than one category here, particularly when articles reporting development of new apparatus also reported research using it; no article in Table 5 was classified more than once.

basic research for clinical advance, only 26 percent of our consultants and only 24 percent of advisers on key articles were basic scientists.[3,5]

In the long run, data and conclusions from any single study should stand, fall, or be modified not by anecdotes or gut reactions, but by confirmation or refutation by better studies with improved design and more objective methods. We believe that a $2 billion industry might well put more of its annual budget into research on improving its main product, which in this case is discovery and its application.

Summary and conclusions

There has been much expert testimony before congressional committees and much national debate on the relative value of targeted in contrast to nontargeted and of applied in contrast to basic biomedical research. Most of it has been based on anecdotal evidence and little or none on an objective analysis of research in broad fields of medicine and surgery. This is understandable because for-instances are easy to come by, whereas research on research is unusually difficult and time consuming. Because we believe that national biomedical science policy should be based on research on the nature of discovery and its application, we have devoted several years to analyzing how and why lifesaving advances have come about in cardiovascular and pulmonary diseases. The advances that we studied were open-heart surgery, blood vessel surgery, treatment of hypertension, management of coronary artery disease, prevention of poliomyelitis, chemotherapy of tuberculosis and acute rheumatic fever, cardiac resuscitation and cardiac pacemakers, oral diuretics (for treatment of high blood pressure or of congestive heart failure), intensive care units, and new diagnostic methods. We screened more than 4000 scientific articles published in these fields, selected 2500 of these for further consideration, and then analyzed 529 of those that we (and 140 consultants) considered to be essential for the clinical advances.

Our analysis showed the following. (i) Of 529 key articles, 41 percent of all work judged to be essential for later clinical advance was not clinically oriented at the time it was done; the scientists responsible for these key articles sought knowledge for the sake of knowledge. (ii) Of the 529 articles, 61.7 percent described basic research (defined as research to determine mechanisms by which living organisms – including humans – function, or mechanisms by which drugs act); 21.2 percent reported other types of research; 15.3 percent were concerned with development of new apparatus, techniques, operations, or procedures; and 1.8 percent were review articles or reported synthesis of the data of others. Our data show that clinical advance requires different types of research and development and not one to the exclusion of another. Thus the problem is not either-or, but a question of how much support to one type and how much to another. Our data compel us to conclude (i) that a generous portion of the nation's biomedical research dollars should be used to identify and then to provide long-term support for creative scientists whose main goal is to learn how living organisms function, without regard to the immediate relation of their research to specific human diseases, and (ii) that basic research, as we have defined it, pays off in terms of key discoveries almost twice as handsomely as other types of research and development combined.

We believe that much more research needs to be done on the nature of research and its application so that data from objective studies can be applied to all aspects of biomedical research. Because the very nature of research on research, particularly if it is prospective rather than retrospective, requires long periods of time, we recommend that an independent, highly competent group be established with ample, long-term support to conduct and support retrospective and prospective research on the nature of scientific discovery, to analyze the causes of long and short lags between discovery and clinical application and to suggest and test means of decreasing long lags, and to evaluate present and proposed mechanisms for the support of biomedical research and development.

References and Notes

1. C. W. Sherwin and R. S. Isenson, *First Interim Report on Project Hindsight* (Office of Director of Defense Research and Engineering, Washington, D.C., 30 June 1966, revised 13 October 1966).

2. J. A. Shannon, in *Research in the Service of Man: Biomedical Knowledge, Development and Use* (Document 55, U.S. Senate, 90th Congress, 1st session, 1967), pp. 72–85; M. B. Visscher, in *Applied Science and Technological Progress* (National Academy of Sciences Report, Washington, D.C., 1967), pp. 185–206; *Technology in Retrospect and Critical Events in Science* (National Science Foundation, Washington, D.C., 1968), prepared by Illinois Institute of Technology; K. W. Deutsch, J. Platt, D. Senghass, *Science* **171**, 450 (1971); G. Holton, *Grad. J.* **9**, 397 (1973); *Interactions of Science and Technology in the Innovative Process: Some Case Studies* (National Science Foundation Report NSF C667, Washington, D.C., 1973), prepared by Battelle Laboratories; E. H. Kone and H. J. Jordan, Eds., *The Greatest Adventure: Basic Research That Shapes Our Lives* (Rockefeller Univ. Press, New York, 1974).

3. Of these, 70 were clinicians, 37 were basic medical scientists, and 33 were engineers, science administrators (in industry, government, or universities), or science writers.
4. Some consultants did not designate such contributions as key articles. We did, however, because we knew of a number of instances in which the final step was "inevitable" but no one seemed willing to take it (for example, vascular surgery was inevitable by 1910 but was not applied until 1939).
5. Bias could also enter into our selection of reviewers of tables. Thirty-two reviewers were physicians, surgeons, or medical or surgical specialists; 10 were basic medical scientists. All were highly knowledgeable in the field that they reviewed.
6. Supported by contract 1-HO-1-2327 from the National Heart and Lung Institute and grants from the Commonwealth Fund and The Burroughs Wellcome Fund.

QUESTIONS FOR DISCUSSION

1. Can creativity be learned? If so, can it be taught?
2. Why is a paradigm vital to progress in science, even though it may inhibit radical breakthroughs?
3. If a wide range of knowledge and experience is vital to creativity, what is the importance of specialization and expertise in the details of a specific field?

RECOMMENDED SUPPLEMENTAL READING

Science and Human Values, 2nd ed., J. Bronowski, New York: Harper and Row, 1965, pp. 3–24.

The Double Helix, James D. Watson, New York: Atheneum Publishers, 1968.

The Structure of Scientific Revolutions, Thomas Kuhn, Chicago, IL: University of Chicago Press, 1970.

"Reflections on the Ambiguity of Science," Robert S. Cohn, in Leroy S. Rouner (ed.), *Foundations of Ethics,* vol. 4, Notre Dame, IN: University of Notre Dame Press, 1983, pp. 223–234.

PART II

The Roots of Honor and Integrity in Science

INTRODUCTION

The essence of science is the pursuit and transmission of knowledge, an endeavor that depends upon honesty, objectivity, intellectual freedom, and trust over generations, across disciplines, and across national borders. As every researcher depends on the validity of others' previous work, and because no single individual can master every dimension of any field, the practical demands of science reinforce an inherently moral social contract among researchers.

Bentley Glass outlines this social contract and how it can help investigators resist the temptation to seek glory and self-aggrandizement at the expense of their colleagues or the truth. Because the truth belongs to everyone, individual researchers must share their findings openly. Because everyone is capable of error, scientists must approach their own research critically and that of others with an open mind. Ideally, competition should enhance the integrity of science because all researchers must rely on colleagues to verify, interpret, and expand upon their work. Thus the truest mark of success in science is the recognition of one's peers.

In ''Making and Breaking the Rules of Science,'' Alexander Kohn examines this social contract and the costs to science and society of deviating from it. Maintaining scientific integrity goes beyond simply avoiding unacceptable behavior to a personal dedication to honesty, which must be reinforced by ongoing professional consideration of the conceptual and ethical goals and foundations of science.

3
The ethical basis of science

Bentley Glass

It has been said that science has no ethical basis, that it is no more than a cold, impersonal way of arriving at the objective truth about natural phenomena. This view I wish to challenge, since it is my belief that by examining critically the nature, origins, and methods of science we may logically arrive at a conclusion that science is ineluctably involved in questions of values, is inescapably committed to standards of right and wrong, and unavoidably moves in the large toward social aims.

Human values have themselves evolved. Man arose after some two billions of years of organic evolution, during which species after species originated, flourished, and fell, or occasionally became the progenitors of species that were new and better adapted, on the basis of the evolutionary scheme of values. Fitness, like it or not, in the long run meant simply the contribution of each trait and its underlying genes to survival. High mortality or sterility led to extinction; good viability and fertility enabled a gene or a trait, an individual or a species, to be perpetuated. Man's own values grew out of his evolutionary origins and his struggle against a hostile environment for survival. His loss of certain unnecessary structures, such as bodily hair once clothing was invented; the homeostatic regulation of his body temperature and blood pressure, breathing, and pre-dominant direction of blood flow; his embryonic and fetal growth inside the mother and his prolonged dependence upon maternal lactation; the slow maturation that enabled his brain to enlarge so greatly; the keen vision so necessary to the hunter using his weapons – all of these and many other important human characteristics that contributed to the social nature of man and cemented the bonds of family and tribe arose adventitiously, were improved step by step, and endured because they promoted human survival. Our highest ethical values – the love of the mother for her child and of the man for his mate, the willingness to sacrifice one's own life for the safety of the family or tribe, and the impulse to care for the weak, the suffering, the helpless – all of these too had the same primitive beginnings.

But these ethical values are always, in the evolutionary scheme of things, relative, and never absolute. Whenever the environment becomes changed, the adaptiveness of existing traits becomes maladjusted, and the forces of natural selection lead to a realignment of the genotype, an alteration of the external features and modes of behavior, a modification of the species. What was once good is so no longer. Something else, in terms of repro-ductive fitness, has become better.

Finally, a crude, embryonic form of science entered the scheme of things, a method of observing and reporting accurately to other persons the movements of the stars, the

From *Science*, 1965, 150, 1254–1261. © AAAS.

planets, and the sun and moon, the behavior and migrations of the food animals, the usefulness of certain seeds for food and of certain stems for fibers, the poisonous properties of others. For generations all such practical lore was transmitted only by word of mouth, but the day came when useful knowledge could be written down and preserved inviolate from the forgetfulness and the twists of memory. These were the first simple steps in the development of science: observation, reporting, written records, communication. To such must be added the processes of human reasoning, at first mostly by analogy, so often wrong; then by improved analysis, by deduction from an established truth, or by induction of an established truth from a multitude of observations.

Seen aright, science is more than the instrument of man's increasing power and progress. It is also an instrument, the finest yet developed in the evolution of any species, for the malleable adaptation of man to his environment and the adjustment of his environment to man. If the human species is to remain successful, this instrument must be used more and more to control the nature and the rate of social and technological change, as well as to promote it. In this sense, at least, science is far more than a new sense organ for comprehending the real relations of natural phenomena and the regularities we call "laws of nature." It is also man's means of adjustment to nature, man's instrument for the creation of an ideal environment. Since it is preeminently an achievement of social man, its primary function is not simply that of appeasing the individual scientist's curiosity about his environment – on the contrary it is that of adjusting man to man, and of adjusting social groups in their entirety to nature, to both the restrictions and the resources of the human environment.

Ethics is a philosophy of morals, a moral system that defines duty and labels conduct as right or wrong, better or worse. The evolutionist is quite prepared to admit the existence of right and wrong in terms of the simple functions of biological structures and processes. The eye is for seeing, an evolutionary adaptation that enables an animal to perceive objects at a distance by means of reflected light rays. Sight conveys information about food, water, danger, companionship, mating, the whereabouts and doings of the young ones, and other vitally important matters. Should one not then say, "To see is right; not to see is wrong"? Similarly, the mind reasons as it does because in the countless ages of evolutionary development its characteristic mental processes led to successful coping with the exigencies of life. Humans whose mental processes, because of different genes, too often led them to wildly erroneous conclusions did not so often leave children to reason in similar ways. It is thus right to be guided by reason, wrong to distrust it. Does it not follow, finally, from consideration of the social role and function of science, that it is *right* to utilize science to develop and regulate human social life, adjustment to change, and rate of social transformation? Conversely, it is *wrong* – morally and ethically wrong – not to do so. We must use whatever light and whatever reason we have to chart our course into the unknown.

Those who distrust science as a guide to conduct, whether individual or social, seem to overlook its pragmatic nature, or perhaps they scorn it for that very reason. Rightly understood, science can point out to us only probabilities of varying degrees of certainty. So, of course, do our eyes and ears, and so does our reason. What science can do for us that otherwise we may be too blind or self-willed to recognize is to help us to see that what is right enough for the individual may be wrong for him as a member of a social group, such as a family; that what is right for the family may be wrong for the nation; and that what is right for the nation may be wrong for the great brotherhood of man.

Nor should one stop at that point. Man as a species is a member – only one of many members – of a terrestrial community and an even greater totality of life upon earth. Ultimately, what is right for man is what is right for the entire community of life on earth. If he wrecks that community, he destroys his own livelihood. In this sense, coexistence is not only necessary but also right, and science can reveal to us the best ways to harbor our resources and to exploit our opportunities wisely.

The subjectivity of science

From the foregoing description of science as itself an evolutionary product and a human organ produced by natural selection, it may already be guessed that I do not adhere to the view that either the processes or the concepts of science are strictly objective. They are as objective as man knows how to make them, that is true; but man is a creature of evolution, and science is only his way of looking at nature. As long as science is a *human* activity, carried on by individual men and by groups of men, it must at bottom remain inescapably subjective.

Our sensory apparatus and the structure of the human nervous system, within which arise our sensations, grow and develop as they do from the first beginnings in the human embryo because of the particular genetic constitutions we inherit from our parents. First and foremost, we are *human* scientists, not insect scientists, nor even monkey scientists. The long past of our evolutionary history, with its countless selections and rejections of various kinds of genes and combinations of genes, has made us what we are. Try as we will, we cannot break the bonds of our subjective interpretations of the physical events of nature. We are born blind to many realities, and at best can apprehend them only by translating them by means of our instruments into something we can sense with our eyes or ears, into something we can then begin to reason about by developing abstract mental concepts about them, by making predictions on the basis of our hypotheses, and by testing our theories to see whether reality conforms to our notions.

This line of reasoning leads us to the conclusion that the objectivity of science depends wholly upon the ability of different observers to agree about their data and their processes of thought. About quantitative measurements and deductive reasoning there is usually little dispute. Qualitative experiences like color, or inductive and theoretical types of reasoning, leave great room for disagreement. Usually they can be reduced to scientific treatment only if the subjective color can by agreement be translated into some quantitative measurement such as a wavelength, only if the reasoning can be rendered quantitative by use of a calculus of probability. It nevertheless remains a basic fact of human existence that the subjectivity of the individual personality cannot be escaped. We differ in our genes, each of us possessing a genotype unique throughout all past and future human history (unless we happen to possess an identical twin). To the extent that our genes endow us with similar, though not identical, sensory capacities and nervous systems, we may make similar scientific observations, and we may agree to ignore the existence of the variables in our natures that prevent us from ever making exactly the same measurements as someone else or arriving at exactly the same conclusions. But it is perilous to forget our genetic individuality and our own uniqueness of experience. These form the basis of the ineradicable subjectivity of science. In the last analysis science is the common fund of agreement between individual interpretations of nature. What science has done is to refine and extend the methods of attaining agreement. It has not banished the place of the individual observer, experimenter, or theoretician, whose work is perhaps subjective quite as much as objective.

These considerations may seem so obvious as not to require the emphasis just given them. Yet I believe not. Somehow there has crept into our writings about the nature and methods of science a dictum that science is objective while the humanistic studies are subjective, that science stands outside the nature of man. What a profound mistake! Science is ultimately as subjective as all other human knowledge, since it resides in the mind and the senses of the unique individual person. It is constrained by the present evolutionary state of man, by the limitations of his senses and the even more significant limitations of his powers of reason. All that can be claimed for science is that it focuses upon those primary observations about which human observers (most of them) can agree, and that it emphasizes those methods of reasoning which, from empirical results or the successful fulfillment of predictions, most often lead to mental constructs and conceptual schemes that satisfy all the requirements of the known phenomena.

Science, integrity, and intellectual freedom

From a consideration that science is a human activity, inescapably subjective, and a product of biological evolution, it is possible to derive a genuine ethical basis of science. J. Bronowski, in an essay entitled "The Sense of Human Dignity" (*1*, p. 63), has sketched a treatment that serves well for a beginning. The values and duties which are the concern of ethics are social, he affirms. The duties of men hold a society together, he says; and "the problem of values arises only when men try to fit together their need to be social animals with their need to be free men." Philosophy must deal with both the social and individual aspects of value. Most philosophical systems have found this very difficult to do. Thus dialectical materialism swings far to the side of social values and leaves little scope for individual freedom. Positivism and analytic philosophy, as typified by Bertrand Russell and Wittgenstein, on the other hand, emphasize the values of the individual.

Hence, continues Bronowski, because the unit of the positivist or the analyst is one individual man, "positivists and analysts alike believe that the words *is* and *ought* belong to different worlds, so that sentences constructed with *is* usually have a verifiable meaning, but sentences constructed with *ought* never have" (*1*, p. 72).

The issue, then, is simply whether verification can indeed be assumed to be carried out by one man. Bronowski concludes, and I find it impossible to deny, that in the practice of science this supposition is sheer nonsense. Verification depends completely on the existence of records that may be consulted, of instruments that may be used, of concepts that must be understood and be properly utilized. In all these ways, knowledge is a social construct, science a collective human enterprise, and verification is no procedure of the naked, unlettered, resourceless man but an application of the collective tools of the trade and the practiced logic of science to the matter at hand. It is a fallacy to assume that one can test what is true and what is false unaided. But then it must follow that all verification, all science, depends upon communication with others and reliance upon others. Thus we come straight to the *ought* of science, for we must be able to trust the word of others. A full and true report is the hallmark of the scientist, a report as accurate and faithful as he can make it in every detail. The process of verification depends upon the ability of another scientist, of any other scientist who wishes to, to repeat a procedure and to confirm an observation.

Neither the philosophy of dialectical materialism nor that of the individualist accords with the basic nature of man and of scientific truth. The extreme social position leaves no room for the conscience of man and the exercise of intellectual freedom because the community dictates what is right and what a man *ought* to do. Yet the positivist's position is also faulty because "how a man *ought* to behave is a social question, which always involves several people; and if he accepts no evidence and no judgment except his own, he has no tools with which to frame an answer" (*1*, p. 72). Again, "All this knowledge, all our knowledge, has been built up communally; there would be no astrophysics, there would be no history, there would not even be language, if man were a solitary animal" (*1*, p. 73).

"What follows?" asks Bronowski, and answers (*1*, p. 73): "It follows that we must be able to rely on other people; we must be able to trust their word. That is, it follows that there is a principle which binds society together, because without it the individual would be helpless to tell the true from the false. This principle is truthfulness. If we accept truth as a criterion, then we have also to make it the cement to hold society together." Whence he derives the social axiom:

"We OUGHT to act in such a way that what IS true can be verified to be so."

So Bronowski. If his reasoning be accepted, and to me it seems unarguable, we must conclude that the cement of society is nothing less than the basic ethical tenet of science itself. The very possibility of verification, the assurance that one's own conclusions are not dreams, hallucinations, or delusions rests upon confirmation by others, by "competent" observers whom we trust to tell the truth.

The scientist's integrity. Ethics rests upon moral integrity. Science rests upon the scientist's integrity. This is so implicit in all of our science that it is rarely expressed and may be overlooked by novice or layman. Bronowski mentions examples of what happens when this basic moral commandment is violated by a scientist. Lysenko is held up to scorn throughout the world and eventually is deposed (*2*). Kammerer commits suicide (*3*). It is very interesting that both of these notorious examples, and others less well known, such as that of Tower, a quondam professor of biology at the University of Chicago, have related to attempts to "prove" or bolster the theory of the inheritance of acquired characteristics. The singular attractiveness of this theory for violators of scientific integrity is no doubt owing to its social significance, since if true it would offer a quick and easy way for man to control the direction of human evolution and would lessen the obdurate qualities of genes modifiable only by mutation in uncontrollable directions.

It is not so generally recognized by these superficial evolutionary philosophers that, if true, the inheritance of characters produced through modifications of the environment would call in question the value of all evolutionary gains, since the modified characters would themselves have no real genetic permanence and would shift and vary with every change of environment. They also do not recognize one of the most essential aspects of heredity, the protection of the genetic nature against vicissitudes. The reason why death is so necessary a part of life is that the ground must be cleared for fresh life. The reason why the genotype must remain unmodifiable by ordinary environmental causes is because the course of life for every individual involves the cumulative effects of injury, disease, and senescence. The new generation must indeed start *fresh* – that is, free from all the disabilities incurred during life by its parents and remoter ancestors. Evolution through the action of natural selection upon mutations, most of which are harmful and nonadaptive, while only a rare exemplar among them is possibly advantageous, is a process slow in the extreme. But it preserves the gains of the past, and it permits every generation to be born anew, unburdened by decrepitude, to try out its varieties of genotypes in each niche of the environment.

The loss of scientific integrity through deliberate charlatanry or deception is less common than the violation of scholarly honesty through plagiarism. The theft of another man's ideas and the claim that another's discovery is one's own may do no injury to the body of scientific knowledge, if the substance of what is stolen be true. It may even do no harm to the original discoverer, who may be dead or in no need of further credit to advance his own career. It is nevertheless a canker in the spirit of the thief and does damage to the fabric of science by rendering less trustworthy the witness of the scientist.

Plagiarism shades into unacknowledged borrowing. Which of us in fact can render exactly the sources of all his ideas? Psychologists have now amply demonstrated the ease with which self-deception enters into the forgetfulness of borrowed benefits. The wintry wind of man's ingratitude blows only on the donor of benefits forgot. Around the self-deluded recipient blow only the mildest, gentlest zephyrs of spring. The newer patterns of scientific publication and support of research have multiplied a thousandfold the opportunities for the scientist's self-deception. Editors of scientific journals today customarily rely upon referees for opinions regarding the merit of manuscripts submitted for publication. The enormous expansion of scientific activity and the development of hundreds of new specialties have made this referee system necessary. The best referee is of course some other scientist who is working closely on the same scientific problems but is not associated with the author in the actual work – in other words, a competitor, since we must not forget that scientists are people who must earn a living, and since compensation and repute follow productivity and publication. Natural selection is at work among scientists, too! What is most alarming about the workings of the referee system is not the occasional overt lapse of honesty on the part of some referee who suppresses prompt publication of a rival's work while he harvests the fruit by quickly repeating it – perhaps even extending it – and rushing into publication with his own account. What is far more dangerous, I believe, because it is far more insidious and widespread, is the inevitable subconscious germination in the mind of any referee of the ideas he has obtained from the unpublished work of another person. If we are frank with ourselves, none of us can really state where most of the seminal ideas that lead us to a particular theory or line of investigation have been derived. Darwin frankly acknowledged the ideas of Malthus which led him to the Theory of Natural Selection; but although he was one of the most honest of men, and one who was deeply troubled when Alfred Russel Wallace sent him in 1858 the brief paper setting forth his own parallel derivation of Darwin's theory, Darwin nevertheless never made the slightest acknowledgment of the idea of natural selection which he had surely read in the work of Edward Blyth in 1835 and 1837 (4). We may guess that Darwin's reasoning at the time went rather as follows:

Blyth's conception is that natural selection leads to a restriction of hereditary variation in populations. Through elimination of the more variable specimens in a species, nature keeps the species true to type and prevents it from becoming maladapted to its environment. Blyth's Natural Selection is not an evolutionary force at all, but instead is a force for maintenance of the status quo.

Yet it is very hard to understand why, when the full significance of the action of natural selection dawned upon Darwin, he did not reexamine the ideas of Edward Blyth. It should have been perfectly evident to him that the very same force that would eliminate variation and maintain the status quo of the species in a stationary environment would operate quite differently in a changing environment. Will we then ever know the extent to which Darwin was really indebted to Blyth, or how the ideas he probably rejected as invalid actually prepared the way for his reception of Malthus's thoughts in 1838?

The conscientious referee of unpublished scientific manuscripts is similarly a gleaner in the harvest fields of others. The only possible way to avoid taking an unfair advantage would be to refuse to referee any manuscripts that might conceivably have a relationship to one's own research work. The consequences for editors left with piles of unevaluated manuscripts might become desperate, were there not, as I believe, a reasonable solution in the possibility that the role of referee could be limited to scientists who have ceased to do active experimental work themselves. What with the increasing life span and the large number of retired but mentally vigorous older scientists, the supply of competent referees would perhaps be sufficient. To be sure, the criticism may be raised that the older scientific men cannot properly evaluate the significance and merit of really revolutionary new ideas and lines of work. Neither, for the most part, can the young! A combination of older referees in the field and younger ones knowledgeable but not working in the same specialty might solve this difficulty.

What has been said about referees applies with even greater force to the scientists who sit on panels that judge the merit of research proposals made to government agencies or to foundations. The amount of confidential information directly applicable to a man's own line of work acquired in this way in the course of several years staggers the imagination. The most conscientious man in the world cannot forget all this, although he too easily forgets when and where a particular idea came to him. This information consists not only of reports of what has been done in the recent past but of what is still unpublished. It includes also the plans and protocols of work still to be performed, the truly germinal ideas that may occupy a scientist for years to come. After serving for some years on such panels I have reached the conclusion that this form of exposure is most unwise. One simply cannot any longer distinguish between what one properly knows, on the basis of published scientific information, and what one has gleaned from privileged documents. The end of this road is self-deception on the one hand, or conscious deception on the other, since in time scientists who must make research proposals learn that it is better not to reveal what they really intend to do, or to set down in plain language their choicest formulations of experimental planning, but instead write up as the program of their future work what they have in fact already performed. Again, the integrity of science is seriously compromised.

Science and intellectual freedom. The first commandment in the ethical basis of science is complete truthfulness, and the second is like unto it:

Thou shalt neither covet thy neighbor's ideas nor steal his experiments.

The third is somewhat different. It requires fearlessness in the defense of intellectual freedom, for science cannot prosper where there is constraint upon daring thinking, where society dictates what experiments may be conducted, or where the statement of one's conclusions may lead to loss of livelihood, imprisonment, or even death.

This is a hard ethic to live by. It brought Giordano Bruno to the stake in 1600. The recantation of Galileo was an easier way; the timidity of Descartes and Leibniz, who left unpublished their more daring scientific thoughts, was understandably human but even less in the interest of science or, ultimately, of the society that felt itself threatened. Whether in the conflict of science with religion, or with political doctrine (as in Nazi Germany), or with social dogma (as in the Marxist countries), scientists must be willing to withstand attack and vilification, ostracism and punishment, or science will wither away and society itself, in the end, be the loser.

From the beginning the inveterate foe of scientific inquiry has been authority – the authority of tradition, of religion, or of the state – since science can accept no dogma within the sphere of its investigations. No doors must be barred to its inquiries, except by reason of its own limitations. It is the essence of the scientific mind not only to be curious but likewise to be skeptical and critical – to maintain suspended judgment until the facts are in, to be willing always, in the light of fresh knowledge, to change one's conclusions. Not even the "laws" of science are irrevocable decrees. They are mere summaries of observed phenomena, ever subject to revision. These laws and concepts remain testable and challengeable. Science is thus wholly dependent upon freedom – freedom of inquiry and freedom of opinion.

But what is the value of science to man, that it should merit freedom? There are those, indeed, who say that science has value only in serving our material wants. To quote one of them: "Science is a social phenomenon, and like every other social phenomenon is limited by the injury or benefit it confers on the community. . . . The idea of free and unfettered science . . . is absurd." Those were the words of Adolf Hitler, as reported by Hermann Rauschning (5). In Soviet states a similar view is held officially; and in the Western democracies, likewise, not a few scientists as well as laymen have upheld a similar opinion. The British biologist John R. Baker has pointed out that this view shades through others, such as the admission that scientists work best if they enjoy their work, and the supposition that science has value in broadening the outlook and purging the mind of pettiness, to the view that a positive and primary value of science lies in its creative aspect "as an end in itself, like music, art, and literature" (6). "Science aims at knowledge, not utility," says Albert Szent-Györgyi (7); and Alexander von Humboldt wrote in his masterpiece, *Cosmos,* that "other interests, besides the material wants of life, occupy the minds of men" (8).

It is readily demonstrated that the social usefulness of the conclusions of science can rarely be predicted when the work is planned or even after the basic discoveries have been made. John R. Baker, in his book *Science and the Planned State,* has cited numerous examples that show the impracticability of too narrowly planned a program of scientific research. The sphere of investigation must be determined by the investigator's choice rather than by compulsion – by perception of a problem to be solved rather than by a dogma to be accepted blindly. Science must be free to question and investigate any matter within the scope of its methods and to hold and state whatever conclusions are reached on the basis of the evidence – or it will perish. But science is represented only by the individual scientists. These persons must acknowledge the moral imperative to defend the freedom of science at any cost to themselves. Every Darwin needs a Thomas Henry Huxley. Every Lysenko demands his martyred Vavilov, his hundreds of displaced geneticists before he is finally deposed. Modern science, from its very beginnings near the end of the 16th century, became immediately concerned with a major political issue, the freedom of the scientist to pursue the truth wherever it might lead him, even though that conclusion might be highly disturbing to settled religious beliefs or social conventions and practice. The pyre of Bruno and the ordeal of Galileo led directly in spirit to the attacks on Charles Darwin 250 years later and to latter-day instances of the social suppression of scientific findings. The distortion of genetics by racists in Nazi Germany finds a counterpart in the United States. Mendelian genetics in the U.S.S.R. and the nutritive qualities of oleomargarine in Wisconsin share a similar fate. The third commandment then reads:

Thou shalt defend the freedom of scientific investigation and the freedom of publication of scientific opinion with thy life, if need be.

Science and communication. Inasmuch as science is intrinsically a social activity and not a solitary pleasure, another primary aspect of the ethics of science is the communication to the world at large, and to other scientists in particular, of what one observes and what one concludes. Both the international scope of scientific activity and the cumulative nature of scientific knowledge lay upon the individual scientist an overwhelming debt to his colleagues and his forerunners. The least he can do in return, unless he is an ingrate, is freely to make his own contributions a part of the swelling flood of scientific information available to all the world.

There are at least five distinct obligations his indebtedness places upon each scientist. The first of these is the obligation to publish his methods and his results so clearly and in such detail that another may confirm and extend his work. The pettiness and jealousy that lead some scientists, in their effort to stay ahead of the ruck, to withhold some significant step of procedure or some result essential to full understanding of the stated conclusions have no place in the realm of science. In other instances it is sheer laziness or procrastination that is at fault. Whatever the only-too-human reason, science suffers.

A second obligation that is far more frequently neglected is the obligation to see that one's contributions are properly abstracted and indexed, and thus made readily available to workers everywhere. Many scientists ignore this obligation completely. Yet, as the sheer volume of scientific publication passes a half-million and soon a million articles a year, it is obviously insufficient to add one's own leaflet to the mountains of paper cramming the scientific libraries of the world. The need to have scientific findings abstracted and indexed has been fully recognized by such international bodies as the International Council of Scientific Unions: its Abstracting Board has urged every author to prepare an abstract in concise, informative style, to be printed at the head of each scientific paper; and the editors of most scientific journals have now made this a requirement for acceptance and publication of a paper. Nevertheless, few authors prepare their abstracts without a reminder, and few heed the requirements for a concise, informative summary that will permit proper indexing of the major items treated in the paper.

A third obligation is that of writing critical reviews, which will be true syntheses of the knowledge accumulating in some field. I firmly believe that there is no scientific activity today more necessary and at the same time less frequently well done than this one. I have said elsewhere (9):

To be sure, the scientist seeks for facts – or better, he starts with observations. . . . But I would say that the real scientist, if not the scholar in general, is no quarryman, but is precisely and exactly a builder – a builder of facts and observations into conceptual schemes and intellectual models that attempt to present the realities of nature. It is the defect and very imperfection of the scientist that so often he fails to build a coherent and beautiful structure of his work . . .

The creativity of scientific writing lies precisely here. The task of the writer of a critical review and synthesis . . . is not only indispensable to scientific advance – it surely constitutes the essence of the scientific endeavor to be no mere quarryman but in some measure a creator of truth and understanding. The aesthetic element that makes scientist akin to poet and artist is expressed primarily in this broader activity.

The critical nature of the critical review grows from our constant forgetfulness of all this. The young scientist is taught carefully and methodically to be a quarryman or a bricklayer. He learns to use his tools well but not to enlarge his perspective, develop his critical powers, or enhance his skill in communication. The older scientist is too often overwhelmed by detail, or forced by the competition of the professional game to stick to the processes of "original research" and "training." The vastness of the scientific literature makes the search for general comprehension and perception of new relationships and possibilities every day more arduous. The editor of the critical review journal finds every year a growing reluctance on the part of the best qualified scientists to devote the necessary time and energy to this task. Often it falls by default to the journeyman of modest talent, a compiler rather than critic and creator, who enriches the scientific literature with a fresh molehill in which later compilers may burrow.

All this need not be so, but it will remain so without a deeper sense of the obligation of the scientist to synthesize and present his broadest understanding of his own field of knowledge. Tomorrow's science stands on the shoulders of those who have done so, no less than on the shoulders of the great discoverers.

A fourth obligation is communication to the general public of the great new revelations of science, the important advances, the noble syntheses of scientific knowledge. There have always been a few eminent scientists who did not scorn to do this: Thomas Henry Huxley, John Tyndall, and Louis Pasteur set the pattern in the 19th century, and in our own time there have indeed been many who followed their precedent. Yet there seems to be a growing tendency to turn this obligation over to professional science writers who, however good, should not replace the direct, personal, and authoritative appeal of the scientist to the general public. As our culture and civilization become day by day more completely based on scientific discovery and technological application, as human exploration becomes ever more restricted to the endless frontiers of science, every citizen must know whereby he lives and whereupon he leans. A democracy rests secure only upon a basis of enlightened citizens who have imbibed the spirit of science and who comprehend its nature as well as its fruits. In fulfilling the requirement of our age for the public understanding of science the scientist must shirk no duty.

A final obligation in the total purview of scientific communication is the obligation to transmit the best and fullest of our scientific knowledge to each succeeding generation. It is well said that genetic transmission of human characteristics and powers is now far overshadowed by cultural inheritance. The transmission of knowledge is the role of the teacher, and the obligation of the scientist to teach is his last and highest obligation to the society that gives him opportunity to achieve his goals.

To every scientist – to some sooner, to some only late – there comes the realization that one lifetime is too short and that other hands and other minds must carry on and complete the work. Only a few scientists are therefore content to limit their entire energies to exploration and discovery. Research is one end, but the other must be the training of the new generation of scientists, the transmission of knowledge and skill, of insight and wisdom. The latter task is no less necessary, no less worthy. From the beginnings of human history, the exponentially accelerating growth of human power . . . has required each generation to instruct and inform the next.

This is the challenge that faces every teacher of a science as he steps into the classroom or guides the early efforts of an individual student. Here, in this sea of fresh faces – here, amidst the stumblings and fumblings – may be the Newton or Einstein, the Mendel or Darwin of to-morrow. For few – so very few – men are self-taught. The teacher cannot supply the potentialities of his students, but he is needed to see that the potentialities will unfold, and unfold fully. His is not only the task of passing on the great tradition of the past, with its skills and accumulated knowledge; he must also provide breadth and perspective, self-criticism and judgment, in order that a well-balanced scientist may grow to full stature and continue the search.

Of all the resources of a nation, its greatest are its boys and girls, its young men and women. Like other material resources, these can be squandered or dissipated. They are potential greatness, but they are only potentialities. Science creates knowledge and knowledge generates power, but knowledge resides only in the minds of men who first must learn and be taught, and power is tyranny unless it be guided by insight and wisdom, justice and mercy. The greatest of men have been teachers, and the teacher is greatest among men (*10*).

The social and ethical responsibilities of scientists

The scientist escapes lightly – instead of ten commandments only four: to cherish complete truthfulness; to avoid self-aggrandizement at the expense of one's fellow-scientist; fearlessly to defend the freedom of scientific inquiry and opinion; and fully to communicate one's findings through primary publication, synthesis, and instruction. Out of these grow the social and ethical responsibilities of scientists that in the past 20 years have begun to loom ever larger in our ken.

These may be considered under the three heads of proclamation of benefits, warning of risks, and discussion of quandaries. The first of these, the advertisement of the benefits of science, seems to be sufficiently promoted in these days when science is so well supported by government and private agencies and when grants are justified on the basis of social benefits. Every bit of pure research is heralded as a step in the conquest of nuclear or thermonuclear power, space exploration, elimination of cancer and heart disease, or similar dramatic accomplishments. The ethical problem here is merely that of keeping a check-rein on the imagination and of maintaining truthfulness. But the truth itself is so staggering that it is quite enough to bemuse the public.

Since 1945 more and more scientists have become engaged in warning of the great risks to the very future of man of certain scientific developments. First the atomic bomb and then the hydrogen bomb brought swift realization of the possibility of the destruction of all civilization and even the extinction of all human life were a nuclear war to break out. The atomic scientists, conscience-stricken, united to secure civilian control of nuclear energy. Albert Einstein and Bertrand Russell issued an appeal to scientists to warn the world of the tragic consequences of overoptimism and of an unbridled arms race. Joined by a dozen notable scientists, they initiated the "Pugwash" Conferences on Science and World Affairs in 1957. In these conferences scientists of East and West sat down together to talk, in objective scientific terms, of the military and political problems of the world and their resolution. It was not that the scientists at all felt themselves to be more highly qualified than diplomats and statesmen, economists or lawyers, to find solutions of the most difficult and delicate problems of international relations. They acted on two grounds only: that they understood the desperate nature of the situation about which the world must be warned in time; and that they hoped discussions by persons accustomed to argue in objective, scientific terms might pave the way for better understanding and more fruitful negotiation on the part of officials. In the ensuing discussions of the effects of fallout from nuclear weapons tests on persons now living and on the generations yet unborn, scientists played a very important role. In no small measure, I believe, historians of the future will recognize how great a part was played by the scientists in bringing about the partial nuclear weapons test ban. Scientists are now deeply involved in politics, and naturally enough often on both sides of the argument, for although they may agree upon the basic scientific facts which are relevant to the issue, there are rarely enough established facts to clinch the argument and there is always room for differences of opinion in interpreting the facts. In these matters the ethic of the matter requires the scientist to state his opinion on matters of social concern, but at the same time to distinguish clearly between what he states to be fact and what opinion he holds. Moreover, his opinion about matters within his technical sphere of competence is an ''informed'' opinion; his opinion about other matters, even other scientific matters, is that of a layman. He must in all honesty make clear to the public in what capacity he speaks.

Nuclear war is only one of the dire misfortunes that are poised above the head of modern man. The unrestricted and appalling rate of population increase in most countries of the world, if projected just a few decades into the future, staggers the imagination with its consequences. Effective control of the birth rate is the only conceivable answer to effective reduction by modern health measures of the death rate. This is the world problem second in importance at the present time, and must engage the conscience of the scientist.

The problem of the future is the ethical problem of the control of man over his own biological evolution. The powers of evolution now rest in his hands. The geneticist can define the means and prognosticate the future with some accuracy. Yet here we enter the third great arena of ethical discussion, passing beyond the benefits of science and the certain risks to the nebulous realm of quandaries. Man must choose goals, and a choice of goals involves us in weighing values – even whole systems of values. The scientist cannot make the choice of goals for his people, and neither can he measure and weigh values with accuracy and objectivity. There is nonetheless an important duty he must perform, because he and he alone may see clearly enough the nature of the alternative choices, including laissez faire, which is no less a choice than any other. It is the social duty and function of the scientist in this arena of discussion to inform and to demand of the people, and of their leaders too, a discussion and consideration of all those impending problems that grow out of scientific discovery and the amplification of human power. Science is no longer – can never be again – the ivory tower of the recluse, the refuge of the asocial man. Science has found its social basis and has eagerly grasped for social support, and it has thereby acquired social responsibilities and a realization of its own fundamental ethical principles. The scientist is a man, through his science doing good and evil to other men, and receiving from them blame and praise, recrimination and money. Science is not only to know, it is to do, and in the doing it has found its soul.

References

1. J. Bronowski, *Science and Human Values* (Messner, New York, 1956).
2. B. Glass, ''Dialectical materialism and scientific research,'' *Quart. Rev. Biol.* 23, 333–337 (1948); D. I. Greenberg, ''Lysenko: Soviet science writes finis to geneticist's domination of nation's biological research,'' *Science* 147, 716–717 (1965).

3. R. B. Goldschmidt, "Research and politics," *Science* 109, 219–227 (1949).

4. L. C. Eiseley, "Charles Darwin, Edward Blyth, and the Theory of Natural Selection," *Proc. Amer. Phil. Soc.* 103, 94–158 (1959).

5. H. Rauschning, *Hitler Speaks: A Series of Political Conversations with Adolf Hitler on His Real Aims* (Butterworths, London, 1939), pp. 220–221.

6. J. R. Baker, *Science and the Planned State* (Macmillan, New York, 1945).

7. A. Szent-Györgi, *World Digest* 55, 50 (1943).

8. A. von Humboldt, *Cosmos: A Sketch of a Physical Description of the Universe*. E. C. Otté, transl. (Bohn, London, 1849).

9. B. Glass, "The critical state of the critical review article," *Quart. Rev. Biol.* 39, 182–185 (1964).

10. ———, "The scientist and the science teacher," *Amer. Assoc. Univ. Professors Bull.* 50, 267–268 (1964).

4
Making and breaking the rules of science

Alexander Kohn

The exponential growth of science and the increase in the number of practising scientists has been accompanied by the appearance of individuals whose actions do not conform with the ethical standards of the scientific community. Although the extent of this deviant behaviour has not yet been satisfactorily investigated and has still to be determined, there is a feeling of embarrassment and unease in the scientific community. This unease stems from the essential importance of honesty in science. Unlike other professions where honesty is merely regarded as highly desirable, the whole edifice of science is built upon honesty; it is not, as Jacob Bronowski has pointed out in *The Common Sense of Science*, an optional extra or a separate domain. 'The institution of science involves an implicit social contract between scientists so that each can depend on the trustworthiness of the rest . . . the entire cognitive system of science is rooted in the moral integrity of aggregates of individual scientists'(1).

Scientists have therefore been deeply disturbed by the fact that during the past decade many incidents of plagiarism, data falsification, misrepresentation of research results and misuse of public funds for fraudulent research, have been reported in scientific periodicals as well as in the mass media. The latest contribution to the literature on this subject is a book by science reporters Broad and Wade (2), entitled *Betrayers of the Truth*.

Before discussing the various forms of misconduct in science, however, we have to understand the basic rules, the norms of science.

Robert Merton, the pioneer of the sociology of science (3), distinguishes between moral, intellectual and technical norms. He has classified these norms as 'universalism', 'disinterestedness', 'scepticism' and 'communalism'.

Universalism implies that truth should be judged in terms of intellectual criteria, criteria that are considered valid in the particular branch of science, and not in terms of the attributes of the author. Disinterestedness requires that the scientist's activities and efforts be directed towards the extension of scientific knowledge, and not towards the personal interests of an individual or a group of scientists. Scepticism involves testing claims both empirically and logically, and not accepting them on the basis of authority. Communalism requires that science be a product of collaborative effort, dictated by the wish to benefit the community, the society; it thus entails openness and sharing of information.

To these norms, as defined by Merton, one may also add rationality and emotional neutrality (4), and according to Cournand and Zuckerman (5), honesty, objectivity, tolerance, doubt of certitude and unselfish engagement. Mohr (6) presents the following list of normative rules: 'Be honest; never manipulate data; be precise; be fair with regard

From *False Prophets: Fraud & Error in Science & Medicine* (Oxford: Basil Blackwell, 1986), pp. 1–11.

to priority; be without bias with regard to data and ideas of your rival; do not make compromises in trying to solve a problem.'

Kenneth S. Norris of the University of California, Santa Cruz, wraps it all up in a down-to-earth comment: 'Science is a set of rules that keep the scientists from lying to each other.'

Violation of these norms is sometimes loosely termed 'fraud'. Actually, in both everyday and legal language, fraud is defined as criminal deception, or as the use of false representation intended to benefit the deceiver. The scientist who is cheating knowingly, who falsifies or invents research data, or who lies about them, is not strictly fraudulent as long as he is not using the false data to obtain financial support from public or government agencies, or from private funds. Fraud is also committed when, on the basis of false data, the scientist is trying to secure a research job, to prove that public funds have been properly used, or to convince the public or the grantors that a certain procedure, material or drug is acceptable and safe. Fraud is more a problem of the social and biological sciences (the so-called 'soft' sciences) than the 'exact' sciences. This is because in the soft sciences one encounters uncontrollable variables which make the experiments difficult to reproduce; fraudulent results therefore have a better chance of cover-up.

Violation of the norms often gains public notice and is described in the lay press in an exaggerated manner. This creates the impression that such deviant behaviour is much more prevalent in the scientific community than is admitted by scientists themselves (7). Considering the constantly increasing numbers of practising scientists, I would estimate that the number of deviant scientists is extremely small. Broad and Wade (2) consider fraud in science to be a small, but not insignificant feature of scientific research, and this view is supported by Dixon (8): 'Blatant fiddling is probably an uncommon though real component of careerist science.' In serious and well-substantiated cases offending individuals, when found out, are punished by the scientific community by being cast out of the ranks.

During a period in the development of a particular science when clearly defined concepts and laws are widely accepted, it is difficult to cheat. When, however, a field of science enters a state of flux, with concepts changing, old patterns collapsing and new models trying to get hold, the area becomes most vulnerable to deceit. Objectivity becomes difficult, even to specialists. Science in revolution invites new hypotheses. At such transitional stages there are those who have the courage to promulgate unpopular hypotheses selflessly, but there are also opportunists who do not hesitate to flood the field with forged data and results of experiments that have not been carried out. In an atmosphere of change and flux, as we have witnessed in the past few decades, such incidents of forgery and misrepresentation are not isolated. During one such time of change when new concepts were emerging, when the new types of radiation were discovered at the turn of the century, 'discoveries' were also made of non-existent radiations (e.g. N-rays, mitogenetic rays); these were the result of negligent or badly controlled experimentation, however, not of deceit or conscious fraud.

Charles Babbage, the famous English mathematician (1792–1871) and the inventor of the first modern calculating machine, defined various types of scientific misconduct, or methods of leading people astray. One speaks of 'forging' when one records observations that have never been made; in other words, when one lies outright about the experimental data. When data are manipulated so as to make them look better, one deals with 'trimming' (in modern usage also 'massaging data' or 'fudging'). 'Cooking', as defined by Babbage, means choosing only data that fit the researcher's hypothesis best, and discarding those that do not: in this case one tells only a part of the truth (in modern jargon 'finagling').

Let us examine examples of different types of cheating in contemporary science. 'Forging' involves reporting experiments that have never been carried out, but which the researcher may feel he needs for the support of his or her hypothesis. In some cases forgers have not only invented experimental data, but have related these non-existent data to non-existent manuscripts allegedly published or accepted for publication.

Another form of cheating in this category is plagiarism, which consists of using the data or ideas of other investigators without reference to the source, or even verbatim copying of a text written by someone else. A number of plagiarizers obtained the necessary data either from a grant proposal or from a manuscript submitted for publication.

In the 'trimming' category one would include that type of cheating which is based on amplification of an experiment: the investigator described accurately the nature of the experiment and its controls, but reports a greater number of trials than have actually been performed, 'adds' or 'removes' animals to or from experimental or control groups, or misrepresents the variance, although using genuine numbers and means.

One encounters examples of 'cooking' when the researcher omits aberrant values, misreports actual conditions of the experiment or alters ancillary data. A kindred mis-demeanour is omission of whole experiments which yielded negative or contrary results to the hypothesis under test.

A number of questions come to mind relating to the norms of science and deviant behaviour. Is there a system of social control in science and what is its nature? What is the incidence of deviant behaviour in science in comparison with that in other fields of human endeavour? Why is there no systematic effort to study such behaviour? Where should the line be drawn between an error and forgery or plagiarism? Is there any connection between the reward system in science and the incentive for deviant behaviour (1)? I shall hope to suggest answers to these questions.

Perhaps we should look first at the existence of 'social control' in science. One of the first lessons a scientist learns is that faking evidence is the worst sin he can commit; it is a sort of capital crime. He also learns that those who commit such crimes are banished from the scientific community, or at best, held in contempt, suffering resentment and antipathy. A deviant scientist will most likely be barred from holding a position in a research organization or university.

Scientists seek recognition: they want to publish and to see their names in print; they wish to be recognized by their fellow scientists, and if the recognition comes from the higher levels of the scientific hierarchy so much the better; they like to be invited to meetings and conferences, and the smaller the conference and the farther from home the better. Scientists fight fiercely for priority of their discoveries. Jevons (9) states that the major motives for a scientist are recognition from fellow scientists, a permanent drive to work, to be creative and not to violate the ethics of science, and, if possible, to be first with a new discovery.

Nevertheless, scientists may be tempted by power or fortune, even if they do not actually seek them, contrary to popular belief that most scientists are willing to work anonymously for the advancement of knowledge. The international scientific community evaluates and judges the work of its members – from publications, lectures, discussions and sometimes even by the grapevine. It controls the activities of individual scientists by granting recognition to the successful members, and withholding it from those who violate the norms of scientific behaviour.

Any new concepts, hypotheses or proofs which have a bearing on the mainstream of science are examined by other members of the scientific community. They are accepted, modified or rejected (sometimes even ignored). The highest reward for a scientist is peer recognition of the validity and importance of his or her particular truth-claim. Thus the organized system of scepticism has a double function: it improves the quality of scientific investigation and it reduces the extent of possible frauds. This scepticism assumes many forms. First there is the self-imposed careful statistical design of experiments which includes double blind tests, randomization of subjects, use of independent observers and, above all, the requirement that the experiment be reproducible.

The concept of the double blind test is extremely important in biological sciences. If a scientist assumes that procedure or substance A has a specific effect on micro-organisms, plants, or humans, he includes in his test procedure a substance B which is known to be 'neutral', without a demonstrable effect. The conditions of the test are such that A and B are coded and neither the experimenter (or his delegate) nor the subject knows whether A or B has been used in any particular test. The code is broken only after the result of the test has been read and recorded.

As to randomization, if a test is done within a population, the subjects of the study have to be chosen at random (regardless of sex, age, ethnic origin, behavioural traits such as smoking, drinking etc.). Selection of individuals for a study may lead the researcher to mistaken conclusions owing to unrecognized bias in the selection (10).

The use of independent observers is important because each observer may interpret the criteria (in clinical studies, for example) differently and apply his individual interpretation to the collected information. One example of this in practice is the frequently varying or even contradictory opinions of pathologists evaluating pathological slides.

In spite of all these precautions, many a research project, especially in the field of psychology, is burdened by so-called 'experimenter bias'. Even in well-designed and controlled experiments the outcome may be biased in favour of a preset hypothesis, set up by, or known to the experimenter. In addition, the number of repeat experiments a scientist performs is usually smaller when the results of an experiment conform to the hypothesis, than in a situation where the results are not as expected.

The attitude to reproducibility, a key factor in controlling fraud, differs in various sciences. It is usually more stringent in the exact sciences (such as physics and chemistry) than in the social and behavioural sciences. Problems arise because the fact that an experiment is not reproducible does not necessarily mean that the concept on which it is based is wrong, nor that there is an error or deception in it. Gravitational waves provide one example. Joseph Weber, an internationally known physicist from the University of Maryland, constructed special detector antennae to measure the existence of these waves, and positioned the antennae at a distance of 1000 km from each other (in Maryland and Illinois). Through them he detected a coincident significant signal, which he interpreted as evidence for gravitational wave bursts coming from sources outside our solar system (11). Though he regarded these signals as significant and excluded the possibility that they might be due to electromagnetic or seismic effects, other physicists considered them to be 'noise'. Later studies with much more sensitive apparatus have not produced any signals comparable to those observed by Weber. This fact, however, does not necessarily invalidate Weber's work and hypothesis, though it does make other workers suspend judgement until more experiments have been carried out.

Dirac once said that it was more important to have beauty in an equation than to have it conform to experiment. Nevertheless, whenever a number of laboratories encounter difficulties in reproducing an experiment, the original findings may fall under a shadow of doubt. In such cases efforts will be made to clarify the causes of irreproducibility. If all attempts fail, a suspicion of deception may arise and will usually be circulated in closed circles but not in public. Voicing of such suspicion is avoided by senior scientists who do not want to destroy the career of their junior colleagues; junior scientists do not dare to accuse their superiors or professors for more empirical reasons. In short, when faced with irreproducible results, we all tend rather to assume that an error has been made rather than a fraud committed. The attractiveness of any theory in its application to society depends on how relevant it is and how well it fits everybody's preconceptions. If the fit is good, then even if the proofs are shaky, there would be a tendency to accept the theory.

The next question we might ask ourselves is just how widespread is the kind of misconduct we have been talking about? At a meeting of the Society of Sociology of Science held in Philadelphia in 1982, Professor Robert Merton complained that there had been numerous discussions on misconduct in science, but that actual quantitative data on the incidence of fraud were still lacking. This situation remains unchanged and it is therefore very difficult both to state how prevalent deviant behaviour in science is, and to make comparisons with the incidence of fraud in other fields of human endeavour. In distinction from other crimes, deviant behaviour in science is not officially reported by the police or the law courts. Therefore there are no official statistics relating to this type of 'crime'. The main source of information is either self-reporting by individuals (admission of guilt in a scientific journal or at a meeting) or 'whistle-blowing', that is, disclosure of fraud by the scientist's colleagues, collaborators or technicians.

In 1976 the *New Scientist* embarked on a study of cheating in science (12,13). This study was instigated by the affair of Sir Cyril Burt, who was at that time accused of having used nonexistent data in his research on the inheritance of intelligence. *New Scientist* sent out questionnaires to its readers asking two main questions: (a) does intentional bias occur among scientists to the same extent as among non-scientists?; (b) how does one distinguish between deliberate misrepresentation and error or carelessness? The term 'intentional bias' was euphemistically used for intentional manipulation of data. The questionnaire contained additional questions, some of which dealt with the incidence of bias, others with knowledge of such practices.

Of 201 valid questionnaires returned to the editors, 194 reported having known about instances of cheating. About one-third of all cases had come to the knowledge of the reporters either from direct or indirect personal contact. Of all reported cases one-fifth of the perpetrators were actually caught in the act, and an additional fifth confessed to malpractice. The incidence of cheating was higher in research performed by single scientists and it lessened the larger the research group became. There were only 15 incidences of complete fabrication of an experiment that had never been carried out; the rest involved trimming and cooking. As to the fate of the 'intentional biasers' who were caught, only ten percent were actually dismissed from their positions. Other forms of punishment are not described in this study.

It would thus seem that the prevalence of cheating in science is extremely high. It would obviously be a good idea, however, to conduct a much more extensive study of larger populations of practising scientists before accepting the conclusions of *New Scientist* in this matter.

An interesting study on the reliability of published scientific papers was carried out by Dr Richard R. Roberts of the National Bureau of Standards (14). He estimated that at least half of all published scientific papers were unusable or unreliable, although this does not necessarily imply cheating.

Another type of test was initiated by Leroy Wolins of Iowa State University (15). He authorized one of his students to write to 37 authors of psychological papers and ask them for the raw data on which they based their research results. Of the 32 who replied, 21 stated that their data had been either accidentally destroyed, lost, or misplaced. Only nine researchers sent their raw data. Dr Wolins, an expert in statistics, analysed these data and found that only seven sets of results could be statistically analysed. Of these seven, three contained errors that invalidated what had been published as fact.

The studies of *New Scientist,* of Roberts and of Wolins, taken together, would indicate that the prevalence of misconduct in science is greater than the scientific community is willing to admit, but these are very selected studies and do not cover the complete range of scientific activities. They should therefore not be used for extrapolation. The real prevalence of cheating may be smaller or greater.

In order to obtain a proper perspective on this problem, I shall analyse a number of published cases of scientific misdemeanour. First, however, consider the following hypothetical case. In an experiment, ten measurements are made of a parameter changing with time. The recorded values are plotted on a semilogarithmic paper as a straight line (i.e. exponential decay). The experiment is repeated five times. Within the limits of properly used statistical deviations, a straight line is indeed observed. In one of the five experiments, however, one of the points is so aberrant that the straight line relationship in this particular experiment cannot be maintained. The location of this point (rogue value) is statistically incompatible with the line drawn through all the other points.

We are now faced with a crucial question. The straight line relationship fits the particular hypothesis of the experimenter, who now wishes to write up the results and submit them for publication. For obvious reasons (limitation of space) he can use only one graph to demonstrate the point he is trying to make. In such a situation many scientists will choose the best results as an illustration. This would not be considered improper, since insistence on presenting the aberrant datum (the rogue value) would lead only to the obfuscation of the issue. Since most of the research done nowadays is cooperative, it is expected that results will have been discussed by all the partners, who would consider the pros and cons of stressing either the conforming values or the aberrant ones and come to a weighted conclusion based on experience, intuition and the communal mode of thinking. Nevertheless, in the strict ethical sense, the issue is debatable.

The course of action described above may still be considered by some purists as unethical. In practice, I would not condemn it as a misconduct. Few of these cases are 'open and shut'; they should be judged against a background of a great variety of factors.

Scientists who neglect the proscribed and sanctioned methodology (i.e., the use of proper controls) may quite unintentionally become responsible for producing erroneous results, and thus be suspected of falsification. A classic example of such methodologically faulty research was the discovery and the prolonged study of mitogenetic rays in the 1930s and of polywater in the 1960s. In the course of a decade several hundreds of papers on a non-existent ray and on a non-existent compound were published by reputable scientists, who failed to employ proper precautions in their research and in the interpretation of their results.

How can this have happened? Whenever a new scientific claim or discovery is made in a field that is important to the advance of knowledge, has practical technological applications or is of social importance, many people try to reproduce the work. As Merton put it, 'scientific inquiry is in effect subject to rigorous policing, to a degree unparalleled in any other field of human activity' (3). Thus the requirement of reproducibility in scientific research aids in the detection of error or fraud, and is therefore a deterrent to misconduct. Nevertheless, there are situations in which repetition of an experiment is extremely difficult, because of the complicated experimental design, for instance, or because of its prohibitive cost, or because the phenomenon studied is rare and unexpected (such as earthquakes, volcano eruptions). In many cases, however, where the results of an experiment are not a part of a necessary link in the advance of knowledge and only serve to support a generally accepted 'truth', serious scientists will seldom be willing to lose time and money to repeat that particular experiment. Thus, many results that find their way into published literature remain unchecked, whether they are rarely or often quoted. In mathematics, for instance, according to one writer, 'this is a real problem: many published mathematical articles undoubtedly contain serious undetected errors, not because the mistakes are too difficult to find, but because contemporary pure mathematics has become so abstract and fragmented that few people bother to look carefully for error' (16).

According to Luria (17), actual cheating in science is the result of a pathological personality akin to that of a compulsive gambler; anyone in science who willingly distorts or invents data believing he will get away with it must have a disturbed sense of reality. To carry the comparison with a gambler further, such a scientist deludes himself that he can beat the odds and bend reality to his wishes. He has lost the awareness of the futility of cheating in science. A cheating scientist, like a gambler, is unable to respond to normal emotional impulses. 'Enthusiasm that brings the scientist to the laboratory door should be left outside along with umbrella and overshoes', says Luria, and should be replaced by scepticism. As another writer has put it: 'If science is misrepresented to the young as an array of glamorous "spectaculars" the seed is sown for later anticlimactic disillusionment and perhaps even dishonesty' (18).

'Cheating may be like cirrhosis of the integrity. An initial slip made in good faith gives rise to a reaction that magnifies the emotional commitment to the mistaken belief, finally leading to the actual destruction of truth' (17). Despite the centrality of honesty in the scientific enterprise, it is foolish to assume that dishonesty, common in most fields of human activity, should be rare in science. Falsification is inevitable in human society, be it scientific or otherwise. Science, like banking, however, has the ways and the means to keep misconduct in check.

References

1. Zuckerman, H. 1977: Deviant behavior and social control in science. In E. Sagarin (ed.) *Deviance and Social Change,* Beverly Hills: Sage Publications.
2. Broad, W. and Wade, N. 1982: *Betrayers of the Truth. Fraud and Deceit in the Halls of Science.* New York: Simon and Schuster.

3. Merton, R. 1973: The normative structure of science. In N. Storer (ed.) *The Sociology of Science. Theoretical and Empirical Investigations,* Chicago: University of Chicago Press.
4. Barber, B. 1952: *Science and the Social Order.* New York: Free Press.
5. Cournand, A. and Zuckerman, H. 1975: The code of science. In P. Weiss (ed.), *Knowledge in Search of Understanding,* Mt Kisco, New York: Futura Publishing Co., 126–47.
6. Mohr, M. 1979: The ethics of science. *International Science Reviews,* 4:45.
7. Gaston, J. 1978: Disputes and deviant views about the ethos of science. In *The Reward System in British and American Science.* New York: Wiley, 158–84.
8. Dixon, B. 1984: Deniers of the truth. *The Sciences,* 24:23.
9. Jevons, F. R. 1973: *Science Observed.* London: Allen and Unwin.
10. Kleinbaum, D. C., Morgenstern, H. and Kupper, L. L. 1981: Selection bias in epidemiological studies. *American Journal of Epidemiology,* 113:452.
11. Weber, J. 1969: Evidence for the discovery of gravitational radiation. *Physical Review Letters,* 22:1320.
12. Saint John-Roberts, I. 1976: Are researchers trustworthy? *New Scientist,* 71, 2 September: 481.
13. Saint John-Roberts, I. 1976: Cheating in science. *New Scientist,* 72, 26 November: 465.
14. Roberts, R. R. 1977: An unscientific phenomenon. Fraud grows in laboratories. *Science Digest,* June, p. 38.
15. Wolins, L. 1962: Responsibility for raw data. *American Psychologist,* 17:657.
16. Zahler, R. 1976: Errors in mathematical proofs. *Science,* 193: 98.
17. Luria, S. A. 1975: What makes a scientist cheat? *Prism,* May, pp. 16, 18.

QUESTIONS FOR DISCUSSION

1. How is trust related to the concept of "professionalism"? Why does the public *want* to trust scientists?
2. Why are honesty and openness essential to the practical goals of science, as well as to its ethical goals?
3. Is true intellectual freedom possible in science today?

RECOMMENDED SUPPLEMENTAL READING

"Integrity in Science," Lewis M. Branscomb, *American Scientist,* 1985, 73, pp. 421–423.
Honor in Science, 2nd ed., Sigma Xi, New Haven, CT: Sigma Xi, 1986.
"On the Drinking of the Hemlock: Socrates, Semmelweis, and Barbara McClintock," Roger J. Bulger, in Roger J. Bulger (ed.), *In Search of the Modern Hippocrates,* Iowa City, IA: University of Iowa Press, 1987, pp. 93–107.
"On Being a Scientist," National Academy of Sciences, Committee on the Conduct of Science, Washington, DC: National Academy Press, 1989.

PART III

Self-deception in Research: Procedural, Perceptual, and Social Causes

---

INTRODUCTION

"Never fall in love with your hypothesis" is a common warning to young scientists, for love may blind even the most skilled researcher to the shortcomings of an approach or technique. As in all human enterprises, scientists' expectations of their work shape their findings, and the unexpected may be overlooked, ignored, or explained away. Bernard Barber outlines how the substantive theories of science, methodological conceptions, religious ideas, professional standing and specialization, and the sociopolitical affiliations of scientists may make researchers resistant to new discoveries despite their professed self-criticism and objectivity.

William Broad and Nicolas Wade document historical examples of prominent scientists' self-deception, in which dedication to a position in the face of overwhelming evidence to the contrary devastated professional reputations and careers. National and personal pride was a common feature in these cases, where false conclusions appeared to support the hopes and prejudices of the researchers and their communities.

Masking and randomization techniques used in clinical trials help to ensure that researchers' expectations do not unconsciously influence their interpretation of data, and proper use of equipment can remove some of the subjective element of observation. Nonetheless, scientists must also be ready to accept the unhappy possibility that a question to which they have dedicated years of work may be a dead end, and must find value in proving a null hypothesis.

5
Resistance by scientists to scientific discovery

Bernard Barber

In the study of the history and sociology of science, there has been a relative lack of attention to one of the interesting aspects of the social process of discovery – the resistance on the part of scientists themselves to scientific discovery. General and specialized histories of science and biographies and autobiographies of scientists, as well as intensive dis- cussions of the processes by which discoveries are made and accepted, all tend to make, at the most, passing reference to this subject. In two systematic analyses of the social process of scientific discovery and invention, for example – analyses which tried to be as inclusive of empirical fact and theoretical problem as possible – there is only passing reference to such resistance in the one instance and none at all in the second (*1*). This neglect is all the more notable in view of the close scrutiny that scholars have given the subject of resistance to scientific discovery by social groups other than scientists. There has been a great deal of attention paid to resistance on the part of economic, technological, religious, and ideological elements and groups outside science itself (*1–3*). Indeed, the tendency of such elements to resist seems sometimes to be emphasized disproportionately as against the support which they also give to science. In the matter of religion, for example, are we not all a little too much aware that religion has resisted scientific discovery, not enough aware of the large support it has given to Western science? (*4,5*).

The mere assertion that scientists themselves sometimes resist scientific discovery clashes, of course, with the stereotype of the scientist as "the open-minded man." The norm of open-mindedness is one of the strongest of the scientist's values. As Philipp Frank has recently put it, "Every influence of moral, religious, or political considerations upon the acceptance of a theory is regarded as 'illegitimate' by the so-called 'community of scientists.' " And Robert Oppenheimer emphasizes the "importance" of "the open mind," in a book by that title, as a value not only for science but for society as a whole (*6*). But values alone, and especially one value by itself, cannot be a sufficient basis for explaining human behavior. However strong a value is, however large its actual influence on behavior, it usually exerts this influence only in conjunction with a number of other cultural and social elements, which sometimes reinforce it, sometimes give it limits.

This article is an investigation of the elements within science which limit the norm and practice of "open-mindedness." My purpose is to draw a more accurate picture of the actual process of scientific discovery, to see resistance by scientists themselves as a constant phenomenon with specifiable cultural and social sources. This purpose, more- over, implies a practical consequence. For if we learn more about resistance to scientific discovery, we shall know more also about the sources of acceptance, just as we know

From *Science*, 1961, 134, pp. 596–602. © AAAS.

more about health when we successfully study disease. By knowing more about both resistance and acceptance in scientific discovery, we may be able to reduce the former by a little bit and thereby increase the latter in the same measure.

Helmholtz, Planck, and Lister

Although the resistance by scientists themselves to scientific discovery has been neglected in systematic analysis, it would be surprising indeed if it had never been noted at all. If nowhere else, we should find it in the writings of those scientists who have suffered from resistance on the part of other scientists. Helmholtz, for example, made aware of such resistance by his own experience, commiserated with Faraday on "the fact that the greatest benefactors of mankind usually do not obtain a full reward during their life-time, and that new ideas need the more time for gaining general assent the more really original they are" (7–9). Max Planck is another who noticed resistance in general because he had experienced it himself, in regard to some new ideas on the second law of thermodynamics which he worked out in his doctoral dissertation submitted to the University of Munich in 1879. Ironically, one of those who resisted the ideas proposed in Planck's paper, according to his account, was Helmholtz: "None of my professors at the University had any understanding for its contents," says Planck. "I found no interest, let alone approval, even among the very physicists who were closely connected with the topic. Helmholtz probably did not even read my paper at all. Kirchhoff expressly disapproved . . . I did not succeed in reaching Clausius. He did not answer my letters, and I did not find him at home when I tried to see him in person at Bonn. I carried on a correspondence with Carl Neumann, of Leipzig, but it remained totally fruitless" (10, p. 18). And Lister, in a graduation address to medical students, warned them all against blindness to new ideas in science, blindness such as he had encountered in advancing his theory of antisepsis.

Scientists are also human

Too often, unfortunately, where resistance by scientists has been noted, it has been merely noted, merely alleged, without detailed substantiation and without attempt at explanation. Sometimes, when explanations are offered, they are notably vague and all-inclusive, thus proving too little by trying to prove too much. One such explanation is contained in the frequently repeated phrase, "After all, scientists are also human beings," a phrase implying that scientists are more human when they err than when they are right (11). Other such vague explanations can be found in phrases such as "Zeitgeist," "human nature," "lack of progressive spirit," "fear of novelty," and "climate of opinion."

As one of these phrases, "fear of novelty," may indicate, there has also been a tendency, where some explanation of the sources of resistance is offered, to express a psychologistic bias – that is, to attribute resistance exclusively to inherent and ineradicable traits or instincts of the human personality. Thus, Wilfred Trotter, in discussing the response to scientific discovery, asserts that "the mind delights in a static environment," that "change from without . . . seems in its very essence to be repulsive and an object of fear," and that "a little self-examination tells us pretty easily how deeply rooted in the mind is the fear of the new" (12). And Beveridge, in *The Art of Scientific Investigation*, says, "there is in all of us a psychological tendency to resist new ideas" (*13*). A full understanding of resistance will, of course, have to include the psychological dimension – the factor of individual personality. But it must also include the cultural and social dimension – those shared and patterned idea-systems and those patterns of social inter-action that also contribute to resistance. It is these cultural and social elements that I shall discuss here, but with full awareness that psychological elements are contributory causes of resistance.

Because resistance by scientists has been largely neglected as a subject for systematic investigation, we find that there is sometimes a tendency, when such resistance is noted, to exaggerate the extent to which it occurs. Thus, Murray says that the discoverer must *always* expect to meet with opposition from his fellow scientists. And Trotter goes overboard in the same way: "the reception of new ideas tends always to be grudging or hostile. . . . Apart from the happy few whose work has already great prestige or lies in fields that are being actively expanded at the moment, discoverers of new truths always find their ideas resisted" (*12*, p. 26). Such exaggerations can be eliminated by more systematic and objective study.

Finally, in the absence of such systematic and objective study, many of those who have noted resistance have been excessively embittered and moralistic. Oliver Heaviside is reported to have exclaimed bitterly, when his important contributions to mathematical physics were ignored for 25 years, "Even men who are not Cambridge mathematicians deserve justice" (*14*). And Planck's reaction to the resistance he experienced was similar. "This experience," he said, "gave me also an opportunity to learn a new fact – a remarkable one, in my opinion: A new scientific truth does not triumph by convincing its opponents and making them see the light, but rather because its opponents eventually die, and a new generation grows up that is familiar with it" (*10*). Such bitterness is not tempered by objective understanding of resistance as a constant phe-nomenon in science, a pattern in which all scientists may sometimes and perhaps often participate, now on the side of the resisters, now on that of the resisted. Instead, such bitterness takes the moralistic view that resistance is due to "human vanities," to "little minds and ignoble minds." Such views impede the objective analysis that is required.

In his discussion of the Idols – idols of the tribe, of the cave, of the marketplace, and of the theatre – Francis Bacon long ago suggested that a variety of preconceived ideas, general and particular, affect the thinking of all men, especially in the face of innovation. Similarly, more recent sociological theory has shown that while the variety of idea-systems that make up a given culture are functionally necessary, on the whole, for man to carry on his life in society and in the natural environment, these several idea-systems may also have their dysfunctional or negative effects. Just because the established culture defines the situation for man, usually helpfully, it also, sometimes harmfully, blinds him to other ways of conceiving that situation. Cultural blinders are one of the constant sources of resistance to innovations of all kinds. And scientists, for all the methods they have invented to strip away their distorting idols, or cultural blinders, and for all the training they receive in evading the negative effects of such blinders, are still as other men, though surely in considerably lesser measure because of these methods and this special training. Scientists suffer, along with the rest of us, from the ironies that evil sometimes comes from good, that one noble vision may exclude another, and that good scientific ideas occasionally obstruct the introduction of better ones.

Substantive concepts

Several different kinds of cultural resistance to discovery may be distinguished. We may turn first to the way in which the substantive concepts and theories held by scientists at any given time become a source of resistance to new ideas. And our illustrations begin with the very origins of modern science. In his magisterial discussion of the Copernican revolution, Kuhn (3) tells us not only about the nonscientific opposition to the heliocentric theory but also about the resistance from the astronomer-scientists of the time. Even after the publication of *De Revolutionibus,* the belief of most astronomers in the stability of the earth was unshaken. The idea of the earth's motion was either ignored or dismissed as absurd. Even the great astronomer-observer Brahe remained a life-long opponent of Copernicanism; he was unable to break with the traditional patterns of thought about the earth's lack of motion. And his immense prestige helped to postpone the conversion of other astronomers to the new theory. Of course, religious, philosophical, and ideological conceptions were closely interwoven with substantive scientific theories in the culture of the scientists of that time, but it seems clear that the latter as well as the former played their part in the resistance to the Copernican discoveries.

Moving to the early 19th century, we learn that the scientists of the day resisted Thomas Young's wave theory of light because they were, as Gillispie says, faithful to a corpuscular model (15). By the end of the century, when scientists had swung over to the wave theory, the validity of Young's earlier discovery was recognized. Substantive scientific theory was also one of the sources of resistance to Pasteur's discovery of the biological character of fermentation processes. The established theory that these processes are wholly chemical was held to by many scientists, including Liebig, for a long time (16). The same preconceptions were also the source of the resistance to Lister's germ theory of disease, although in this case, as in that of Pasteur, various other factors were important.

Because it illustrates a variety of sources of scientific resistance to discovery, I shall return several times to the case of Mendel's theory of genetic inheritance. For the present, I mention it only in connection with the source of resistance under discussion, substantive scientific theories themselves. Mendelian theory, it seems clear, was resisted from the time of its announcement, in 1865, until the end of the century, because Mendel's conception of the separate inheritance of characteristics ran counter to the predominant conception of joint and total inheritance of biological characteristics (17, 18). It was not until botany changed its conceptions and concentrated its research on the separate inheritance of unit characteristics that Mendel's theory and Mendel himself were independently rediscovered by de Vries, a Dutchman, by Carl Correns, working in Tübingen, and by Erich Tschermak, a Viennese, all in the same year, 1900.

New conceptions about the electronic constitution of the atom were also resisted by scientists when fundamental discoveries in this field were being made at the end of the 19th century. The established scientific notion was that of the absolute physical irreducibility of the atom. When Arrhenius published his theory of electrolytic dissociation, his ideas met with resistance for a time, though eventually, thanks in part to Ostwald, the theory was accepted and Arrhenius was given the Nobel prize for it (19). Similarly, Lord Kelvin regarded the announcement of Röntgen's discovery of x-rays as a hoax, and as late as 1907 he was still resisting the discovery, by Ramsay and Soddy, that helium could be produced from radium, and resisting Rutherford's theory of the electronic composition of the atom, one of the fundamental discoveries of modern physics. Throughout his long and distinguished life in science Kelvin never discarded the concept that the atom is an indivisible unit (*20*).

Let us take one final illustration, from contemporary science. In a recent case history of the role of chance in scientific discovery it was reported that two able scientists, who observed, independently and by chance, the phenomenon of floppiness in rabbits' ears after the injection of the enzyme papain, both missed making a discovery because they shared the established scientific view that cartilage is a relatively inert and uninteresting type of tissue (*21*). Eventually one of the scientists did go on to make a discovery which altered the established view of cartilage, but for a long time even he had been blinded by his scientific preconceptions. This case is especially interesting because it shows how resistance occurs not only between two or more scientists but also within an individual scientist. Because of their substantive conceptions and theories, scientists sometimes miss discoveries that are literally right before their eyes.

Methodological conceptions

The methodological conceptions scientists entertain at any given time constitute a second cultural source of resistance to scientific discovery and are as important as substantive ideas in determining response to innovations. Some scientists, for example, tend to be antitheoretical, resisting, on that methodological ground, certain discoveries. "In Baconian science," says Gillispie, "the bird-watcher comes into his own while genius, ever theorizing in far places, is suspect. And this is why Bacon would have none of Kepler or Copernicus or Gilbert or anyone who would extend a few ideas or calculations into a system of the world" (*15*). Goethe too, as Helmholtz pointed out in his discussion of Goethe's scientific researches, was antitheoretical (*22*). A more recent discussion of Goethe's scientific work also finds him antianalytical and antiabstract (*15*). Perhaps Helmholtz had been made aware of Goethe's antitheoretical bias because his own discovery of the conservation of energy had been resisted as being too theoretical, not sufficiently experimental. German physicists were probably antitheoretical in Helmholtz's day because they feared a revival of the speculations of the Hegelian "nature-philosophy" against which they had fought so long, and eventually successfully.

Viewed in another way, Goethe's antitheoretical bias took the form of a positive preference for scientific work based on intuition and the direct evidence of the senses. "We must look upon his theory of colour as a forlorn hope," says Helmholtz, "as a desperate attempt to rescue from the attacks of science the belief in the direct truth of our sensations" (*22*). Goethe felt passionately that Newton was wrong in analyzing color into its quantitative components by means of prisms and theories. Color, for him, was a qualitative essence projected onto the physical world by the innate biological character and functioning of the human being.

Later scientists also have resisted discovery because of their preference for the evidence of the senses. Otto Hahn, noted for his discoveries in radioactivity, who received the Nobel prize for his splitting of the uranium atom in 1939, reports the following case: "Emil Fischer was also one of those who found it difficult to grasp the fact that it is also possible by radioactive methods of measurement to detect, and to recognize from their chemical properties, substances in quantities quite beyond the world of the weighable; as is the case, for example, with the active deposits of radium, thorium, and actinium. At my inaugural lecture in the spring of 1907, Fischer declared that somehow he could not believe those things. For certain substances the most delicate test was afforded by the sense of smell and no more delicate test could be found than that!" (*23*).

Another methodological source of resistance is the tendency of scientists to think in terms of established models, indeed to reject propositions just because they cannot be put in the form of some model. This seems to have been a reason for resistance to discoveries in the theory of electromagnetism during the 19th century. Ampère's theory of magnetic currents, for example, was resisted by Joseph Henry and others because they did not see how it could be fitted into the Newtonian mechanical model (*24*). They refused to accept Ampère's view that the atom of the Newtonian model had electrical properties which caused magnetic phenomena. And Lord Kelvin's resistance to Clerk Maxwell's electromagnetic theory of light was due, says Kelvin's biographer (*20*), to the fact that Kelvin found himself unable to translate into a dynamical model the abstract equations of Maxwell's theory. Kelvin himself, in the lectures he had given in Baltimore in 1884, had said, "I never satisfy myself until I can make a mechanical model of a thing. If I can make a mechanical model I can understand it. As long as I cannot make a mechanical model all the way through I cannot understand; and that is why I cannot get the electro-magnetic theory" (*20*). Thus, models, while usually extremely helpful in science, can also be a source of blindness.

Scientists' positions on the usefulness of mathematics is a last methodological source of resistance to discovery. Some scientists are excessively partial to mathematics, others excessively hostile. Thus, when Faraday made his experimental discoveries on electro-magnetism Gillispie tells us, few mathematic physicists gave them any serious attention. The discoveries were regarded with indulgence or a touch of scorn as another example of the mathematical incapacity of the British, their barbarous emphasis on experiment, and their theoretical immaturity (*15*). Clerk Maxwell, however, resolved that he "would be Faraday's mathematicus" – that is, put Faraday's experimental discoveries into more mathematical, general, and theoretical a form. Initial resistance was thus overcome. Long ago Augustus De Morgan commented on the antimathematical prejudice of English astronomers of his time. In 1845, he pointed out, the Englishman Adams had, on the basis of mathematical calculations, communicated his discovery of the planet Neptune to his English colleagues. Because they distrusted mathematics, his discovery was not published, and eight months later the Frenchman Leverrier announced and published his simultaneous discovery of the planet, once again on the basis of mathematical calculations. Because the French admired mathematics, Leverrier's discovery was published first, and thus he gained a kind of priority over Adams (*25*).

Mendel was another scientist whose ideas were resisted because of the anti-mathematical preconceptions of the botany of his time. "It must be admitted, however," says his biographer, Iltis, "that the attention of most of the hearers [when he read his classic monograph, "Experiments in Plant-Hybridization," before the Brünn Society for the Study of Natural Science in 1865] was inclined to wander when the lecturer was engaged in rather difficult mathematical deductions; and probably not a soul among them really understood what Mendel was driving at. . . . Many of Mendel's auditors must have been repelled by the strange linking of botany with mathematics, which may have reminded some of the less expert among them of the mystical numbers of the Pythagoreans. . . ." (*18*). Note that the alleged "difficult mathematical deductions" are what we should now consider very simple statistics. And it was not just the audience in Brünn that had no interest in or knowledge of mathematics. Mendel's other biographer, Krumbiegel, tells us that even the more sophisticated group of scientists at the Vienna Zoological-Botanical Society would have given Mendel's theory as poor a reception, and for the same reasons.

In some quarters the antimathematical prejudice persisted in biology for a long time after Mendel's discovery, indeed until after he had been rediscovered. In his biography of Galton, Karl Pearson reports that he sent a paper to the Royal Society in October 1900, eventually published in November 1901, containing statistics in application to a biological problem (*26*). Before the paper was published, he says, "a resolution of the Council [of the Royal Society] was conveyed to me, requesting that in future papers mathematics should be kept apart from biological applications." As a result of this, Pearson wrote to Galton, "I want to ask your opinion about resigning my fellowship of the Royal Society." Galton advised against resigning, but he did help Pearson to found the journal *Biometrika,* so that there would be a place in which mathematics in biology would be explicitly encouraged. Galton wrote an article for the first issue of the new journal, explaining the need for this new agency of "mutual encouragement and support" for mathematics in biology and saying that "a new science cannot depend on a welcome from the followers of the older ones, and [therefore] . . . it is advisable to establish a special Journal for Biometry" (*27*). It seems strange to us now that prejudice against mathematics should have been a source of resistance to innovation in biology only 60 years ago.

Religious ideas

Although we have heard more of the way in which religious forces outside science have hindered its progress, the religious ideas of scientists themselves constitute, after substantive and methodological conceptions, a third cultural source of resistance to scientific innovation. Such internal resistance goes back to the beginning of modern science. We have seen that the astronomer colleagues of Copernicus resisted his ideas in part because of their religious beliefs, and we know that Leibniz, for example, criticized Newton "for failing to make providential destiny part of physics" (*15*). Scientists themselves felt that science should justify God and His world. Gradually, of course, physics and religion were accommodated one to the other, certainly among scientists themselves. But all during the first half of the 19th century resistance to discovery in geology persisted among scientists for religious reasons. The difficulty, as Gillispie has put it on the basis of his classic analysis of geology during this period, "appears to be one of religion (in a crude sense) *in* science rather than one of religion *versus* scientists." The most embarrassing obstacles faced by the new sciences were cast up by the curious providential materialism of the scientists themselves (*5*). When, in the 1840's, Robert Chambers published his *Vestiges of Creation,* declaring a developmental view of the universe, the theory of development was so at variance with the religious views which all scientists accepted that "they all spoke out: Herschel, Whewell, Forbes, Owen, Prichard, Huxley, Lyell, Sedgwick, Murchison, Buckland, Agassiz, Miller, and others" (*5,* p. 133; *28, 29*).

Religious resistance continued and was manifested against Darwin, of course, although many of the scientists who had resisted earlier versions of developmentalism accepted Darwin's evolutionary theory, Huxley being not the least among them. In England, Richard Owen offered the greatest resistance on scientific grounds, while in America and, in fact, internationally, Louis Agassiz was the leading critic of Darwinism on religious grounds (*5, 29, 30*).

In more recent times, biology, like physics before it, has been successfully accommodated to religious ideas, and religious convictions are no longer a source of resistance to innovation in these fields. Resistance to discoveries in the psychological and social sciences that stems from religious convictions is perhaps another story, but one that does not concern us here.

In addition to shared idea-systems, the patterns of social interaction among scientists also become sources of resistance to discovery. Here again we are dealing with elements that, on the whole, probably serve to advance science but that occasionally produce negative, or dysfunctional, effects.

Professional standing

The first of these social sources of resistance is the relative professional standing of the discoverer. In general, higher professional standing in science is achieved by the more competent, those who have demonstrated their capacity for being creative in their own right and for judging the discoveries of others. But sometimes, when discoveries are made by scientists of lower standing, they are resisted by scientists of higher standing partly because of the authority the higher position provides. Huxley commented on this social source of resistance in a letter he wrote in 1852: "For instance, I know that the paper I have just sent in is very original and of some importance, and I am equally sure that if it is referred to the judgment of my 'particular' friend that it will not be published. He won't be able to say a word against it, but he will pooh-pooh it to a dead certainty. You will ask with wonderment, Why? Because for the last twenty years [. . . .] has been regarded as the great authority in these matters, and has had no one tread on his heels, until, at last, I think, he has come to look upon the Natural World as his special preserve, and 'no poachers allowed.' So I must manoeuvre a little to get my poor memoir kept out of his hands" (8, p. 367).

Niels Henrik Abel, early in the 19th century, made important discoveries on a classical mathematical problem, equations of the fifth degree (31). Not only was Abel himself unknown but there was no one of any considerable professional standing in his own country, Norway (then part of Denmark), to sponsor his work. He sent his paper to various foreign mathematicians, the great Gauss among them. But Gauss merely filed the leaflet away unread, and it was found uncut after his death, among his papers. Ohm was another whose work, in this case experimental, was ignored partly because he was of low professional standing. The researches of an obscure teacher of mathematics at the Jesuit Gymnasium in Cologne made little impression upon the more noted scientists of the German universities.

Perhaps the classical instance of low professional standing helping to create resistance to a scientist's discoveries is that of Mendel. The notion that Mendel was "obscure," in the sense that his work did not come to the attention of competent and noted professionals in his field, can no longer be accepted. First of all, the proceedings volume of the Brünn society in which his monograph was printed was exchanged with proceedings volumes of more than 120 other societies, universities, and academies at home and abroad. Copies of his monograph went to Vienna and Berlin, to London and Petersburg, to Rome and Uppsala (18). In London, according to Bateson, the monograph was received by the Royal Society and the Linnaean Society (32). Moreover, we know from the extensive correspondence between them – correspondence which was later published by Mendel's rediscoverer, Correns – that Mendel sent his paper to one of the distinguished botanists of his time, Carl von Nägeli of Munich (*15, 17, 18*). Von Nägeli resisted Mendel's theories for a number of reasons: because his own substantive theories about inheritance were different and because he was unsympathetic to Mendel's use of mathematics, but also because he looked down, from his position of authority, upon the unimportant monk from Brünn. Mendel had written deferentially to von Nägeli, in letters that amounted to small monographs. In these letters, Mendel addressed von Nägeli most respectfully, as an acknowledged master of the subject in which they were both interested. But von Nägeli was the victim of his own position as a scientific pundit. Mendel seemed to him a mere amateur expressing fantastic notions, or at least notions contrary to his own. Von Nägeli's letters to Mendel seem unduly critical to present readers, more than a little supercilious. Nevertheless, the modest Mendel was delighted that the great man had even deigned to reply and sent cordial thanks for the gift of von Nägeli's monograph. On both sides, von Nägeli was defined as the great authority, Mendel as the inferior asking for consideration his position did not warrant. Ironically, Mendel took von Nägeli's advice, to change from experiments on peas to work on hawkweed, a plant not at all suitable at that time for the study of inheritance of separate characteristics. The result was that Mendel labored in a blind alley for the rest of his scientific life.

Nor was von Nägeli unique. Others, such as W. O. Focke, Hermann Hoffman, and Kerner von Marilaun, also dismissed Mendel's work because he seemed "an insignificant provincial" to them. Focke did list Mendel's monograph in his own treatise, *Die Pflanzenmischlinge,* but only for the sake of completeness. Focke paid much more attention to those botanists who had produced quantitatively large and apparently more important contributions – men such as Kölreuter, Gärtner, Wichura, and Wiegmann, of higher professional standing (*33*). Certainly, in this case, quantity of publication was inadequate as a measure of professional worth. Focke's listing of Mendel served only to bring his work, directly and indirectly, to the attention of Correns, de Vries, and von Tschermak after they had independently rediscovered the Mendelian principle of inheritance.

Mendel met with resistance from the authorities in his field after his discovery was published. But sometimes men of higher professional standing sit in judgment on lesser figures *before* publication and prevent a discovery's getting into print. This can be illustrated by an incident in the life of Lord Rayleigh. For the British Association meeting at Birmingham in 1886, Rayleigh submitted a paper under the title, "An Experiment to show that a Divided Electric Current may be greater in both Branches than in the Mains." "His name," says his son and biographer, "was either omitted or accidentally detached, and the Committee 'turned it down' as the work of one of those curious persons called paradoxers. However, when the authorship was discovered, the paper was found to have merits after all. It would seem that even in the late 19th century, and in spite of all that had been written by the apostles of free discussion, authority could prevail when argument had failed!" (*34*). So says the fourth Baron Rayleigh, and we may wonder whether his remark does not still apply, some 75 years later.

Professional specialization

Another social source of resistance is the pattern of specialization that prevails in science at any given time. On the whole, of course, as with any social or other type of system, such specialization is efficient for internal and environmental purposes. Specialization concentrates and focuses the requisite knowledge and skill where they are needed. But occasionally the negative aspect of specialization shows itself, and innovative "outsiders" to a field of specialization are resisted by the "insiders." Thus, when Helmholtz announced his theory of the conservation of energy, it met with resistance partly because he was not a specialist in what we now think of as physics. Referring in the later years of his life to the opposition of the acknowledged experts, Helmholtz said he met with such a remark as this from some of the older men: "This has already been well known to us; what does this young medical man imagine when he thinks it necessary to explain so minutely all this to us?" (*8*, p. *97*). To be sure, on the other side, medical specialists have a long history of resisting scientific innovations from what they define as "the outside." Pasteur met with violent resistance from the medical men of his time when he advanced his germ theory. He regretted that he was not a medical specialist, for the medical men thought of him as a mere chemist poaching on their scientific preserves, not worthy of their attention. In France, even before Pasteur, Magendie had met with resistance for attempting to introduce chemistry into medicine (*35*). If medicine now listens more respectfully to nonmedical science and its discoveries, it is partly because many nonmedical scientists have themselves become experts in a variety of medical-science specialties and so are no longer "outsiders."

Societies, "schools," and seniority

Scientific organizations, as we may safely infer from their large number and their historical persistence, serve a variety of useful purposes for their members. And of course scientific publications are indispensable for communication in science. But occasionally, when organizations or publications are incompetently staffed and run, they may serve as another social source of resistance to innovation in science. There have been no scholarly investigations into the true history of our scientific organizations and publications, but something is known and points in the direction I have suggested. In the early 19th century, for example, even the Royal Society fell on bad days. Lyons tells us that a contemporary, Granville, "severely criticized the shortcomings of the Society" during that period (*36*). Granville gave numerous instances in which the selection or rejection of papers by the Committee of Papers was the result of bad judgment. Sometimes the paper had not been read by any Fellow who was an authority on the subject with which it dealt. In other cases, none of the members of the committee who made the judgment could have had any expert opinion in the matter. It was such an incompetent committee, for example, that resisted Waterston's new molecular theory of gases when he submitted a paper making this contribution. The referee of the Royal Society who rejected the paper wrote on it, "The paper is nothing but nonsense." As a result, Waterston's work lay in utter oblivion until rescued by Rayleigh some 45 years later (*12*, p. 26). Many present-day misjudgments of this kind probably occur, although the multiplicity of publication outlets now provides more than one chance for a significant paper ignored by the incompetent to appear in print.

The rivalries of what are called "schools" are frequently alleged to be another social source of resistance in science. Huxley, for example, is reported to have said, two years before his death, " 'Authorities,' 'disciples,' and 'schools' are the curse of science; and do more to interfere with the work of the scientific spirit than all its enemies" (*37*). Murray suggests that the supposed warfare between science and theology is equaled only by the warfare among rival schools in each of the scientific specialties. Unfortunately, just what the term *school* means is usually left unclear, and no empirical evidence of anything but the most meager and unsystematic character is ever offered by way of illustration (*38*). No doubt some harmful resistance to discovery, as well as some useful competition, comes out of the rivalry of "schools" in science, but until the concept itself is clarified, with definite indicators specified, and until research is carried out on this more adequate basis, we can only feel that "there is something there" that deserves a scholarly treatment it has not yet received.

That the older resist the younger in science is another pattern that has often been noted by scientists themselves and by those who study science as a social phenomenon. "I do not," said Lavoisier in the closing sentences of his memoir *Reflections on Phlogiston* (read before the Academy of Sciences in 1785), "expect my ideas to be adopted all at once. The human mind gets creased into a way of seeing things. Those who have envisaged nature according to a certain point of view during much of their career, rise only with difficulty to new ideas. It is the passage of time, therefore, which must confirm or destroy the opinions I have presented. Meanwhile, I observe with great satisfaction that the young people are beginning to study the science without prejudice. . . . " (*15*). Or again, Hans Zinsser remarks in his autobiography, "That academies and learned societies – commonly dominated by the older foofoos of any profession – are slow to react to new ideas is in the nature of things. For, as Bacon says, *scientia inflat,* and the dignitaries who hold high honors for past accomplishment do not usually like to see the current of progress rush too rapidly out of their reach" (*39*).

Now of course the older workers in science do not always resist the younger in their innovations, nor can it be physical aging in itself that is the source of such resistance as does occur. If we scrutinize carefully the two comments I have just quoted and examine other, similar ones with equal care, we can see that *aging* is an omnibus term which actually covers a variety of cultural and social sources of resistance. Indeed, we may put it this way, that as scientists get older they are more likely to be subject to one or another of the several cultural and social sources of resistance I have analyzed here. As a scientist gets older he is more likely to be restricted in his response to innovation by his substantive and methodological preconceptions and by his other cultural accumulations; he is more likely to have high professional standing, to have specialized interests, to be a member or official of an established organization, and to be associated with a "school." The likelihood of all these things increases with the passage of time, and so the older scientist, just by living longer, is more likely to acquire a cultural and social incubus. But this is not always so, and the older workers in science are often the most ardent champions of innovation.

After this long recital of the cultural and social sources of resistance, by scientists, to scientific discovery, I need to emphasize a point I have already made. That some resistance occurs, that it has specifiable sources in culture and social interaction, that it may be in some measure inevitable, is not proof either that there is more resistance than acceptance in science or that scientists are no more open-minded than other men. On the contrary, the powerful norm of open-mindedness in science, the objective tests by which concepts and theories often can be validated, and the social mechanisms for ensuring competition among ideas new and old – all these make up a social system in which objectivity is greater than it is in other social areas, resistance less. The development of modern science demonstrates this ever so clearly. Nevertheless, some resistance remains, and it is this we seek to understand and thus perhaps to reduce. If "the edge of objectivity" in science, as Charles Gillispie has recently pointed out, requires us to take physical and biological nature as it is, without projecting our wishes upon it, so also we have to take man's social nature, or his behavior in society, as it is. As men in society, scientists are sometimes the agents, sometimes the objects, of resistance to their own discoveries (*40*).

References and Notes

1. S. C. Gilfillan, *The Sociology of Invention* (Follet, Chicago, 1935): B. Barber. *Science and the Social Order* (Free Press, Glencoe, Ill., 1952), chap. 9.
2. P. G. Frank, in *The Validation of Scientific Theories*, P. G. Frank, Ed. (Beacon Press, Boston, 1957); J. Rossman, *The Psychology of the Inventor* (Inventors Publishing Co., Washington, D.C., 1931), chap. 11; R. H. Shryock, *The Development of Modern Medicine* (Univ. of Pennsylvania Press, Philadelphia, 1936), chap. 3; B. J. Stern, in *Technological Trends and National Policy* (Government Printing Office, Washington, D.C., 1937); V. H. Whitney, *Am. J. Sociol.* **56**, 247 (1950); J. Stamp, *The Science of Social Adjustment* (Macmillan, London, 1937), pp. 34 ff.; A. C. Ivy, *Science* 108, 1 (1948).
3. T. S. Kuhn, *The Copernican Revolution* (Harvard Univ. Press, Cambridge, Mass., 1957).
4. A. N. Whitehead, *Science and the Modern World* (Macmillan, New York, 1947), chap. 1; R. K. Merton, *Osiris* **4**, pt. 2 (1938).
5. C. C. Gillispie, *Genesis and Geology* (Harvard Univ. Press, Cambridge, Mass., 1951).
6. R. Oppenheimer, *The Open Mind* (Simon and Schuster, New York, 1955).
7. Quoted from von Helmholtz's *Vorträge und Reden* in R. H. Murray (*8*).
8. R. H. Murray, *Science and Scientists in the Nineteenth Century* (Sheldon, London, 1825).
9. Lord Kelvin also commented on the "resistance" to Faraday. In his article on "Heat" for the 9th edition of the *Encyclopaedia Britannica* he made a comment on the circumstance "that fifty years passed before the scientific world was converted by the experiments of Davy and Rumford to the rational conclusion as to the nonmateriality of heat: 'a remarkable instance of the tremendous inefficiency of bad logic in confounding public opinion and obstructing true philosophic thought.' " [S. P. Thompson, *The Life of William Thomson, Baron Kelvin of Largs* (Macmillan, London, 1910)].
10. M. Planck, *Scientific Autobiography*, F. Gaynor, trans. (Philosophical Library, New York, 1949).
11. See D. L. Watson, *Scientists are Human* (Watts, London, 1938).
12. W. Trotter, *Collected Papers* (Humphrey Milford, London, 1941).
13. W. I. B. Beveridge, *The Art of Scientific Investigation* (Random House, New York, rev. ed., 1959).
14. H. Levy, *Universe of Science* (Century, New York, 1933), p. 197.
15. C. C. Gillispie, *The Edge of Objectivity* (Princeton Univ. Press, Princeton, N.J., 1960).
16. R. Vallery-Radot, *The Life of Pasteur*, R. L. Devonshire, trans. (Garden City Publishing Co., New York, 1926), pp. 175, 215.
17. I. Krumbiegel, *Gregor Mendel und das Schicksal Seiner Entdeckung* (Wissenschaftliche Verlagsgesellschaft, Stuttgart, 1957).
18. H. Iltis, *Life of Mendel*, E. Paul and C. Paul, trans. (W. W. Norton, New York, 1932).
19. J. J. Thomson, *Recollections and Reflections* (Bell, London, 1936), p. 390.
20. S. P. Thompson, *The Life of William Thomson: Baron Kelvin of Largs* (Macmillan, London, 1910).
21. B. Barber and R. C. Fox, *Am. J. Sociol.* **64**, 128 (1958).
22. H. von Helmholtz, *Popular Scientific Lectures* (Appleton, New York, 1873).

23. O. Hahn, *New Atoms, Progress and Some Memories* (Elsevier, New York, 1950), pp. 154–155.

24. T. Coulson, *Joseph Henry: His Life and Work* (Princeton Univ. Press, Princeton, N.J., 1950), p. 36.

25. S. E. De Morgan, *Memoir of Augustus De Morgan* (Longmans, Green, London, 1882).

26. K. Pearson, *The Life, Letters and Labours of Francis Galton* (Cambridge Univ. Press, Cambridge, England, 1924), vol. 3, pp. 100, 282–283.

27. *Biometrika*, **1**, 7 (1901–02).

28. That scientists were religious also, and in the same way, in America can be seen in A. H. Dupree *(29)*.

29. A. H. Dupree, *Asa Gray* (Harvard Univ. Press, Cambridge, Mass., 1959).

30. E. Lurie, *Louis Agassiz: A Life in Science* (Univ. of Chicago Press, Chicago, 1960).

31. O. Ore, *Niels Henrik Abel: Mathematician Extraordinary* (Univ. of Minnesota Press, Minneapolis, 1957).

32. R. A. Fisher, *Ann. Sci.* **1**, 116 (1933).

33. H. F. Roberts, *Plant Hybridization Before Mendel* (Princeton Univ. Press, Princeton, N.J., 1929), pp. 210–211.

34. R. J. Strutt, *John William Strutt, Third Baron Rayleigh* (Arnold, London, 1924), p. 228.

35. J. M. D. Olmstead, *François Magendie, Pioneer in Experimental Physiology and Scientific Medicine in the 19th Century* (Schuman, New York, 1944), pp. 173–175.

36. H. Lyons, *The Royal Society, 1661–1940* (Cambridge Univ. Press, Cambridge, England, 1944), p. 254.

37. C. Bibby, *T. H. Huxley: Scientist, Humanist, and Educator* (Horizon, New York, 1959), p. 18.

38. For the best available sociological essay, see F. Znaniecki, *The Social Role of the Man of Knowledge* (Columbia Univ. Press, New York, 1940), chap. 3.

39. H. Zinsser, *As I Remember Him: The Biography of R. S.* (Little, Brown, Boston, 1940), p. 105.

40. For invaluable aid in the preparation of this article I am indebted to Dr. Elinor G. Barber. The Council for Atomic Age Studies of Columbia assisted with a grant for typing expenses.

6
Self-deception and gullibility

William Broad and Nicholas Wade

In 1669 the distinguished English physicist Robert Hooke made a wonderful discovery. He obtained the long-sought proof of Copernicus' heliocentric theory of the solar system by demonstrating stellar parallax – a perceived difference in position of a star due to the earth's motion around the sun. One of the first to use a telescope for this purpose, Hooke observed the star Gamma Draconis and soon reported to the Royal Society that he had found what he was looking for: the star had a parallax of almost thirty seconds of arc. Here at last was impeccable experimental proof of the Copernican theory.

This heartening triumph of empirical science was only momentarily dashed when the Frenchman Jean Picard announced he had observed the star Alpha Lyrae by the same method but had failed to find any parallax at all. A few years later England's first Astronomer Royal, the brilliant observer John Flamsteed, reported that the Pole Star had a parallax of at least forty seconds.

Hooke and Flamsteed, outstanding scientists of their day, are leading lights in the history of science. But they fell victim to an effect that to this day has continued to trap many lesser scientists in its treacherous coils. It is the phenomenon of experimenter expectancy, or seeing what you want to see. There is indeed a stellar parallax, but because of the vast distance of all stars from earth, the parallax is extremely small – about one second of arc. It cannot be detected by the relatively crude telescopes used by Hooke and Flamsteed.[1]

Self-deception is a problem of pervasive importance in science. The most rigorous training in objective observation is often a feeble defense against the desire to obtain a particular result. Time and again, an experimenter's expectation of what he will see has shaped the data he recorded, to the detriment of the truth. This unconscious shaping of results can come about in numerous subtle ways. Nor is it a phenomenon that affects only individuals. Sometimes a whole community of researchers falls prey to a common delusion, as in the extraordinary case of the French physicists and N-rays, or – some would add – American psychologists and ape sign language.

Expectancy leads to self-deception, and self-deception leads to the propensity to be deceived by others. The great scientific hoaxes, such as the Beringer case and the Piltdown man discussed in this chapter, demonstrate the extremes of gullibility to which some scientists may be led by their desire to believe. Indeed, professional magicians claim that scientists, because of their confidence in their own objectivity, are easier to deceive than other people.

From William Broad and Nicholas Wade, *Betrayers of the Truth* (New York: Simon & Schuster, 1982), 107–125. Copyright 1982 by William Broad and Nicholas Wade. Reprinted by permission of Simon & Schuster.

Self-deception and outright fraud differ in volition – one is unwitting, the other deliberate. Yet it is perhaps more accurate to think of them as two extremes of a spectrum, the center of which is occupied by a range of actions in which the experimenter's motives are ambiguous, even to himself. Many measurements that scientists take in the laboratory admit judgment factors to enter in. An experimenter may delay a little in pressing a stopwatch, perhaps to compensate for some extraneous factor. He can tell himself he is rejecting for technical reasons a result that gives the ''wrong'' answer; after a number of such rejections, the proportion of ''right'' answers in the acceptable experiments may acquire a statistical significance that previously was lacking. Naturally it is only the ''acceptable'' experiments that get published. In effect, the experimenter has selected his data to prove his point, in a way that is in part a deliberate manipulation but which also falls short of conscious fraud.

The ''double-blind'' experiment – in which neither doctor nor patients know who is receiving a test drug and who a placebo – has become standard practice in clinical research because of the powerful effects of the doctor's expectancy, to say nothing of the patients'. But the habit of ''blinding'' the experimenter has not become as universal in science as perhaps it should. A dramatic demonstration of experimenter expectancy has been provided in a series of studies by Harvard psychologist Robert Rosenthal. In one of his experiments he gave psychology students two groups of rats to study. The ''maze-bright'' group of rats, the students were told, had been specially bred for its intelligence in running mazes. The ''maze-dull'' group were genetically stupid rats. The students were told to test the maze-running abilities of the two groups. Sure enough, they found that the maze-bright rats did significantly better than the maze-dull rats. In fact there was no difference between the maze-bright and maze-dull animals: all were the standard strain of laboratory rats. The difference lay only in the students' expectancies of each group. Yet the students translated this difference in their expectancies into the data they reported.[2]

Perhaps some of the students consciously invented data to accord with the results they thought they should be getting. With others, the manipulation was unconscious and much more subtle. Just how it was done is rather hard to explain. Perhaps the students handled more gently the rats they expected to perform better, and the treatment enhanced the rats' performance. Perhaps in timing the run through the maze the students would unconsciously press the button on the stopwatch a fraction too early for the maze-bright rats and a fraction too late for the maze-dull animals. Whatever the exact mechanism, the researchers' expectations had shaped the result of the experiment without their knowledge.

The phenomenon is not just a pitfall for laboratory scientists. Consider the situation of a teacher administering IQ tests to a class. If he has prior expectations about the children's intelligence, are these likely to shape the results he gets? The answer is yes, they do. In an experiment similar to that performed on the psychology students, Rosenthal told teachers at an elementary school that he had identified certain children with a test that predicted academic blooming. Unknown to the teachers, the test was just a standard IQ test, and the children identified as ''bloomers'' were chosen at random. At the end of the school year, the children were retested, by the teachers this time, with the same test. In the first grade, those who had been identified to the teachers as academic bloomers gained fifteen IQ points more than did the other children. The ''bloomers'' in the second grade gained ten points more than the controls. Teachers' expectancies made no or little difference in the upper grades. In the lower grades, comments Rosenthal, ''the children have not yet acquired those reputations that become so difficult to change in the later grades and which give teachers in subsequent grades the expectancies for the pupil's performance. With every successive grade it would be more difficult to change the child's reputation."[3]

A particularly fertile ground for scientific self-deception lies in the field of animal-to-man communication. Time and again, the researcher's expectation has been projected onto the animal and reflected back to the researcher without his recognizing the source. The most famous case of this sort is that of Clever Hans, a remarkable horse that could apparently add and substract and even solve problems that were presented to it. He has acquired immortality because his equine spirit returns from time to time to haunt the laboratories of experimental psychologists, announcing its presence with ghostly laughter that its victims are almost always the last to hear.

Hans's trainer, a retired German schoolteacher named Wilhelm Von Osten, sincerely believed that he had taught Hans the ability to count. The horse would tap out numbers with his hoof, stopping when he had reached the right answer. He would count not just for his master but for others as well. The phenomenon was investigated by a psychologist, Oskar Pfungst, who discovered that Von Osten and others were unconsciously cuing the equine prodigy. As the horse reached the number of hoof taps corresponding to the correct answer, Von Osten would involuntarily jerk his head. Perceiving this unconscious cue, Hans would stop tapping. Pfungst found that the horse could detect head movements as slight as one-fifth of a millimeter. Pfungst himself played the part of the horse and found that twenty-three out of twenty-five questioners unwittingly cued him when to stop tapping.

Pfungst's celebrated investigation of the Clever Hans phenomenon was published in English in 1911, but his definitive account did not prevent others from falling into the same trap as Von Osten. Man's age-old desire to communicate with other species could not so easily be suppressed. By 1937 there were more than seventy "thinking" animals, including cats and dogs as well as horses. In the 1950's the fashion turned to dolphins. Then came an altogether new twist in the dialogue between man and animals. The early attempts to teach speech to chimpanzees had faltered because of the animals' extreme physical difficulty in forming human sounds. Much greater progress was made when Allen and Beatrice Gardner of the University of Nevada taught American Sign Language to their chimpanzee Washoe.

Washoe and her imitators readily acquired large vocabularies of the sign language and, even more significantly, would string the signs together in what appeared to be sentences. Particularly evocative was the apes' reported use of the signs in apposite novel combinations. Washoe was said to have spontaneously made the signs for "drink" and "fruit" on seeing a watermelon. Gorilla Koko reportedly described a zebra as a "white tiger." By the 1970's the signing apes had become a flourishing subfield of psychological research.

Then came a serious crisis in the form of an ape named Nim Chimpsky, in honor of the well-known linguist Noam Chomsky. Nim's trainer, psychologist Herbert Terrace, found he learned signs just like the other chimps, and started using them in strings. But were the strings of signs proper sentences or just a routine that the crafty ape had learned would induce some appropriate action in its human entourage? Certain features in Nim's linguistic development threw Terrace into a crisis of doubt. Unlike children of his age, Nim suddenly plateaued in his rate of acquisition of new vocabulary. Unlike children, he rarely initiated conversation. He would string signs together, but his sentences were lacking in syntactic rigor: Nim's longest recorded utterance was the sixteen-sign declarative pronouncement, "Give orange me give cat orange me eat orange give me eat orange give me you."

Terrace was eventually forced to decide that Chimpsky, and indeed the other pointing pongids, were not using the signs in a way characteristic of true language. Rather, they were probably making monkeys out of their teachers by imitating or Clever Hansing them. Nim's linguistic behavior was more like that of a highly intelligent, trained dog than of the human children he so much resembled in other ways.

The critics began to move in on the field. "We find the ape 'language' researchers replete with personalities who believe themselves to be acting according to the most exalted motivations and sophisticated manners, but in reality have involved themselves in the most rudimentary circus-like performances," wrote Jean Umiker-Sebeok and Thomas Sebeok.[4] At a conference in 1980, Sebeok was even more forthright: "In my opinion, the alleged language experiments with apes divide into three groups: one, outright fraud; two, self-deception; three, those conducted by Terrace. The largest class by far is the middle one."[5] The battle is not yet over, but the momentum at present lies with the critics. Should they prove correct, the whole field of ape language research will slide rapidly into disrepute, and the ghost of Clever Hans will once again enjoy the last laugh.

Researchers' propensity for self-delusion is particularly strong when other species enter the scene as vehicles for human imaginings and projections. But scientists are capable of deluding themselves without any help from other species. The most remarkable known case of a collective self-deception is one that affected the community of French physicists in the early 1900's. In 1903 the distinguished French physicist René Blondlot announced he had discovered a new kind of rays, which he named N-rays, after the University of Nancy, where he worked.

In the course of trying to polarize X-rays, discovered by Röntgen eight years earlier, Blondlot found evidence of a new kind of emanation from the X-ray source. It made itself apparent by increasing the brightness of an electric spark jumping between a pair of pointed wires. The increase in brightness had to be judged by eye, a notoriously subjective method of detection. But that seemed to matter little in view of the fact that other physicists were soon able to repeat and extend Blondlot's findings.

A colleague at the University of Nancy discovered that N-rays were emitted not just by X-ray sources but also by the nervous system of the human body. A Sorbonne physicist noticed that N-rays emanated from Broca's area, the part of the brain that governs speech, while a person was talking. N-rays were discovered in gases, magnetic fields, and chemicals. Soon the pursuit of N-rays had become a minor industry among French scientists. Leading French physicists commended Blondlot for his discovery. The French Academy of Sciences bestowed its valuable Leconte prize on him in 1904. The effects of N-rays "were observed by at least forty people and analyzed in some 300 papers by 100 scientists and medical doctors between 1903 and 1906," notes an historian of the episode.[6]

N-rays do not exist. The researchers who reported seeing them were the victims of self-deception. What was the reason for this collective delusion? An important clue may be found in the reaction to an article written in 1904 by the American physicist R. W. Wood. During a visit to Blondlot's laboratory, Wood correctly divined that something peculiar was happening. At one point Blondlot darkened the laboratory to demonstrate an experiment in which N-rays were separated into different wavelengths after passing through a prism. Wood surreptitiously removed the prism before the experiment began, but even with the centerpiece of his apparatus sitting in his visitor's pocket, Blondlot obtained the expected results. Wood wrote a devastating account of his visit in an English scientific journal. Science is supposed to transcend national boundaries, but Wood's critique did not. Scientists outside France immediately lost interest in N-rays, but French scientists continued for several years to support Blondlot.

"The most astonishing facet of the episode," notes the French scientist Jean Rostand, "is the extraordinarily great number of people who were taken in. These people were not pseudo-scientists, charlatans, dreamers, or mystifiers; far from it, they were true men of science, disinterested, honorable, used to laboratory procedure, people with level heads and sound common sense. This is borne out by their subsequent achievements as Professors, Consultants and Lecturers. Jean Bacquerel, Gilbert Ballet, André Broca, Zimmern, Bordier – all of them have made their contribution to science."[7]

The reason why the best French physicists of their day continued to support Blondlot after Wood's critique was perhaps the same as the reason for which they uncritically accepted Blondlot's findings in the first place. It all had to do with a sentiment that is supposed to be wholly foreign to science: national pride. By 1900 the French had come to feel that their international reputation in science was on the decline, particularly with respect to the Germans. The discovery of N-rays came just at the right time to soothe the self-doubts of the rigid French scientific hierarchy. Hence the Academy of Sciences, faced after the Wood exposé with almost unanimous criticism from abroad and strong skepticism at home, chose nonetheless to rally round Blondlot rather than ascertain the truth. The members of the academy's Leconte prize committee, which included the Nancy-born Henri Poincaré, chose Blondlot over the other leading candidate, Pierre Curie, who had shared the Nobel prize the year before.

Most historians and scientists who have written about the N-ray affair describe it as pathological, irrational, or otherwise deviant. One historian who is not part of this consensus is Mary Jo Nye. To seek an understanding of the episode, she chose to examine "not the structure of Blondlot's psyche, but rather the structure of Blondlot's scientific community, its organization, aims and aspirations around 1900." Her conclusion, in brief, is that the episode arose from at most an exaggeration of the usual patterns of behavior among scientific communities. The N-ray affair, she says, "was not 'pathological,' much less 'irrational' or 'pseudo-scientific.' The scientists involved in the investigations and debate were influenced in a normal, if sometimes exaggerated, way by traditional reductionist scientific aims, by personal competitive drives, and by institutional, regional, and national loyalties."[8]

That a whole community of scientists can be led astray by nonrational factors is a phenomenon that bears some pondering. To dismiss it as "pathological" is merely to affix a label. In fact the N-ray affair displays in extreme form several themes endemic to the scientific process. One is the unreliability of human observers. The fact is that all human observers, however well trained, have a strong tendency to see what they expect to see. Even when subjectively assessed qualities such as the brightness of a spark are replaced by instruments such as counters or print-outs, observer effects still enter in. Careful studies of how people read measuring devices has brought to light the "digit preference phenomenon" in which certain numbers are unconsciously preferred over others.[9]

Theoretical expectation is one factor that may distort a scientist's observation. The desire for fame and recognition may prevent such distortions from being corrected. In the case of N-rays, a nexus of personal, regional, and national ties combined to carry

French physicists far away from the ideal modes of scientific inquiry, and not only that, but to persist in gross error for long after it had been publicly pointed out.

Do scientists take adequate steps to protect themselves from experimental pitfalls of this nature? "Blinded" studies, in which the researcher recording the data does not know what the answer is supposed to be, are a useful precaution but are not sufficient to rule out self-deception. So pervasive are the coils of self-deception in the biological sciences that a foolproof methodology is hard to devise. Theodore X. Barber compiled a manual of pitfalls in experimental research with human subjects, which he concluded with the following poignant postscript: "Before this text was mailed to the publisher, it was read critically by nine young researchers or graduate students. After completing the text, three of the readers felt that, since there were so many problems in experimental research, it may be wiser to forsake experimentation in general (and laboratory experiments in particular) and to limit our knowledge-seeking attempts to other methods, for example, to naturalistic field studies or to participant observation."[10]

The bedrock of science is observation and experiment, the empirical procedures that make it different from other kinds of knowledge. Yet observation turns out to be most fallible when it is most needed: when an experimenter's objectivity falters. Take the case of the eighteenth-century savant Johann Jacob Scheuchzer, who set out to find evidence that mankind at the time of Noah had been caught up in a terrible flood. Find it he did, and Scheuchzer hailed the skeletal remains of his flood man as *Homo diluvii testis*. Examination years later showed the fossil to be a giant amphibian, long ago extinct.

Twentieth-century science has not escaped the danger to which Scheuchzer fell victim. When the American astronomer Adriaan van Maanen announced in 1916 that he had observed rotations in spiral nebulae, the result was accepted because it confirmed a prevailing belief that the nebulae were nearby objects. Later work by Edwin Hubble, van Maanen's colleague at the Mount Wilson Observatory, showed that, to the contrary, the spiral nebulae are galaxies at an immense distance from our own, and that they do not rotate in the manner described by van Maanen. What made van Maanen's eyes deceive him?

The standard explanation, promulgated in such publications as the *Dictionary of Scientific Biography,* is that "the changes he was attempting to measure were at the very limits of precision of his equipment and techniques."[11] But random error of the sort suggested cannot explain the fact that van Maanen over the course of a decade reported many nebulae to be rotating in the same direction (unwinding rather than winding up). The subjectivity of scientific observers has prompted a historian of the van Maanen affair, Norriss Hetherington, to comment that "today science holds the position of queen of the intellectual disciplines. . . . The decline of the dominance of theology followed from historical studies that revealed the human nature and thus the human status of theology. Historical and sociological studies that begin to investigate a possible human element of science similarly threaten to topple the current queen."[12]

Self-deception is so potent a human capability that scientists, supposedly trained to be the most objective of observers, are in fact peculiarly vulnerable to deliberate deception by others. The reason may be that their training in the importance of objectivity leads them to ignore, belittle, or suppress in themselves the very nonrational factors that the hoaxster relies on. The triumph of preconceived ideas over common sense has seldom been more complete than in the case of Dr. Johann Bartholomew Adam Beringer.

A physician and learned dilettante of eighteenth-century Germany, Beringer taught at the University of Würzburg and was adviser and chief physician to the prince-bishop. Not content with his status as a mere healer and academician, he threw himself into the study of "things dug from the earth," and began a collection of natural rarities such as figured stones, as fossils were then called. The collection assumed a remarkable character in 1725, when three Würzburg youths brought him the first of a series of extraordinary stones they had dug up from nearby Mount Eivelstadt.[13]

This new series of figured stones was a treasure trove of insects, frogs, toads, birds, scorpions, snails, and other creatures. As the youths brought further objects of their excavations to the eager Beringer, the subject matter of the fossils became distinctly unusual. "Here were leaves, flowers, plants, and whole herbs, some with and some without roots and flowers," wrote Beringer in a book of 1726 describing the amazing discovery. "Here were clear depictions of the sun and moon, of stars, and of comets with their fiery tails. And lastly, as the supreme prodigy commanding the reverent admiration of myself and of my fellow examiners, were magnificent tablets engraved in Latin, Arabic, and Hebrew characters with the ineffable name of Jehovah."

Shortly after the publication of his book, historical accounts relate, Beringer discovered on Mount Eivelstadt the most unusual fossil of all, one that carried his own name.

An official inquiry was held, at Beringer's request, to discover who was responsible for perpetrating the hoax. One of the young diggers turned out to be in the employ of two of Beringer's rivals, J. Ignatz Roderick, professor of geography, algebra, and analysis at the University of Würzburg, and the Honorable Georg von Eckhart, privy councillor and librarian to the court and to the university. Their motive had been to make Beringer a laughingstock because "he was so arrogant."

What also emerged at the inquiry was that the hoaxsters, apparently fearful that things might go too far, had tried to open Beringer's eyes to the prank before the publication of his book. They started a rumor that the stones were fakes, and when that didn't work they had him told directly. Beringer could not be persuaded that the whole thing was a massive piece of fakery; he went ahead and published his book.

Even within Beringer's lifetime, the legend of the "lying stones" began to gain momentum. By 1804, James Parkinson in his book *Organic Remains of a Former World* mentioned the debacle and drew out a lesson: "It plainly demonstrates, that learning may not be sufficient to prevent an unsuspecting man, from becoming the dupe of excessive credulity. It is worthy of being mentioned, on another account: the quantity of censure and ridicule, to which its author was exposed, served, not only to render his contemporaries less liable to imposition; but also more cautious in indulging in unsupported hypotheses."[14]

Parkinson was not the only observer to comment on the salutary effect of hoaxes in promoting skepticism. In 1830, in his book *Reflections on the Decline of Science in England*, Charles Babbage remarked: "The only excuse which has been made for them is when they have been practised on scientific academies which had reached the period of dotage." By way of example he noted how the editors of a French encyclopedia had credulously copied the description of a fictitious animal that a certain Gioeni claimed to have discovered in Sicily and had named after himself, *Gioenia sicula*.[15]

When hoaxes go awry, it is often for want of occasion, not of gullibility on the part of the intended victims, as in the case of the Orgueil meteorite, a shower of stones that fell near the village of Orgueil, France, on the night of May 14, 1864. A few weeks earlier, Louis Pasteur had started a furious debate in France by delivering the famous lecture before the French Academy in which he derided the long-standing theory of spontaneous generation, which held that life-forms can develop from inanimate matter. Noticing that the material of the Orgueil meteorite became pasty when exposed to water, a hoaxster molded some seeds and particles of coal into a sample of the meteorite and waited for them to be discovered by Pasteur's opponents. The hoaxster's motive was presumably to let them adduce the seeds as evidence for life spontaneously generating in outer space, whereupon he would pull the rug out from under them by announcing the hoax.

What went wrong with the scheme was that the doctored fragment was never examined during the debate. Though other pieces of the meteorite were intensively studied at the time, the hoaxster's carefully prepared fragment lay unexamined in a glass display jar at the Musée d'Histoire at Montauban, France, for ninety-eight years. When its turn at last came, in 1964, the incentive for belief had disappeared, and the forgery was immediately recognized as such.[16]

Had the fragment been studied at the time, the hoax would doubtless have been successful. When the conditions are right, there is no limit to human gullibility, as was proved by the remarkable incident of the Piltdown man.

British national pride in the early years of the twentieth century suffered from a matter of serious disquiet. The Empire was at its height, the serenity of the Victorian era was still aglow, and to educated Englishmen it was almost self-evident that England had once been the cradle, as it was now the governess, of world civilization. How then to explain that striking evidence of early man – not just skeletal remains but Paleolithic cave paintings and tools as well – was coming to light in France and Germany but not in Britain? The dilemma was exacerbated in 1907 with the discovery near Heidelberg, Germany, of a massive, early human jawbone. It seemed depressing proof that the first man had been a German.

The discovery of the Piltdown man was made by Charles Dawson, a lawyer who maintained a quiet practice in the south of England and dabbled in geology. A tireless amateur collector of fossils, Dawson noticed a promising-looking gravel pit on Piltdown Common, near Lewes in Sussex. He asked a laborer digging there to bring him any flints he might find. Several years later, in 1908, the laborer brought him a fragment of bone that Dawson recognized as part of a thick human skull. Over the next three years further bits of the skull appeared.

In 1912 Dawson wrote to his old friend Arthur Smith Woodward, a world authority on fossil fishes at the geology department of the British Museum of Natural History, saying he had something that would top the German fossil found at Heidelberg. Woodward made several visits with Dawson to the Piltdown gravel pit. On one of these expeditions, Dawson's digging tool struck at the bottom of the pit and out flew part of a lower jaw. Close examination led Woodward and Dawson to believe that it belonged to the skull they had already reconstructed.

In great excitement, Smith Woodward took everything back to the British Museum, where he put the jaw and cranium together, filling in missing parts with modeling clay and his imagination. The result was truly remarkable. The assembled skull became the "dawn man" of Piltdown. Kept secret until December 1912, it was unveiled before a full house at the Geological Society in London, where it created a sensation. Some skeptics suggested that the human skull and apelike jaw did not belong together; others pointed out that two characteristically abraded molar teeth were not enough to prove the jaw was human. But these objections were ignored, and the find was accepted as a great and genuine discovery.[17]

The talk in clubs and pubs could note with satisfaction the new proof that the earliest man was indeed British. The Piltdown skull was also of scientific interest because it seemed to be the "missing link," the transitional form between ape and man that was postulated by Darwin's still controversial theory of evolution. Subsequent excavations at the gravel pit were not disappointing. A whole series of new fossils emerged. The clinching evidence came from a pit a few miles away – the discovery a few years later of a second Piltdown man.

Yet some were troubled by the Piltdown finds, among them a young zoologist at the British Museum, Martin A. C. Hinton. After a visit to the site in 1913, Hinton concluded that the whole thing was a hoax. He decided to smoke out the tricksters by planting clearly fraudulent fossils and watching the reactions. He took an ape tooth from the collection at the museum and filed it down to match the model canine tooth that Smith Woodward had fashioned out of clay. Hinton had the obvious forgery placed in the pit by an accomplice and sat back to wait for it to be discovered and the entire Piltdown collection to be exposed.

The tooth was discovered, but nothing else went right with Hinton's plan. All involved with the "discovery" seemed delighted and soon notified the nation about the new find. Hinton was astonished that his scientific colleagues could be taken in by so transparent a fake, and he suffered the additional mortification of seeing Charles Dawson, whom he suspected to be the culprit, acquiring kudos for his handiwork. He decided to try again, only this time with something so outrageous that the whole country would laugh the discoverers to scorn.

In a box in the British Museum he found a leg bone from an extinct species of elephant. He proceeded to carve it into an extremely appropriate tool for the earliest Englishman – a Pleistocene cricket bat. He took the bat to Piltdown, buried it, and waited for the laughter.

It was a long wait. When the bat was unearthed, Smith Woodward was delighted. He pronounced it a supremely important example of the work of Paleolithic man, for nothing like it had ever been found before. Smith Woodward and Dawson published a detailed, serious description of the artifact in a professional journal but stopped short of calling it an actual cricket bat.[18] Hinton was astonished that none of the scientists thought of trying to whittle a bit of bone, fossil or fresh, with a flint edge. If they had, they would have discovered it was impossible to imitate the cuts on the cricket bat. "The acceptance of this rubbish completely defeated the hoaxsters," notes a historian of the Piltdown episode.[19] "They just gave up, and abandoned all attempts to expose the whole business and get it demolished in laughter and ridicule." Perhaps Hinton and friends should have considered planting a bone on which the name Smith Woodward had been carved.

Piltdown man retained its scientific luster until the mid–1920's and the discovery of humanlike fossils in Africa. These indicated a very different pattern of human evolution to that suggested by the Piltdown skull. Instead of a human cranium with an apelike jaw, the African fossils were just the reverse – they had humanlike jaws with apelike skulls. Piltdown became first an anomaly, then an embarrassment. It slipped from sight until modern techniques of dating showed in the early 1950's that the skull and its famous jaw were fakes: an ape jaw, with filed-down molars, and a human skull had each been suitably stained to give the appearance of great age.

Circumstantial evidence pointed to the skull's discoverer, Dawson, as the culprit. But many have doubted that he could have been the instigator; although he was best placed to salt the gravel pit, he probably lacked access to the necessary fossil collections as well as the scientific expertise to assemble fossils of the right age for the Piltdown gravel. Indeed, the real mystery is not who did it but how a whole generation of scientists could have been taken in by so transparent a prank. The fakery was not expert. The tools were poorly carved and the teeth crudely filed. "The evidences of artificial abrasion immediately sprang to the eye. Indeed so obvious did they seem it may well be asked – how was it that they had escaped notice before," remarked anthropologist Le Gros Clark.[20]

The question is one that the victims always ask in retrospect yet seldom learn to anticipate. A group of scientists particularly plagued by tricksters and charlatans are parapsychologists, researchers who apply the scientific method to the study of telepathy, extrasensory perception, and other paranormal phenomena. Because parapsychology is widely regarded as a fringe subject not properly part of science, its practitioners have striven to be more than usually rigorous in following correct scientific methodology.

The founder of parapsychology, J. B. Rhine, made great strides in putting the discipline on a firm scientific footing. As a mark of its growing scientific acceptability, the Parapsychological Association in 1971 was admitted to the American Association for the Advancement of Science. The field seemed to be making solid headway toward the goal of scientific acceptability. Noting this progress with satisfaction, Rhine in 1974 commented on the decline of fraudulent investigators: "As time has passed our progress has aided us in avoiding the admission of such risky personnel even for a short term. As a result, the last twenty years have seen little of this cruder type of chicanery. Best of all, we have reached a stage at which we can actually look for and to a degree choose the people we want in the field." Rhine also warned against the danger of relying on automatic data recording as a means of avoiding the pitfalls of subjective measurement: "Apparatus can sometimes also be used as a screen to conceal the trickery it was intended to prevent," he noted.[21]

Less than three months after his article had appeared, Rhine's Institute for Parapsychology in Durham, North Carolina, was rocked by a scandal that involved Walter J. Levy, a brilliant young protégé whom Rhine had planned to designate his successor as director of the institute.

Levy had developed a highly successful experiment for demonstrating psychic ability in rats: through psychokinetic powers, the animals could apparently influence an electric generator to activate electrodes implanted in the pleasure centers of the brain. For more than a year the experiment had given positive results, and Rhine urged Levy to have it repeated in other labs. The work, however, quickly took a turn for the worse; results fell back to the chance level.

At this point one of the junior experimenters noticed that Levy was paying more than usual attention to the equipment. He and others decided to check out their suspicions by observing their senior colleague from a concealed position. They saw Levy manipulating the experimental apparatus so as to make it yield positive results. To Rhine's credit, he published an article recounting the whole episode.[22] "Right from the start the necessity of trusting the experimenter's personal accuracy or honesty must be avoided as far as possible," he concluded.

Most parapsychologists have training in a conventional scientific discipline, and they bring their scientific training to bear on the study of the paranormal. The competence with which the study is conducted is probably a measure of that training. But if so, scientists have not shown themselves to be highly successful in dealing with the unexpected problems of the occult world. Their subjects, those who claim occult powers, have invariably followed one of two patterns when put under systematic observation: either their powers "fade" or they are exposed as tricksters. That background might lead parapsychologists to approach new claimants with a certain degree of skepticism. But when the Israeli mentalist Uri Geller toured the United States demonstrating his psychic powers, the parapsychologists gave an enormous boost to his claims by confirming them in the laboratory.

Harold Puthoff and Russell Targ, two laser physicists at the Stanford Research Institute, wrote a scientific article corroborating Geller's ability to guess the number on a die concealed in a metal box. The article was accepted and published by *Nature,* a leading scientific journal.[23] Other scientists, such as the English physicist John Taylor of London University, endorsed Geller's psychic abilities. It fell to a professional magician, not a scientist or a parapsychologist, to explain to the public what was behind the Geller phenomenon. James Randi, of Rumson, New Jersey, showed audiences that he could duplicate all Geller's feats, but by simple conjury. "Any magician will tell you that scientists are the easiest persons in the world to fool," says mathematical columnist Martin Gardner.[24] Geller, note two students of deception, "prefers scientists as witnesses and will not perform before expert magicians, and for good reason. Scientists, by the very nature of their intellectual and social training, are among the easiest persons for a conjuror to deceive. . . ."[25]

For an extreme example of gullibility among some of America's best physicists and engineers, consider the remarkable case of the Shroud of Turin Research Project, a group of scientists devoted to studying a relic that believers say is the true burial cloth of Christ. Members of the group work at the Los Alamos National Laboratory, where America's nuclear weapons are designed, and at other military research centers. "The great majority of them are, or until recently were, engaged in the design, manufacture, or testing of weapons, from simple explosives to atomic bombs to high-energy 'killer' lasers," notes an admiring article.[26]

In their spare time the scientists study the Shroud of Turin with the most modern scientific instruments. Though careful not to say it is genuine, they say they cannot prove it is a fake, leaving the strong impression that it is the real thing. They add that there are features of the shroud that cannot be explained by modern technology; its image, of a full-length crucified man, was not painted, they say, because there is no sign of pigment. It is a reverse image, like a photographic negative, and encodes three-dimensional information. From what they tell reporters, they seem to favor a short intense burst of light, presumably from inside the body, as the cause of the image.

But consider some brief facts about the Shroud of Turin: (i) it first came to light in about 1350, at a time when medieval Europe was swamped with purported Holy Land relics of all kinds; (ii) the bishop of Troyes, France, in whose diocese it first appeared, "discovered the fraud and how the said cloth had been cunningly painted, the truth being attested by the artist who had painted it," according to a letter written to the Pope in 1389 by one of the bishop's successors; (iii) traces of two medieval pigments have been discovered in particles lifted off the shroud.[27] The negative image with its three-dimensional encoded information is simply the result of an artist trying to paint an image as it might be expected to register on a cloth covering a dead body. He put in shading to indicate the body's contours, and used so dilute a pigment that even modern tests mostly fail to reveal it. How did a group of the nation's elite bomb designers get so far along the road of persuading themselves (and numerous reporters) that they had a miracle on their hands?

"In entering upon any scientific pursuit," said the nineteenth-century astronomer John Herschel, "one of the student's first endeavours ought to be to prepare his mind for the reception of truth, by dismissing, or at least loosening, his hold on all such crude and hastily adopted notions respecting the objects and relations he is about to examine, as may tend to embarrass or mislead him." Good advice but hard to follow, as the long and continuing history of self-deception and gullibility in science repeatedly shows.

The frequency of scientific self-deception and hoaxes takes on special significance when it is remembered that the skeptical frame of mind is supposedly an essential part of the scientist's approach to the world. The scientific method is widely assumed to be a powerful and self-correcting device for understanding the world as it is and making sense of nature. What is the scientific method, and what are the flaws that make this adamantine armor so strangely vulnerable to the unexpected?

Notes

1. It is interesting to note that historians espousing the conventional ideology of science have tried to save appearances by assuming that Hooke and Flamsteed were observing another phenomenon, known as stellar aberration, which they innocently mistook for the stellar parallax. This explanation will not wash. Stellar aberration is an apparent displacement similar to which a raindrop seen from a moving car seems to fall slantwise instead of straight down. It was discovered in 1725 by James Bradley in the very course of trying to repeat Hooke's observation of the stellar parallax. Bradley himself specifically stated that Hooke's data could not be measurements of stellar aberration. Hooke's observations were "really very far from being either exact or agreeable to the phenomena," Bradley reported. "It seems that Hooke found what he expected to find," notes Norriss Hetherington of the University of California, Berkeley, in an account of this episode ("Questions About the Purported Objectivity of Science," unpublished MS).
2. Robert Rosenthal, *Experimenter Effects in Behavioral Research* (Appleton-Century-Crofts, New York, 1966), pp. 158–179.
3. *Ibid.*, pp. 411–413.
4. Jean Umiker-Sebeok and Thomas A. Sebeok, "Clever Hans and Smart Simians," *Anthropos,* 76, 89–166, 1981.
5. Nicholas Wade, "Does Man Alone Have Language? Apes Reply in Riddles, and a Horse Says Neigh," *Science,* 208, 1349–1351, 1980.
6. Mary Jo Nye, "N-rays: An Episode in the History and Psychology of Science," *Historical Studies in the Physical Sciences,* 11:1, 125–156, 1980.
7. Jean Rostand, *Error and Deception in Science* (Basic Books, New York, 1960), p. 28.
8. Nye, *op. cit.,* p. 155.
9. Rosenthal, *op. cit.,* pp. 3–26.
10. Theodore Xenophon Barber, *Pitfalls in Human Research* (Pergamon Press, New York, 1973), p. 88.
11. Richard Berendzen and Carol Shamieh, "Maanen, Adriann van," *Dictionary of Scientific Biography* (Charles Scribner's Sons, New York, 1973), pp. 582–583.

12. Norriss S. Hetherington, ''Questions About the Purported Objectivity of Science,'' unpublished MS.
13. Melvin E. Jahn and Daniel J. Woolf, *The Lying Stones of Dr. Johann Bartholomew Adam Beringer* (University of California Press, Berkeley, 1963).
14. *Ibid.*
15. Charles Babbage, *Reflections on the Decline of Science in England* (Augustus M. Kelley, New York, 1970).
16. Edward Anders *et al.*, ''Contaminated Meteorite,'' *Science*, 146, 1157–1161, 1964.
17. J. S. Weiner, *The Piltdown Forgery* (Oxford University Press, London, 1955).
18. Charles Dawson and Arthur Smith Woodward, ''On a Bone Implement from Piltdown,'' *Quarterly Journal of the Geological Society*, 71, 144–149, 1915.
19. L. Harrison Matthews, ''Piltdown Man: The Missing Links,'' *New Scientist*, a ten-part series, beginning April 30, 1981, pp. 280–282.
20. Quoted in Stephen J. Gould, *The Panda's Thumb* (W. W. Norton, New York, 1980), p. 112.
21. J. B. Rhine, ''Security Versus Deception in Parapsychology,'' *Journal of Parapyschology*, 38, 99–121, 1974.
22. J. B. Rhine, ''A New Case of Experimenter Unreliability,'' *Journal of Parapsychology*, 38, 215–225, 1974.
23. Russell Targ and Harold Puthoff, ''Information Transmission Under Conditions of Sensory Shielding,'' *Nature*, 251, 602–607, 1974.
24. Martin Gardner, ''Magic and Paraphysics,'' *Technology Review*, June 1976, pp. 43–51.
25. Umiker-Sebeok and Sebeok, *op. cit.*
26. Cullen Murphy, ''Shreds of Evidence,'' *Harper's*, November 1981, pp. 42–65.
27. Walter C. McCrone, ''Microscopical Study of the Turin 'Shroud,' '' *The Microscope*, 29, 1, 1981.

QUESTIONS FOR DISCUSSION

1. Both science and religion seek to explain the nature and function of reality. How do the rules of evidence vary between these two fields? How do they overlap?
2. Can a researcher ever be absolutely objective, or does the individual always become a part of the observation?
3. How does peer review guard against self-deception and subjective interpretation of data? How can peer review fall prey to these same forces?

RECOMMENDED SUPPLEMENTAL READING

The Betrayers of the Truth, William Broad & Nicholas Wade, New York: Simon & Schuster, 1982.
The Limits of Science, Peter Medawar, New York: Oxford University Press, 1984.
''The Tomato Effect: Rejection of Highly Efficacious Therapies,'' James S. Goodwin & Jean M. Goodwin, *Journal of the American Medical Association*, 1984, 251, pp. 2387–2390.

PART IV

The Responsible Conduct of
Biological Research

INTRODUCTION

Several cases of alleged scientific misconduct involving prominent scientists have been recurrent front-page news in the past decade, eroding the public's confidence in the scientific establishment. The actual pervasiveness of misconduct among scientists is unknown. Are we seeing the tip of an iceberg of misconduct or a media creation?

The National Institutes of Health has defined scientific misconduct as "fabrication, falsification, plagiarism, or other practices that seriously deviate from those that are commonly accepted within the scientific community for proposing, conducting, or reporting research."[1] The various institutions that receive federal funds for research are now establishing policies and mechanisms to investigate charges of suspected instances of misconduct.

In order for the process of normal science to advance, certain steps are followed in a scientific experiment. The scientist must assess what has been accomplished by others; develop an appropriate hypothesis; design and execute the experiments necessary to test it; record, process, and analyze the data obtained; and publish the results. High-quality execution is necessary at each step to ensure the integrity of the resulting product. It is important to define the normal range of acceptable behavior at each of these stages, for although fabrication, falsification, and plagiarism may be measurable phenomena, questions remain about how to define and assess practices that "seriously deviate" from those commonly accepted in scientific research.

The National Academy of Sciences' (NAS) report on responsible science attempts to define misconduct and identify other questionable research practices. Although the NAS does not identify questionable laboratory practices as misconduct, the report points out that poor data management and failure to observe safety regulations are detrimental to the research process. Students need to learn to manage data and safety hazards responsibly to become competent investigators; while discussion of these issues belongs in a book on research methodology rather than one on ethics, competence could be considered an ethical requirement for professional scientists.

To ensure that suspected misconduct is reported and dealt with fairly, safeguards for the rights and reputations of the accused and accuser need to be clearly established. Still to be determined as well is the most appropriate body to investigate alleged misconduct: individual research institutions, professional societies, Congress? The other duties of each of these groups could both facilitate and hinder such inquiries. More generally, it would be useful to identify the pressures that may lead researchers to deviate from identified norms, and to reflect on the nature of an environment that would encourage responsible action among scientists.

Note

1. Federal Register, August 8, 1989, p. 32446.

7

The pathogenesis of fraud in medical science

Robert G. Petersdorf

Recently I had a disquieting experience. A young faculty member about to be appointed in a clinical department was discovered to have submitted several papers containing fraudulent data to several reputable journals. Up to this shocking discovery he had not been suspected of malfeasance. In fact, he was considered somewhat of a "child prodigy." He had done superbly in medical school and was excellently trained; during his fellowship he wrote over 30 papers. When he was proposed for his initial faculty appointment, he had authored in excess of 100 papers.

In assembling the proposal for this man's academic appointment, a senior member of the department reviewed some of these publications. The data of several control groups were the same in several papers: normally, different experiments should have different controls. The senior faculty member consulted with the coauthors. They had never seen the papers. Technicians in the laboratory could not recall the experiments. The data books could not be found. No purchase orders for the animals used in the experiments could be found. The grants to which the work had been credited had not contained enough money to purchase the animals used in the work that was published. When the young investigator was confronted with these doubts, he denied all the allegations but was unable to marshal proof that the allegations were false. His letter of resignation from the faculty followed shortly thereafter.

One might think that the episode ends here. Although a full investigation has corroborated the fraud in some papers, others need to be reviewed. The investigation will need to be continued: to protect the coauthors; to salvage the reputations of the research fellows who worked with the culpable investigator (but who can give them back the years of fellowship?); and to protect the granting agencies.

The "pre-med syndrome"

How have we gotten into this sorry mess? Believe it or not, it probably began with the "pre-med syndrome," painfully familiar to many in medical education. It begins with fierce competition in college, excessive emphasis on grades, and the rise of students who become 22-hour-a-day study machines. The syndrome was analyzed in detail in the May 1985 issue of *The Washington Monthly* (1). Some quotes from this article are instructive.

A recent study of 400 medical students by doctors at two Chicago medical schools revealed that 88% of the subjects had cheated at least once while they were pre-meds. The researchers found

From *Annals of Internal Medicine*, 1986, 104, pp. 252–254. Reproduced with permission.

widespread cynicism among their subjects as demonstrated by frequent agreement with statements such as "people have to cheat in this dog-eat-dog world."

The majority of students continued to cheat in medical school:

The most disturbing finding was that there was a continuum from cheating in college to cheating in medical school in didactic areas to cheating in clerkships and patient care. Cheating in medical school may be a predictor to cheating in practice.

The culture in which we train our young promotes cheating:

From crib notes in organic chemistry to Medicare fraud and fudged results in medical research, the connection may be there.

The large size of science

A second factor in the pathogenesis of scientific fraud is the very size of science itself. Despite some recent erosion of research budgets, they are much greater in absolute terms than ever before. The department of medicine that I chaired for 15 years, from 1964 to 1979, serves as an example (2). During this 15-year period the research budget quintupled while the teaching load only tripled. This increase in the research enterprise was accompanied by an increase in the size of graduate training programs. The number of housestaff tripled, the number of graduate students and postdoctoral fellows increased markedly, and the number of clinical fellows increased most of all.

In fellowship training groups in internal medicine, as many as 18 fellows in a group is not unusual. Despite claims that more than 50% of these clinical fellows go into academic medicine – claims that I have never believed even in the days of training grants – I have real doubts as to whether we need so many persons in advanced training, either for the academy or for practice. In fact, there is now good evidence that we do not need them for practice, where there is a surfeit of almost all types of specialists and subspecialists (3). The penchant for procreation among directors of clinical programs and among trainers of basic scientists knows no bounds; they feel that they have a right to generate the intellectual progeny of the future, whether that progeny becomes an overpopulation or not.

What are the consequences of big science? First, there is the inability to say grace over the large research groups that now exist. Thus these groups have an intermediate layer of junior faculty, many of whom are relatively inexperienced in training people and supervising research. It also results in group projects. There are not enough good ideas to go around to keep the excessive number of trainees busy. As a consequence, group projects abound with the inevitable result, the multiauthored paper. Characteristic of the multiauthored paper is that it is often not completely reviewed, and usually not in detail by every author. A few decades ago the department chair read every paper emanating from his department. This is clearly no longer possible, but now even division heads do not read the papers, as some in whose divisions fraud has occurred now ruefully admit.

Competition

A third factor in the pathogenesis of fraud is competition itself – not necessarily the competition to be first in press but, more often, the competition for grants. The progressive funding of grants with higher priorities does not connote that the science is necessarily better. It only means that competition for the research dollar is greater. Getting new grants or successful renewals requires productivity, and productivity, in turn, requires training of new people who can then publish more papers.

There is also competition for position, and our system of academic promotions is the prime example. Promotions committees count and weigh papers but do not read them. The reported research is usually narrow in scope, and the promotions committees quite often are unable to understand the nature of the work. It is much easier, therefore, for them to judge quantity not quality. Unfortunately, it is also far easier to judge quantity or quality of research than excellence in teaching and excellence in clinical care.

Academic personnel policies such as tenure exacerbate competition. Tenure appointments are guarded with jealousy and are made with a sense of false elitism, and tenure is often based on faulty criteria. Competition among young faculty for the scarce tenured slot returns the faculty to the days of the "pre-med syndrome." Tenure as a personnel policy in medical schools assures only a small fraction of the faculty member's income (4). The good do not need it and the mediocre use it as a shield. Tenure tends to perpetuate mediocrity.

Some academicians contend that the intense competition, both professional and economic, in science makes an occasional instance of research fraud inevitable. I do not share this fatalistic attitude. I believe firmly that the committed scientist cannot alter the truth. But even if some research fraud is inevitable, it is probably preventable, if not by the sponsoring institution, then by the principal investigator himself.

In this era of big science, principal investigators must be more careful in screening their associates. All too often younger investigators are invited to join a laboratory because the funds are available to support them or because they provide an extra pair of hands to do the work. Principal investigators must learn to contain the size of their laboratories. I have from time to time seen the size of a laboratory equated with the quality of work emanating from it. In science, as in all else, big is sometimes beautiful, but often it is not.

Original research data need to be checked at several levels; graduate students, postdoctoral fellows, and junior and senior faculty members must check and cross-check the raw data and not just the computer printouts, graphs, or figures that are often an intermediate product of research. Although data books may clutter the laboratory, they must be retained so that in case of doubt they will be available for review. Multiauthored papers require input and checking by all persons named as authors and not just the senior author. Heads of divisions, departments, institutes, and schools should be sufficiently familiar with the laboratories under their administrative purview so that they will be able to launch an investigation of alleged fraud when such an investigation is needed.

Conclusions

Medical science today is too competitive, too big, too entrepreneurial, and too much bent on winning. Gone is the threadbare gentility when science depended on philanthropy for its support and was carried out by a solo investigator with perhaps one fellow and one technician (5). That era is gone if for no other reason than our science today is technically so sophisticated. But while science may be less genteel, less threadbare, and less fun, none of these is an excuse for fraud or lesser abuses. Those who have chosen science for a career have, in a sense, taken an oath to discover and disseminate the truth, much as physicians have sworn the Oath of Hippocrates. Beyond these individual commitments, the institutions in which science is performed – the medical schools, research institutes, and universities – need to create an environment in which truth prevails. They must have mechanisms (6) in place to ferret out untruths and to set their house in order, when untruths are discovered.

References

1. Barrett PM. The premed machine. *The Washington Monthly* 1985;May:41–51.
2. Petersdorf RG. The evolution of departments of medicine. *N Engl J Med* 1980;**303**:489–96.
3. Petersdorf RG. Is the establishment defensible? *N Engl J Med.* 1983;**309**:1053–7.
4. Petersdorf RG. The case against tenure in medical schools. *JAMA.* 1984;**251**:920–4.
5. Petersdorf RG. Academic medicine: no longer threadbare or genteel. *N Engl J Med.* 1981;**304**:841–3.
6. Petersdorf RG. Preventing and investigating fraud in research [Editorial]. *J Med Educ.* 1982;**57**:880–1.

8
Pressure to publish and fraud in science

Patricia K. Woolf

Q. Is there pressure to publish in today's science?

A. Yes, there is.

Q. Is pressure to publish bad for science?

A. Bad or good, we're stuck with it. Since its birth, modern science has had an ethos that called for communications; scientists have felt some pressure to make their results known. Publication is an established way of doing so.

Q. Should there be pressure to publish?

A. Why not? If the public has paid for research, they are entitled to evidence that research has been done.

Q. Are publications the product of research? Doesn't the public pay for new knowledge and ideas?

A. Yes, that's the ideal, but not all experiments work. The public is really paying for a good-faith effort by highly skilled people who collectively have a pretty good chance of coming up with some information that is an advance.

Q. How do we know which scientific results represent advances in scientific knowledge?

A. That's where publication comes in; information known only to the discoverer cannot be evaluated and become knowledge. Some say it isn't even science until it is published. Research reports are evaluated by editors and referees before they are published, and then publication allows other scientists to further evaluate and use the results.

Q. Why is there so much concern about pressure to publish?

A. Many persons in science are worried that their important but complicated system of communication is in jeopardy. Because of undue pressure it may not be working the way it's supposed to.

Q. Why is it complicated?

A. Publication is no longer just a way to communicate information. It has come to be a way of evaluating scientists; in many cases it is the primary factor in professional advancement.

Q. Is that so bad? If articles are refereed, doesn't that ensure a breadth of professional judgment?

A. Some say that the quantity of published papers has become more important for evaluation than the quality of ideas they contain.

Q. Is that true?

From *Annals of Internal Medicine*, 1986, 104, pp. 254–56. Reproduced with permission. The author acknowledges grant support from the Rockefeller Foundation.

A. It's hard to say. The evidence is anecdotal. Promotion and granting committees meet in secret; according to a dean in a major medical school, "Confidentiality fans the flames of paranoia." There are no systematic studies of these deliberations, but some reputable people have criticized the system. We need more systematic information about the relation of publications to professional advancement.

Q. Why are they so critical if the facts are not known?

A. Their experience has led them to be concerned about science. And they are worried that careerism is damaging a very important national resource – our research establishment.

Q. Is there that much pressure to publish?

A. It depends on what sort of pressure you mean.

Q. Is there more than one kind of pressure to publish?

A. There are at least two sorts: the pressure the scientist feels from the tradition of science, and the pressures from institutions.

Q. Are these pressures the same?

A. How could they be? Institutions and their departments may have different standards for promotion. Requirements are often implicit rather than explicit, and frequently they are misunderstood. Some research fields publish more heavily than others.

Q. Why have so many of the recently disclosed frauds been found in medical schools?

A. No one knows for sure. Their research environments are highly competitive. The heroic nature of their quest directly affects issues of life and death, so there are greater economic and social rewards in medical science. Another possibility is that some fraud occurs in all science, but it is more likely to be detected in a rapidly growing research area like biomedicine.

Q. Is there more pressure on medical scientists than on others?

A. Some say there is. Medical researchers often have clinical responsibilities in addition to teaching, research, writing, and applying for research funds.

Q. Have any studies measured psychological pressures on scientists?

A. I haven't found any in a search of the literature. One study currently underway at a major medical school is trying to find out if persons who are up for promotion really understand the promotion and tenure procedures of the institution.

Q. How can we measure the amount of pressure being put on scientists by institutions?

A. One way is to look at the amount of publishing done by practicing research scientists in our best institutions.

Q. Aren't you just counting papers again?

A. It's not the best way of determining research outcomes, but if becoming a full professor at a good university takes an exorbitant amount of publishing, we probably have a problem on our hands.

Q. How many papers does the average scientist publish?

A. A study by King and colleagues (1) showed that in 1977 the average number of articles published per physical scientist was 0.20/year, up from 0.17/year in 1965. The average number per life scientist in 1977 was 0.40/year, up from 0.30 in 1965. In this period only the social sciences showed a big decline; the average number of papers per social scientist was 0.22/year, down from 0.60 in 1965 (1). But these data include industrial or government scientists who may not be actively publishing. A better definition of scientist is probably a "publishing scientist." Price and Gursey (2) have determined that among publishing scientists, the average productivity is 1 paper per scientist per year.

Q. What are the rates of publication of scientific faculty in our major universities?

A. They differ among disciplines. In a study of the faculty of nine distinguished universities, rates ranged from 1.8 publications per scientist per year in physics to a high of 2.7 publications per scientist per year in biochemistry. Astronomy, chemistry, and microbiology were the other specialties studied. Publication records of over 1000 faculty members were examined (3).

Q. What about medical schools?

A. There are many medical schools whose faculty publish very little. In the 1973–1975 period the average rate of publication for privately controlled medical schools was 250 papers per year and for publicly controlled medical schools, 150 papers per year (4).

Q. What do federal granting agencies expect from their investments in research? Is there unreasonable pressure to produce simply to satisfy these requirements? On the average, how many papers per grant per year are produced?

A. The Office of Program Planning and Evaluation of the National Institutes of Health (NIH) has examined the literature output of NIH-supported research. A recent study of faculty in departments of medicine shows that one third of M.D. faculty are not significantly engaged in research at all (5). The NIH makes between 5000 and 6000 competitive grants per year. The average length of the grants is 3.2 years and that amounts to roughly 16,000 to 20,000 grants in force. In the same period and with the predicted lag of 3 years between a grant award and its resultant publication, 16,000 to 20,000 papers per year are produced. These figures are subject to a possible 20% to 30% increase, because at different periods some journals were not included in the survey. But that amounts to 1 or 1.3 papers per grant year (6; Gee H. Personal communication).

Q. If you double that to 2 or even 3 papers a year per grant, would that be too much pressure on a scientist?

A. It doesn't seem like it.

Q. If these institutional expectations are relatively modest, why is fraud associated with pressure to publish?

A. There are two principal reasons. First, several of the most spectacular frauds have taken place in laboratories where the number of papers published every year significantly exceeded the norm. Second, many of the persons involved have mentioned pressure as a factor. The newspapers usually report that view, and pressure has come to be a stock explanation.

Q. Could we look at those two factors separately?

A. That's sensible. "Pressure" has come to be a convenient explanation, for two reasons. The reports of these events have shown how shocked scientists are to discover that one of their colleagues was not playing by the rules. They may explain that fault using a psychological excuse that focuses on the flawed personality of an individual person and not on science in general; it is a less severe condemnatory judgment than, for instance, moral turpitude.

Q. Is that what's called medicalizing the deviance?

A. Yes, it seems to isolate the problem and let the other scientists off the hook. But then questions began to be asked about where the pressure comes from.

Q. Does that bring us round to the publishing practices in laboratories where fraud was discovered?

A. Let's look at just a few. The first of the major recent scandals, that of William

Summerlin at the Memorial Sloan-Kettering Cancer Center, was in the research group supervised by Robert A. Good. In the 5 years before 1975, Good had published 342 papers, an average of 68/year (16 as first author, 325 as coauthor with at least 136 coauthors). Several other frauds were associated with medical research groups that have been extremely prolific. In the period 1975 to 1980, which preceded the discovery of fraud in their laboratories, Eugene Braunwald had published 171 papers, an average of 29/year. Philip Felig had published 191 papers, an average of 31/year. Ephraim Racker, who is not on a medical faculty, had published an average of 16/year (7).

Q. How do these pockets of prolific publication compare with similar departments in similar institutions?

A. These scientists have made important contributions, significant far beyond the numbers of their publications. Therefore, comparisons with average productivity have limited value. But, yes, their average levels of publishing are significantly higher.

Q. Should we be worried about such prolific publishing?

A. There is reason for concern on several levels. Simple time-and-motion studies lead to the conclusion that when an author's productivity is extremely high, his participation in each paper has to be low. Or at least there is no clear way of telling which articles the author contributed to significantly. These prolific scientists are clearly operating in ways very different from those in the mainstream of science. One can argue that excellent science has always been out of the mainstream, but when there are significant deleterious effects on younger coworkers in their laboratories and eventual effects on scientific research in the United States as a whole, we have a responsibility to question the wisdom of those research and publishing practices.

References

1. King DW, McDonald DD, Roderer NK. *Scientific Journals in the United States*. Stroudsburg, Pennsylvania: Hutchinson Ross Publishing Company; 1981:62.
2. Price D, Gursey S. Studies in scientometrics: Part I. Transience and continuance in scientific authorship. In: International Forum on Information and Documentation. Moscow: International Federation for Documentation; 1975:17–24.
3. Frame JD. Quantitative indicators for evaluation of basic research programs/projects. *IEEE Trans Eng Manage*. 1983;30:106–12.
4. McAllister PR, Narin F. Characterization of the research papers of U.S. medical schools. *J Am Soc Inform Sci. 1983;*34:123–31.
5. Beaty HN, Babbott D, Higgins EJ, Jolly P, Levey GS. Research activities of faculty in academic departments of medicine. *Ann Intern Med*. 1986;104:90–7.
6. Analysis of research publications supported by NIH and NIGMS. In: *NIH Program Evaluation Report*. Bethesda, Maryland: National Institutes of Health; 1980.
7. *Science Citation Index Source Index*. Philadelphia: Institute for Scientific Information; 1970–80.

9

Science, statistics, and deception

John C. Bailar III

In science, lying is condemned, even by some of its few practitioners. Deliberate or careless deception short of lying, however, seems to be universally accepted and sometimes even promoted as a part of the culture of science. I do not suggest that scientists as a group are careless, venal, or otherwise depraved: they may even be above the human average in developing and adhering to detailed, albeit tacit, standards of professional conduct. Those who are clearly violators are drummed out of our ranks, loudly and publicly. But what about less clearcut deception?

My thesis is that our professional norms are incomplete and that several kinds of widely accepted practices (Table) should also be widely recognized as potentially deceptive and harmful. Some of these practices also have much value, but at timeos they are inappropriate and improper and, to the extent that they are deceptive, unethical.

The scientific method is fundamentally concerned with the processes of inference, generally from data that are necessarily inaccurate to some degree, incomplete, drawn from small samples, or not quite appropriate for a specific task. Inference – that is, drawing conclusions or making deductions from imperfect data – provides most of the excitement and intellectual ferment of science. Scientific rewards are probably more closely related to valid inferences established than to such related activities as imaginative hypotheses formulated, elegant experiments designed and conducted, or new methods developed. The rewards for publishing a first-class inference can include income, position and power, professional status, and the respect of colleagues. Such rewards may sometimes count for more than self-respect and the joy of discovery. We must therefore be attentive to scientific norms and activities that may distort the processes of inference.

An example of a deceptive practice is the statistical testing (such as the calculating of p values) of *post hoc* hypotheses. It is widely recognized that t-tests, chi-square tests, and other statistical tests provide a basis for probability statements only when the hypothesis is fully developed before the data are examined in any way. If even the briefest glance at a study's results moves the investigator to consider a hypothesis not formulated before the study was started, that glance destroys the probability value of the evidence at hand. Certainly, careful and unstructured review of data for unexpected clues is a critical part of science. Such review can be an immensely fruitful source of ideas for new, before-the-fact hypotheses that can be tested in the correct way with other new or existing data, and sometimes findings may be so striking that independent confirmation by a proper statistical test is superfluous. Statistical "tests" are also used sometimes in nonprobability ways as rough measures of the size of an effect, rather than to test

From *Annals of Internal Medicine*, 1986, 104, pp. 259–260. Reproduced with permission.

Table 1. *Some practices that distort scientific inferences*

Failure to deal honestly with readers about non-random error (bias)
Post hoc hypotheses
Multiple comparisons and data dredging
Inappropriate statistical tests and other statistical procedures
Fragmentation of reports
Low statistical power
Suppressing, trimming, or "adjustng" data; or undisclosed repetition of "unsatisfactory" experiments
Selective reporting of findings

hypotheses. (An example is the column of p values that sometimes accompanies a table comparing the pretreatment characteristics of patient groups in a randomized clinical trial.) When either the test itself or the reporting of the test is motivated by the data, a probability statement such as "$p < 0.05$" is deceptive and hence damaging to inference.

Other potential problems are the selective reporting of findings and the reporting of a single study in multiple fragments. These practices can obscure critical aspects of an investigation, so that readers will misjudge the evidential value of the data presented. Such reporting may be deceptive, whether deliberately or accidentally. On the other hand, these practices sometimes have positive value that should be preserved. For example, they can facilitate the tasks of both the investigator and the user when a demand for a monolithic analysis might seriously delay or frustrate the progress of both.

"Negative" conclusions of low statistical power – that is, reporting that no effect was found when there was little chance of detecting the effect – can also distort inference, especially when investigators do not report on statistical power. The concept of power is formally defined in terms of the random variability of results that is inherent in a specific combination of data structure, sample size, statistical models, and analytic method; but I believe that the concept should be substantially broadened to include the likelihood that a particular effect would be detected and reported if it were present to some specified degree. Such an analysis rarely accompanies "negative" findings, and readers may be left with an unjustified sense that an effect not demonstrated is an effect not present. Again, however, there are counterarguments: a report with low power may be better than no report (and no power), or meta-analysis (1) of several low-power reports may come to stronger conclusions than any one of them alone. Reporting negative studies of low power can create ethical problems, but those problems may be largely mitigated if the low power is accurately and clearly reported as well. Too many scientists resist the objective reporting of this kind of weakness in their work, and pressure for "strong" results may be greatest during the formative years of graduate training and career entry. Thus we may be training new scientists in unethical methods.

Despite the occasionally useful roles of these and other practices listed in Table 1, each can seriously distort the processes of inference and should therefore be an object of concern. Where the practices have legitimate applications, they should, of course, be used; but even then they should be fully and explicitly disclosed by the investigator, justified in some detail, and accepted with caution by readers. A combination of restraint in their overall use, limiting their use to clearly appropriate situations, providing full disclosure and justification, and maintaining the readers' skepticism will help to diminish the frequency and severity of ethical problems. Full disclosure here means more than a few words buried in the fine print of a Methods section; it means not just that the author send a message, but that the author also work to ensure that the message is received and correctly interpreted by readers. There are parallels here to the evolving requirements for informed consent by experimental subjects.

Pressures to publish can be great and may account for many of the abuses suggested by Table 1. I fear that even the constrained use of these potentially damaging practices will leave attractive loopholes for an army of ambitious practitioners of science, each feeling great pressure to publish, who will rush in to explain why his or her situation is different, why full disclosure is inappropriate, and so forth. I am convinced that science, scientists, and society as a whole would benefit from substantially broader concepts, ultimately based on the need to protect the processes of inference, about ethical standards and violations in science.

Reference

1. Louis TA, Fineberg HV, Mosteller F. Findings for public health from meta-analysis. *Annu Rev Public Health*. 1985;6:1–20.

10
Methods, definitions, and basic assumptions

Panel on Scientific Responsibility and the Conduct of Research, National Academy of Sciences

Evaluating available data

The panel sought to develop a report that would address conflicting perspectives and priorities basic to enhancing integrity in the research process. An examination of empirical studies on research behaviors yielded few significant insights.[1]

The panel also concluded that existing social studies of the U.S. scientific research enterprise are not adequate to support conclusions about the relative effectiveness of various alternatives for fostering the integrity of the research process. For example, the value of formal and informal educational approaches in fostering responsible research practices has, to the panel's knowledge, not been systematically addressed. And although some research institutions in recent years have adopted formal guidelines designed to foster responsible practices, the experience with research guidelines is limited.[2]

The panel also found barriers to obtaining data on specific incidents of misconduct. Confidential institutional reports are not available if misconduct cases are under appeal or are subject to litigation, if the institutions have negotiated private settlements with the subjects of misconduct complaints, if there are findings of no misconduct, or if the misconduct has been judged to be not significant enough to warrant penalties. Those involved in handling or evaluating misconduct cases are usually not at liberty to discuss their findings. Those who have been parties at interest in misconduct cases may have a biased view of specific actions. An increasing amount of litigation in misconduct cases has further complicated the collection and analysis of primary data.

Thus many of the panel's findings and recommendations are derived from informed judgments based on discussions with persons knowledgeable about the research process and about factors that affect the contemporary research environment. The panel also met with individuals who have both knowledge of and a broad range of perspectives on the significance of the reported cases of misconduct in science. The panel's overall outlook and opinions are based on general ethical principles that are well accepted by scientists and by society.

Defining terms – articulating a framework for fostering responsible research conduct

In the opening paragraphs of this chapter, the panel defined the term "integrity of the research process" as the adherence by scientists and their institutions to honest and

Reprinted with permission from *Responsible Science: Ensuring the Integrity of the Research Process, Volume I*, c. 1992 by the National Academy of Sciences. Published by National Academy Press, Washington, DC.

verifiable methods in proposing, performing, evaluating, and reporting research activities. This term is sometimes thought to be synonymous with "integrity of science," but the terms of reference are different.[3] Science is not only a body of information, composed of current knowledge, theories, and observations, but also the process by which this body of knowledge is developed. Furthermore, the scientific process is a social enterprise that involves individuals and institutions engaged in developing, certifying, and communicating research results. Throughout this report the panel focuses on the integrity of the research process as defined above.

Misconduct in science is commonly referred to as fraud.[4] But most legal interpretations of the term "fraud" require evidence not only of intentional deception but also of injury or damage to victims. Proof of fraud in common law requires documentation of damage incurred by victims who relied on fabricated or falsified research results. Because this evidentiary standard seemed poorly suited to the methods of scientific research, "misconduct in science" has become the common term of reference in both institutional and regulatory policy definitions.

However, "misconduct in science" as commonly used is an amorphous term, often covering a spectrum of both significant and trivial forms of misbehavior by scientists. The absence of a clear, explicit definition that focuses on actions highly detrimental to the integrity of the research process has impeded the development of effective institutional oversight and government policies and procedures designed to respond to such actions. Varying definitions of misconduct in science have also impeded comparison of the results of survey studies. If, for example, survey respondents apply the term "misconduct in science" to a broad range of behaviors that extend beyond legal or institutional definitions, their responses weaken the significance of reported survey results.

In order to provide policy guidance for scientists, research institutions, and government research agencies concerned about ensuring the integrity of the research process as well as addressing misconduct in science, the panel developed a framework that delineates three categories of behaviors in the research environment that require attention. These categories are (1) misconduct in science, (2) questionable research practices, and (3) other misconduct.

The panel seeks to accomplish several goals by proposing these three categories. Foremost is a precise definition of misconduct in science aimed at identifying behaviors that scientists agree seriously damage the integrity of the research process. For example, although using inadequate training methods or refusing to share research data or reagents are not desirable, such actions generally are regarded as behaviors that are not comparable to the fabrication of research data. In the same manner, sexual harassment and financial mismanagement are illegal behaviors regardless of whether scientists are involved, but these actions are different from misconduct in science because they do not compromise, in a direct manner, the integrity of the research process.

Unethical actions of all types are intolerable, and appropriate actions by the research community to address such problems are essential. But the panel believes that there are risks inherent in developing institutional policies, procedures, and programs that treat all of these behaviors without distinction. Inappropriate actions by government and institutional officials can create an atmosphere that disturbs effective methods of self-regulation and harms pioneering research activities. In particular, many scientists are concerned that the term "misconduct in science," which has been construed as including "serious deviations from accepted practices" (as currently defined in government regulations), could be defined in such a way that it could be applied inappropriately to the activities of honest scientists engaged in creative research efforts.

The panel recognizes that this framework may not satisfy all scientists, lawyers, or policymakers. Its primary purpose is to advance the quality of policy and educational discussions about distinctions between different kinds of troubling behavior within the research environment, and to allow scientists, institutional officers, and public officials to focus their attention and their efforts toward prevention on substantive issues rather than discrepancies in terminology. Thus the framework of definitions proposed in this report should be viewed as a tool for use in a sustained effort by the research community to strengthen the integrity of the research process, to promote responsible research conduct, and to clarify appropriate methods to address instances of misconduct in science. The three categories will need to be refined through continued dialogue, criticism, and experience.

In developing its framework of definitions, the panel adopted an approach that evaluates how seriously the various behaviors compromise the integrity of the research process. The panel also considered other criteria, such as intent to deceive. The panel concluded that while intention is important, especially in the adjudication of allegations of misconduct in science, intention is often hard to establish and does not provide, by itself, an adequate basis for separating actions that seriously damage the integrity of the research process from questionable research practices or other misconduct.[5,6]

Misconduct in science

Misconduct in science is defined as fabrication, falsification, or plagiarism, in proposing, performing, or reporting research. Misconduct in science does not include errors of judgment; errors in the recording, selection, or analysis of data; differences in opinions involving the interpretation of data; or misconduct unrelated to the research process.

Fabrication is making up data or results, falsification is changing data or results, and plagiarism is using the ideas or words of another person without giving appropriate credit.

By proposing this precise definition of misconduct in science, the panel is in unanimous agreement that the core of the definition of misconduct in science should consist of fabrication, falsification, and plagiarism. The panel unanimously rejects ambiguous language such as the category ''other serious deviations from accepted research practices'' currently included in regulatory definitions adopted by the Public Health Service and the National Science Foundation (DHHS, 1989a; NSF, 1991b). Although government officials have often relied on scientific panels to define ''other serious deviations,'' the vagueness of this category has led to confusion about which actions constitute misconduct in science. In particular, the panel wishes to discourage the possibility that a misconduct complaint could be lodged against scientists based solely on their use of novel or unorthodox research methods. The use of ambiguous terms in regulatory definitions invites exactly such an overexpansive interpretation.

In rejecting the ''other serious deviations'' category, the panel considered whether a different measure of flexibility should be included in its proposed definition of misconduct in science, so as to allow the imposition of sanctions for conduct similar in character to fabrication, falsification, and plagiarism. Some panel members believe that the definition should also encompass other actions that directly damage the integrity of the research process and that are undertaken with the intent to deceive. For example, misuse of the peer-review system to penalize competitors, deceptive selection of data or statistical analysis, or encouragement of trainees to practice misconduct in science might not always constitute a form of fabrication, falsification, or plagiarism. Yet such actions could, in some circumstances, damage the integrity of the research process sufficiently to constitute misconduct in science.

All members of the panel support the basic definition of misconduct in science proposed above, but the panel did not reach final consensus on whether additional flexibility was needed to address as misconduct in science other practices of an egregious character similar to fabrication, falsification, and plagiarism. These issues deserve further consideration by the scientific research community to determine whether the panel's definition of misconduct in science is flexible enough to include all or most actions that directly damage the integrity of the research process and that were undertaken with the intent to deceive.

Questionable research practices

Questionable research practices are actions that violate traditional values of the research enterprise and that may be detrimental to the research process. However, there is at present neither broad agreement as to the seriousness of these actions nor any consensus on standards for behavior in such matters. Questionable research practices do not directly damage the integrity of the research process and thus do not meet the panel's criteria for inclusion in the definition of misconduct in science. However, they deserve attention because they can erode confidence in the integrity of the research process, violate traditions associated with science, affect scientific conclusions, waste time and resources, and weaken the education of new scientists.

Questionable research practices include activities such as the following:

- Failing to retain significant research data for a reasonable period;
- Maintaining inadequate research records, especially for results that are published or are relied on by others;
- Conferring or requesting authorship on the basis of a specialized service or contribution that is not significantly related to the research reported in the paper;[7]
- Refusing to give peers reasonable access to unique research materials or data that support published papers;
- Using inappropriate statistical or other methods of measurement to enhance the significance of research findings;[8]
- Inadequately supervising research subordinates or exploiting them; and
- Misrepresenting speculations as fact or releasing preliminary research results, especially in the public media, without providing sufficient data to allow peers to judge the validity of the results or to reproduce the experiments.

The panel wishes to make a clear demarcation between misconduct in science and questionable research practices – the two categories are not equivalent, and they require different types of responses by the research community and research institutions. However, the relationship between these two categories is not well understood. It may be difficult to tell, initially, whether alleged misconduct constitutes misconduct in science or a questionable research practice. In some cases, for example, scientists accused of plagiarism have testified about an absence of appropriate training methods for properly citing the work of others. The selective use of research data is another area where the boundary between fabrication and creative insight may not be obvious.

The panel emphasizes that scientists, individually and collectively, need to take questionable research practices seriously because when tolerated, such practices can encourage an environment that fosters misconduct in science. But questionable practices are not equivalent to misconduct in science, and they are not appropriate subjects for investigations directed to misconduct.

Other misconduct

Certain forms of unacceptable behavior are clearly not unique to the conduct of science, although they may occur in a laboratory or research environment. Such behaviors, which are subject to generally applicable legal and social penalties, include actions such as sexual and other forms of harassment of individuals; misuse of funds; gross negligence by persons in their professional activities; vandalism, including tampering with research experiments or instrumentation;[9] and violations of government research regulations, such as those dealing with radioactive materials, recombinant DNA research, and the use of human or animal subjects. Industry-university relationships, and the resultant possibility of conflicts of interest, also raise issues that require special attention.

In these cases, recognized legal and institutional procedures should be in place to address complaints and to discourage behavior involving forms of misconduct that are not unique to the research process. Allegations of harassment, for example, should be handled by officials designated to implement personnel or equal opportunity regulations. Allegations of misuse of research funds should be addressed by those responsible for the financial integrity of the research institutions involved. The panel concluded that such behaviors require serious attention but lie outside the scope of the charge for this study.

On some occasions, however, certain forms of ''other misconduct'' are directly associated with misconduct in science. Among these are cover-ups of misconduct in science, reprisals against whistle-blowers, malicious allegations of misconduct in science, and violations of due process protections in handling complaints of misconduct in science. These forms of other misconduct may require action and special administrative procedures.

Understanding causes and evaluating cures

The causes of misconduct in science are undoubtedly diverse and complex. Individual scientists, institutional officials, and scholars in the social studies of science over the past decade have suggested that various factors lead to or encourage misconduct in science, but the influence of any individual factor or combination of suggested factors has not been examined systematically.

Two alternate, possibly complementary, hypotheses have been advanced for considering the causes of misconduct in science and formulating methods for prevention and treatment. Many observers have explained the problem of misconduct in science as one that results primarily from character or personality flaws, from environmental stimuli in the research system, or from some interaction of both:[10]

1. *Misconduct in science is the result of individual pathology.* Misconduct in science is commonly viewed as the action of a psychologically disturbed individual. An analysis

by Bechtel and Pearson (1985) of 12 cases of deviant behavior reported in the 1970s and early 1980s supported the hypothesis that scientists who engage in deviant behavior are commonly individuals who operate alone and who conceal their misconduct.[11]

2. *Factors in the modern research environment contribute to misconduct in science.* But although the "bad person" approach to explaining deviant behavior in science has had strong support within the scientific community, Bechtel and Pearson and others have questioned whether this hypothesis alone adequately explains the phenomenon of misconduct in science.

A broad range of factors in the research environment have been suggested as possible causes of misconduct in science. Such factors include (a) funding and career pressures of the contemporary research environment (such as the pressure to publish; NSB, 1988); (b) inadequate institutional oversight; (c) inappropriate forms of collaborative arrangements between academic scientists and commercial firms; (d) inadequate training in the methods and traditions of science;[12] (e) the increasing scale and complexity of the research environment, leading to the erosion of peer review, mentorship, and educational processes in science; and (f) the possibility that misconduct in science is an expression of a broader social pattern of deviation from traditional norms. In addition, it has been noted that some areas of research, such as biological and clinical research, do not yet proceed from explicit scientific laws and also make extensive use of empirical observations not related to theory. Moreover, the characteristics of certain research materials in these fields inhibit the replication of research findings as a vehicle for self-correction.

The panel has reviewed various suggestions about possible causes of misconduct in science but makes no judgment about the significance of any one factor. The panel believes that speculations about individual pathology or about environmental factors as the primary causes have not been verified; misconduct in science is probably the result of a complicated interaction of psychological and environmental factors. Moreover, although one or more such factors may contribute to specific cases of misconduct in science, the panel has not discerned a broad trend that would highlight any single factor as a clear generic cause.

Regardless of the causes of deviant behavior, the panel is concerned that some "cures" for misconduct in science would damage the research process itself. The uncertainty of evidence about external factors as causes means that recommending policy solutions for treating and preventing the problem of misconduct in science is problematic. As a result, efforts to foster integrity in the research process and to reduce the occurrence of misconduct in science should be evaluated systematically to identify steps that prove to be effective.

Starting from logical assumptions

The integrity of the research process has sometimes been called into question by sensationalized reports about specific cases of misconduct in science.[13] But because misconduct in science seems infrequent, many scientists have suggested that it does not present a serious problem. According to this view, when misconduct occurs in an important field of research, incorrect information will be corrected or eventually replaced by correct results through the work of others.

The panel agrees that confirmed cases of misconduct in science are rare. Nevertheless, the panel believes that every case of misconduct in science is serious and requires action for the following reasons:

1. *Misconduct is wrong.*   One can object to misconduct in science simply on ethical grounds, since it often involves actions that betray personal and public trust and the search for truth. Misconduct in science, if not properly addressed, can undermine the reasons for doing and supporting science itself.

2. *Misconduct in science wastes time and resources.*   Misconduct can mislead scientists and waste the efforts of those who try to build on reported results. It requires substantial effort to correct false claims. Plagiarism can discourage scientists who see their contributions stolen or misrepresented by others and can damage honest reputations and the intellectual audit trail that affects the history of science.

3. *Misconduct can lead to injuries and harmful consequences.*   Significant harm can result if false claims influence public health or technical or political decisions. Although mechanisms of self-correction may expose false claims, they are not designed to detect or deter misconduct in science. False information relating to medical procedures, for example, may lead to mistreatment of patients. Falsehoods should be publicly corrected, as soon as possible, to prevent such damage. We should not wait for the slow corrective action of further research. Similar comments apply in other areas of science in which false reports may have adverse practical consequences.

The time interval between the release and application of initial research reports in medical treatment, commercial products, services, and public policy decisions is diminishing. Resources for replicative research may not be available in some areas of research. Thus correction of research results, through replicative or related research efforts, is not a panacea; neither is it always timely.

4. *Misconduct by scientists, and weak institutional responses to these incidents, can lead to counter-productive regulation and control.*   The image of scientists cheating in their laboratories is deeply disturbing to scientists themselves and to members of the public who have generally held scientists in high esteem. Even a few well-publicized cases of misconduct in science, particularly when such cases involve prominent individuals at respected institutions, have stimulated legal and administrative demands for accountability that divert funds and attention from scholarly purposes, interfere with the traditional autonomy granted to science, and malign the status of reputable scientists and their institutions.

5. *Misconduct in science can undermine public support of science.*   Misconduct is one part of a larger public examination of scientific and educational institutions. Public confidence in the methods by which scientists maintain the integrity of the research process can be eroded when misconduct occurs in a social environment that is already disturbed by, for example, reports of misuse of the indirect costs associated with research funds, and other behaviors that violate public trust.

On the basis of these assumptions, the panel concluded that actions designed both to foster the integrity of the research process and to respond to misconduct in science are both timely and warranted.

NOTES

1. Some good examples of studies of scientific practice and the social organization of science include Traweek (1988), Hull (1988), Latour (1987), Latour and Woolgar (1979), Hackett and Chubin (1990), and Hackett (1990).
2. It is the panel's hope that the base of knowledge will be augmented by additional data derived

from systematic evaluation of experiences in fostering responsible research practices. See also in Volume II of this report the background paper on this topic prepared for the panel by Nicholas Steneck.

3. A discussion of the dimensions of integrity in science is included in chapters 1 and 12 in Holton (1988).

4. Discussions focused initially on "scientific fraud" but encountered difficulties with the legal definition of the word "fraud." Government regulations and institutional policies have adopted terms such as "research misconduct," "scientific misconduct," and "misconduct in science," but these terms are subject to a variety of interpretations.

   For early discussions about the relationship between fraud and misconduct in science, see Andersen (1988). See also the discussion on "fraud" and "misconduct" on p. 32447 in Department of Health and Human Services (1989a).

   Some scientists object to the terms "scientific fraud" or "misconduct in science" because the fabrication and falsification of research results are deceptive acts that are not in themselves science. However, the social, political, and legal framework in which scientists must operate requires that we admit to the possibility of deliberate falsehoods that may masquerade as science.

5. Some institutional policies make *intention* or *deception* an explicit part of their definition of misconduct in science, whereas other policies assume, implicitly, that intention is part of the common understanding of actions, such as falsification, fabrication, and plagiarism, that constitute misconduct in science. See, for example, the definitions in the policies for addressing allegations of misconduct in science included in Volume II of this report.

6. Another approach considered by the panel in defining behaviors that violate the integrity of the research process was to deal only with misconduct in science and questionable research practices and to omit "other misconduct" as a category for a framework of definitions. Although the panel chose to focus on behaviors that directly compromise the integrity of the research process, it also wanted to recognize the public dimensions of discussions about misconduct in science. Thus the panel concluded that issues such as conflict of interest, mismanagement of funds, and the harassment of colleagues on the basis of race or gender must necessarily be recognized in a framework of definitions intended to categorize behavior that adversely affects the conduct of scientific research. These forms of "other misconduct" deserve serious and sustained analysis on their own merits, but such an examination was beyond the resources and scope of this particular study.

7. It is possible that some extreme cases of noncontributing authorship may be regarded as misconduct in science because they constitute a form of falsification. These would include only cases in which an individual who has made *no* identifiable contribution to a research paper is named, or seeks to be named, as a co-author.

8. See Bailar (1986).

9. The fourth report of the NSF inspector general (NSF, 1991a) describes a misconduct case involving tampering with other researchers' experiments. This type of case would not constitute misconduct in science under the panel's definition. An allegation of this type of incident should be addressed under regulations governing vandalism or destruction of property.

10. As noted in Bechtel and Pearson (1985), several leading figures in the scientific community have advocated the "disturbed individual" theory.

    For discussions of the impact of reward systems and social controls on deviant behavior in science, see the analysis by Zuckerman (1977). For a historical perspective, see Gaston (1978).

11. The authors concluded that the deviant behavior in these cases, usually faking scientific experiments and data, was displayed by single individuals who acted alone. They observed that many of these individuals held positions of high social status and respectability within their professions and that the scientists involved also made elaborate efforts to conceal their illegitimate behavior.

12. It has been suggested that research physicians whose sole degree is an M.D. have not been adequately exposed to the scientific methods and skills that are the foundation of a Ph.D. program.
13. See Broad and Wade (1982).

QUESTIONS FOR DISCUSSION

1. Why has the federal government taken such an interest in the ethical conduct of research in the past several years?
2. In these days of scientific specialization, what institutional policies and procedures might be established that could improve self-regulation among researchers and decrease the potential for misconduct in the laboratory?
3. What is the proper role, if any, for legally enforceable, governmental regulations in the conduct of research? What are the likely effects of such regulation?

RECOMMENDED SUPPLEMENTAL READING

U.S. Office of Technology Assessment, *Regulatory Environment for Science,* Washington, DC: U.S. Department of Commerce, 1986.

"Policies and Procedures for Dealing with Possible Misconduct in Science," Department of Health and Human Services (DHHS), *NIH Guide for Grants and Contracts,* 1986, 15 (July 18), pp. 1–37.

"Research Data Management," Paul Gilchrist, in Wm. C. McGaghie & J. J. Frey (eds.), *Handbook for the Academic Physician,* New York: Springer-Verlag, 1986, pp. 251–276.

"The Integrity of the Scientific Literature," Walter W. Stewart & Ned Feder, *Nature,* 1987, 325, pp. 207–214.

"On Analysing Scientific Fraud," Eugene Braunwald, *Nature,* 1987, 325, 215–16.

"OSI: Why, What, and How," Jules V. Hallum & Suzanne W. Hadley, *ASM News,* 1990, 56 (12), pp. 647–251.

"Misconduct in Science: Recurring Issues, Fresh Perspectives," American Association for the Advancement of Science (AAAS), Executive summary of a conference, November 15–16, 1991, Washington, DC.

PART V

The Ethics of Authorship and Publication

INTRODUCTION

Science depends on a lively exchange of ideas and information through a vast and growing professional literature. Defining the roles of its contributors, rarely examined in the past, is crucial, particularly as responsibility for preventing and detecting fraudulent claims in publication is now a matter of deep professional and public concern.

What makes an author an author? The answer seems self-evident: an author is someone who writes a paper. Clearly, some scientific papers list more authors than could have been involved in the process of writing per se. Do other contributors warrant being identified as authors? Should the source of a study's working hypothesis be given authorship credit? What about individuals who facilitate the study's funding, provide laboratory space, or open the study to their patients?

The International Committee of Medical Journal Editors' "Guidelines on Authorship" state that anyone listed as an author should have participated sufficiently in the work to take public responsibility for its content; along with credit for the piece comes accountability for its quality, originality, and validity.

Edward Huth argues that much unjustified authorship is due to tenure policies that reward the *number* of papers that researchers publish, rather than their *quality*. The corresponding practices of dividing the findings of a single investigation into several publishable conclusions, or republishing old data in new formats, weaken the literature even as they strengthen researchers' vitae.

Ideally, the potential abuse of authorship and wasteful publication is preventable through peer review, in which papers are judged by experts for their contribution to a particular field. As Arthur E. Baue notes, however, reviewers' valuable efforts get little recognition, and a variety of forces may make it hard for them to provide a balanced assessment of a colleague's work.

Editing a journal requires particular professional responsibility. Editors must set their journals' goals, limits, and formal standards, choose and assign appropriate reviewers, and keep sufficiently abreast of their fields that their material is timely and thought-provoking without being premature, incomplete, or unnecessarily provocative. Nonetheless, only the combined efforts of authors, reviewers, and editors can ensure the integrity and value of the literature on which scientific advancement relies.

11
An ethical code for scientists

Ward Pigman and Emmett B. Carmichael

A new phenomenon of our present-day society is the obviously important role played by science. Only a short time ago science was considered by many "practical" men as a plaything of inconsequential importance in contributing to the welfare of society. Although the significance of science was becoming more generally evident before World War II, this war demonstrated to the public in general and to legislators and businessmen in particular that science, especially basic science, is much more than a scholarly pursuit – that it is a vital force for the advancement or destruction of society. Science is now "big business." As a result, the scientist cannot and must not remain a scholarly recluse divorced from the remainder of society. His behavior and that of society toward him will greatly influence the progress of science and, to an increasing extent, that of society itself.

During its long period of development, science has evolved a code of professional tradition and ethics, largely in an unwritten form. This code, really the foundation of the scientific method in many of its aspects, has to a considerable extent been responsible for the achievements of science. Polanyi's (*12*) description of the effect of disregard for scientific traditions is applicable to many of our modern industrial and research organizations:

Those who have visited the parts of the world where scientific life is just beginning, know of the backbreaking struggle that the lack of scientific tradition imposes on the pioneers. Here research work stagnates for lack of stimulus, there it runs wild in the absence of any proper directive influence. Unsound reputations grow like mushrooms: based on nothing but commonplace achievements, or even on mere empty boasts. Politics and business play havoc with appointments and the granting of subsidies for research. However rich the fund of local genius may be, such environment will fail to bring it to fruition.

The important achievements of science and its contributions to our civilization seem adequate proof of the basic validity of these traditions. On the other hand, conditions of scientific work have changed greatly, and obviously the traditions must be interpreted in terms of prevailing conditions. Science has emerged from a period in which the predominant effort was made by individuals, sometimes of almost an amateur status, to a period marked by the development of large research groups, many in the pursuit of research for profit. As a result, it is timely for the scientist to consider his professional traditions and to relate them in terms of the structure of modern scientific work.

From *Science*, 1950, 111, pp. 643–647. © AAAS.

These traditions are essentially an unwritten code of professional ethics. As pointed out by Leake (9), the term ''professional ethics'' as used generally includes the attitude of the individual scientist to society and to other scientists. It will be so used here. This concept of professional ethics inextricably involves social obligations, questions of etiquette, and adherence to accepted traditions. Claude Bernard (1) has contributed one of the better discussions of the ethical qualities needed in scientists, and the relationship of these qualities to the scientific method, although his remarks apply in the main to medicine and physiology.

Some of our professional organizations have established formal written codes of professional ethics.* In the medical field numerous papers and books have been written on the subject. One of the first extensive codifications was that of Percival (9) (1803), but the general precepts of Hippocrates (circa 500 B.C.) have modern acceptance. A major consideration at the first meeting of the American Medical Association in 1847 was the formulation of a code of professional ethics (9). The present code provides means for enforcement by its members. There has been some discussion of the professional responsibilities of industrial chemists (6) and a code has been proposed for this group (7). Scientific groups generally, however, have not formalized their traditions but have passed them on by example and by word of mouth as an informal part of the graduate student's training.

This failure of scientists as a group to consider ethics is revealed in the fact that *Chemical Abstracts,* since it was founded in 1907, listed only four references under ethics in its indices. It is true that professional codes at best can only express an ideal; their acceptance and application will depend upon the individual scientists. We believe, however, that the scientist's position in the world today makes it extremely important that his time-proved traditions be reconsidered in terms of modern circumstances and possibly written into a formal code. We believe that such an action would maintain the advance of science, increase its public support, and improve the professional relations of scientists. Improved professional relations would better morale and increase productivity among research men. Mills (10) has pointed out the social implications of ethical behavior in the distribution of research grants.

The planning of an ethical code for scientists should take into account first the scientist's general obligations as a member of society, and beyond that his special obligation as a scientist to protect society – here, there are many problems related to warfare, to the health and general well-being of mankind, and to nationalism versus internationalism. Such a code should preserve the scientist's ethical traditions and incorporate the scientific method. It should state the scientist's obligation to explain the nature and purposes of science, and the policies in dealing directly with the public. It should clarify the scientist's attitudes toward patents and secrecy restrictions. It should affirm the scientist's obligations to individuals – to his employer, his associates, other scientists, and his assistants and graduates – and scientists' obligation as a group to other professions.

We have merely indicated the scope of the problem. To deal with it fully in all its

*American Medical Association, *Principles of Medical Ethics* (14); American Dental Association, *Principles of Ethics* (15); American Associatin of University Professors, *Statements of Principle in Academic Freedom and Tenure* (16); American Institute of Chemical Engineers, *Constitution*, Article VIII (17); Engineers' Council for Professional Development, *Canons of Ethics for Engineers* (18). ''The Geneticists' Manifesto'' adopted at the Seventh International Congress of Genetics, held at Edinburgh in 1939. Published in *The Journal of Heredity*, September, 1939. Reprints distributed by American Genetics Association (19).

phases would require the efforts of scientists in many different fields of study and kinds of employment. Some of these phases have already received considerable attention. Because the results of atomic research have such unmistakable implications for society, attention has been paid to the scientist's attitude on the use of his discoveries, particularly for military purposes, and to the necessity of his being socially conscious (*3, 4, 5, 8, 10, 13*). Other phases of the problem have received little or no public consideration.

Many of the scientist's obligations are reciprocal in the sense that the scientist has grown to expect certain conditions for his work, and to a considerable extent these conditions affect the quality of his work. Sometimes his obligations are conflicting. He may at times be faced with the dilemma of obligations to his employer that conflict with obligations to the public as a whole. What should his attitude be when his employer's immediate interest causes harm to the general public? Suppose that his employer is a company that is pouring waste products into a stream and he knows that at a reasonable cost this pollution could be greatly minimized. Should he assume, as a lawyer does, that his primary obligation is to his client, and become an automatic defender of the company's position? Or should he consider that he has duties to society greater than those to the company?

A group of very pressing problems is presented in the application of traditions related to the authorship and publication of scientific researches. In the early days of science most articles carried the name of only one worker, whereas multiple authorship is now most common and sometimes ten or more persons may be involved. As a detailed example of the need for a code of professional ethics, we will discuss some of the problems involved in authorship.

General obligations of authors

Quality of papers. Everyone will agree that scientific articles should be of good quality, should be original in content, and should describe all work in a reproducible fashion. These are fundamental requirements of the scientific method and yet most scientists would admit that many research articles are published that are deficient in some or all of these respects.

Claude Bernard (*2*) has described the importance of adequate details:

In scientific investigation, minutiae of method are of the highest importance. The happy choice of an animal, an instrument constructed in some special way, one reagent used instead of another, may often suffice to solve the most abstract and lofty questions. . . . the greatest scientific truths are rooted in details of experimental investigation which form, as it were, the soil in which these truths develop.

Even casual inspection will show that many articles are not written so that the work can be repeated. Traditional procedure is often ignored in reporting new compounds; occasional articles will not give analyses of new compounds or the compounds will be poorly described so that their identity is questionable. Scientific journals lack space to print all the good material they receive today, and understandably urge authors to shorten their articles, but great care is needed to avoid eliminating important details.

Direct responsibility to prior work. The traditions of science demand that any report of scientific work must consider prior work, integrate it in the general subject, and cite proper references to it. Frequent violations of this principle must be familiar to all scientists. One of us has previously called attention to an instance of this type, particularly in relation to the naming of methods (*11*).

The basic concept behind this principle, even more fundamental than professional courtesy, is that frequently the solution to a problem may already be in the literature and needless repetition is economic waste. Thorough literature searching can be defended from an economic standpoint alone. In order to speed the incorporation of new work into the general body of basic knowledge, each author has the responsibility of assisting in the integration of his work with that of previous workers.

To many scientists, establishment of priority for new discoveries is important, and organizations that seek patent protection for their work may set up involved and expensive procedures to establish the date of discovery. Is this a tradition that should be continued? Some scientific journals do not carry the date a manuscript was submitted, and few indicate whether essential changes of content have been made after that date. "Letters to the Editor" may require careful controls to prevent abuses.

Criticism and disagreement. The scientific method requires that all research work be open to critical examination and testing by researchers in the field. It also requires that dissenting theories and results be treated with tolerance, and not suppressed merely because they disagree with currently accepted ideas. Many scientists would add that mistakes and errors should be publicly acknowledged.

The widespread violation of these principles today is affecting not only the progress of science but our economy as well. Many commercial research organizations keep closed files of their researches as a matter of policy, in the belief that they will have an advantage over their competitors. Most of them do not realize that lack of criticism of the worker by qualified colleagues in his own field fosters the carrying out and perpetuation of poor or erroneous work, the continued employment and promotion of unqualified workers, and the perpetuation of poor research policies. Criticism by members of the worker's organization and by consultants is usually inadequate because of the influence of personal motives and lack of knowledge in the specific field. Objections to excessive secrecy in military research should take into account this principle as a primary consideration.

Classical examples of the value of scientific controversy are well known. When properly conducted, such debates lead to clarification and advancement of knowledge. But improperly conducted, they lead to enduring feuds, and because of this possibility, there is a tendency among editors of journals to suppress scientific polemics. A continuation or extension of this trend will be a severe blow to the scientific method. However, as stated by Wise (*13*),

the research worker should not permit himself to become embittered or involved in useless polemics. . . . It simply means that his criticisms must be objective and that they must not descend to the plane of personalities. He must show that he is dealing with a set of data, not with an enemy.

Property rights of the scientist in his work. A currently controversial problem of the application of scientific tradition involves the rights of a researcher to his work. The decision to try to publish or reveal his research once was the sole right of the scientist. Now, with the investigator receiving financial support from others in most cases, the final decision is tending to fall on the provider of the funds. In the extreme case, what is there to prevent someone in authority from taking over the work of an associate and passing it off as his own work? What should an editor of a scientific journal do if he receives for publication a suitable manuscript from an established worker and simultaneously a letter from the supporting group saying that it should not be published? Should the supporting group be required to provide satisfactory and convincing grounds? By tradition and perhaps even by legal mandate, the rights of an artist to certain phases of the disposition of his work have been affirmed. Should these not apply equally to the scientist, whose application of his science is often an art?

At least one established graduate institution has the policy that all doctoral theses are published solely in the names of the individual graduate students. In certain instances, the idea was suggested by a member of the faculty, who carried out some preliminary work, supervised the principal research, drew or helped draw the conclusions, rewrote the thesis and wrote the final published version. Is this an example of acceptable ethics?

Publicity. Some scientists violently oppose general publicity and popularization of their work. Others seek publicity, and some even condone or support erroneous and misleading publicity. What should be the attitude of the scientist? Does he owe the public a duty to attempt to explain the purpose and significance of his work? Should chicanery and excessive or misleading publicity on the part of scientists and nonscientists be exposed as a function of scientific societies? It is of interest that the *Principles of Medical Ethics* includes a considerable discussion of the impropriety of advertising and publicity-seeking and that AMA members are required to advise the public against misrepresentation. A firm stand on this issue by scientists generally might be of considerable help in establishing the professional status of the scientist in the public mind.

Multiple authorship

With the change in status of research, owing to its being produced not by independent individuals but by several dependent workers or even large groups, the scientific tradition in respect to the etiquette of authorship needs reinterpretation or extension. The responsibilities involved in multiple authorship or group research must be analyzed.

"Senior" authorship and order of names. To many scientists, the order of the authors' names on a publication has a significance. Is this a tradition that should be preserved, clarified, and enforced, or is it an outmoded, unessential form of etiquette? In current publications, the application seems uncertain and haphazard. Should the concept of the "senior author" (the first one listed) be preserved? If so, should the senior author be the person highest in the administrative rank, the one who has done most of the laboratory work, the one who has written the paper, the one who furnished the original idea, or the one whose technical skill and thoughts have carried along the research?

Administrators and financial supporters. In publications, what consideration should be given to administrators and financial supporters? Some scientists might say that they should be indicated as authors only when their contribution to the actual solution of the problem has been substantial, continuous, and of a high level. Probably most scientists would agree that mere general administrative supervision of a project or even the suggestion of the original idea for the project is insufficient for an authorship. Certainly no one should be granted authorship of any type merely because he has seniority or is in charge of a laboratory. We cite as an example a man serving as technical liaison between a company and a research organization who insisted that his name be included as an author, before he would ask for supporting funds for the research, although his total contribution was limited to this action.

Graduate students and technical assistants. Criteria are necessary for assessing the role of graduate students and technical assistants in relation to authorship. Should not senior authorship for a graduate student be limited to those instances in which a real contribution, beyond adequate laboratory work, has been made? On the other hand, is it not the duty of the directing professor to encourage the student to his maximum performance, rather than use him as a laboratory assistant? If a technical assistant is to be given authorship of any type, more than an adequate performance of routine methods should be required of him.

Group projects. An example of the large group projects that characterize modern science is the penicillin research during World War II. Industrial organizations provide many more examples. Frequently there is no attempt on the part of administrators to set up the program so that the work of individual investigators is kept discrete. The improved quality of work resulting from the establishment of definite responsibility might be the basis for making a definite statement in regard to this problem. The interpretation of the scientific tradition in terms of modern group research is an extremely important and as yet unexplored field.

Preparation of manuscripts. The published paper is the final record of the finished research work, and the medium through which the information is made generally available and useful. With the present shortage of publication space, the preparation of the manuscript becomes more important than ever. Rigid adherence to established scientific traditions on the part of authors and editors becomes increasingly essential.

To many persons, the preparation of a research paper may seem to be a routine matter, but actually it requires a high order of skill and technical knowledge and an acquaintance with scientific traditions. In many researches the actual preparation of the manuscript, the integration of the findings with the prior related work, consideration of the significance of the data, and arrangements for publication may require a considerable portion of the time and skill required for the entire project. Possibly the actual preparation of the manuscript should be a factor in defining the responsibilities of the senior author. Laboratory workers without a good background of knowledge, and research administrators without close daily contact with the laboratory work and a thorough knowledge of the field probably should be discouraged from actual preparation of the manuscript. On the other hand, simple manuscript revision, in spite of the poor writing ability of many scientists, should not generally be made the basis for authorship of a research paper. Still another problem is determining the duties and responsibilities of the referees of scientific articles.

The interpretation of scientific traditions, and their formal codification, if that is to be accomplished, are essentially a task for scientists. As this discussion demonstrates, the problems of interpretation are manifold and if they are not solved they may severely hinder the progress of science. The harm done may not only be general but may apply particularly to industrial research of the group type. Incidental effects of the code, but of considerable importance, would be the great improvement in morale among scientific workers, the improvement in the quality of scientific work, the assistance it would give to editors of scientific journals and research administrators, and the basis it would provide for exposing poor work and even instances of chicanery. It would be of great assistance in the training of graduate students in the scientific method. The preparation of a formal code of professional ethics should be of considerable value in establishing the professional status of the scientist in the public mind. It seems more than a coincidence that the groups that already have formal statements of their social and professional responsibilities and have definite rules of professional behavior are those definitely accepted by the public as having professional status.

As we have pointed out, violations of professional ethics on the part of scientists are frequent and familiar to all scientists. Sometimes they are deliberate violations for personal power or gain. Frequently, they are the results of carelessness or unfamiliarity of research administrators or research workers with the established traditions. They may even result from excessive pressure of work, a condition that appears common in industrial research. Some violations are the result of misguided attempts by editors and reviewers of scientific journals to shorten articles.

Is not the time opportune for our scientific organizations, or some agency of Unesco, to consider the manner of the application of scientific traditions to the newly developed conditions of scientific research? We suggest that the establishment of a definite code of professional ethics and conduct by our major scientific groups would have profound and favorable effects for science, society, and the scientist.

A mere statement of principles would be of help. An extensive codification and attempt to discipline or expose gross violations might be desirable. Our societies have various ways and means of enforcing regulations. Exclusion from membership and control of publications and means of publicity are powers that could be used to control unscrupulous and continuous violations. There may appear to be an anomaly in scientists' establishing a formal code of ethics to preserve traditions that include independence in their work, but this merely reflects an anomaly in present conditions of scientific work. It seems far better for scientists to affirm such a code positively than to be regimented to an increasing extent without any control over the conditions under which they must work. A. V. Hill (8) puts the problem as follows:

The important thing is not a creed "which except a man believe faithfully he cannot be saved." What matters is that scientific men should argue and discuss the matter of scientific ethics as one of infinite importance to themselves and the rest of mankind with the same honesty, humility and resolute regard for the facts they show in their scientific work.

If they do, then something will surely crystallize out from their discussion, and I have faith enough in the goodness and wisdom of most scientific men to believe that the result on the whole will be good and wise. It may in the end be embodied in a new Hippocratic Oath; or it may be absorbed in trade union rules for the scientific profession; or ethical behavior in science may just come to be accepted as an honorable obligation as unbreakable as that of accuracy and integrity.

We add that all problems will not be solved, but science is expanding and moving. The rate of progress will be profoundly affected by the consideration that is given to the maintenance and proper application of time-proved scientific traditions as the conditions of scientific work change.

References

1. Bernard, Claude. *An introduction to the study of experimental medicine.* Trans. by H. C. Greene. New York: Macmillan Co., 1927.

2. *Ibid.*, p. 14.
3. Blakeslee, A. F. *Science,* 1940, **92,** 589.
4. Carlson, A. J. *Science,* 1946, **103,** 377.
5. Condon, E. U. *Science,* 1946, **103,** 415.
6. Fernelius, W. C. *Chem. Eng. News,* 1946, **24,** 1664.
7. Gehrke, W. H., Aneshansley, C. H., and Rothemund, P. *Chem. Eng. News,* 1947, **25,** 2562.
8. Hill, Archibald V. *Chem. Eng. News,* 1946, **24,** 1343.
9. Leake, C. D. (Ed.) *Percival's medical ethics.* Baltimore: Williams & Wilkins, 1927.
10. Mills, C. A. *Science,* 1948, **107,** 127.
11. Peoples, S. A. and Carmichael, E. B. *Science,* 1945, **102,** 131.
12. Polanyi, M. *Sci. Mon.,* 1945, **60,** 141.
13. Wise, L. E. *Paper Industry & Paper World,* 1946, **28,** 1299.
14. *A.M.A. Directory,* 1942, p. 14.
15. *A.D.A. Directory,* 1947, p. 2.
16. *Bull. A. A. U. P.,* 1949, **35,** 66.
17. *A. I. C. E. Constitution,* Art. VIII.
18. Engineers' Council for Professional Development, Oct. 25, 1947.
19. *J. Hered.,* Sept. 1939.

12
Guidelines on authorship

International Committee of Medical Journal Editors

At its last meeting the International Committee of Medical Editors (the Vancouver group) drew up the following guidelines on authorship and on other contributions that should be acknowledged. The committee also expanded the section on information to be given in the covering letter to include details of any conflict of interest and clarify the position of the author responsible for final approval of proofs. These guidelines will be incorporated into the Uniform Requirements for the Submission of Manuscripts to Biomedical Journals (1) when it is next revised.

Guidelines on authorship

Each author should have participated sufficiently in the work to take public responsibility for the content. This participation must include: (*a*) conception or design, or analysis and interpretation of data, or both; (*b*) drafting the article or revising it for critically important intellectual content; and (*c*) final approval of the version to be published. Participation solely in the collection of data does not justify authorship.

All elements of an article (*a, b,* and *c* above) critical to its main conclusions must be attributable to at least one author.

A paper with corporate (collective) authorship must specify the key persons responsible for the article; others contributing to the work should be recognised separately (see Acknowledgments and other information).

Editors may require authors to justify the assignment of authorship.

Acknowledgments of contributions that fall short of authorship

At an appropriate place in the article (title page, footnote, or appendix to the text; see journal's requirements) one or more statements should specify: (*a*) contributions that need acknowledging but do not justify authorship, (*b*) acknowledgments of technical help, (*c*) acknowledgments of financial and material support, and (*d*) financial relationships that may constitute a conflict of interest.

Persons who have contributed intellectually to the paper but whose contribution does not justify authorship may be named and their contribution described – for example, "advice," "critical review of study proposal," "data collection," "participation in clinical trial." Such persons must have given their permission to be named.

From *British Medical Journal*, 1985, 291 (Sept. 14), p. 722.

Technical help should be acknowledged in a separate paragraph from the contributions above.

Financial or material support from any source must be specified. If a paper is accepted it may also be appropriate to include mention of other financial relationships that raise a conflict of interest, but initially these should be outlined in the covering letter.

Information to be included in the covering letter

Manuscripts must be accompanied by a covering letter. This must include: (*a*) information on prior or duplicate publication or submission elsewhere of any part of the work; (*b*) a statement of financial or other relationships that might lead to a conflict of interests; (*c*) a statement that the manuscript has been read and approved by all authors; and (*d*) the name, address, and telephone number of the corresponding author, who is responsible for communicating with the other authors about revisions and final approval of the proofs.

The manuscript must be accompanied by copies of any permissions to reproduce published material, to use illustrations of identifiable persons, or to name persons for their contributions.

Reference

1. International Committee of Medical Journal Editors. Uniform requirements for manuscripts submitted to biomedical journals. *Br Med J* 1962;284:1766–70.

13

Peer and/or peerless review:
Some vagaries of the editorial process

Arthur E. Baue

Review and judgment by one's peers seem to be inherently if not a perfect system, at least the best of any alternatives. It is the basis of our jury system. It is the most common way to evaluate and provide support for research. It is thought to be the hallmark of a good ''peer-reviewed'' scientific journal. A jury, however, is formed publicly, the names of study section members are published, and both of these groups act collectively. Reviewers or referees for journals function individually and anonymously. Also, there are peers and there are experts. Experts may hardly be peers or peers expert.

The peer review system for scientific journals has been criticized because it is slow, expensive, and time consuming for many scientists; it also is anonymous, which allows for the possibility of elitism, bigotry, prejudice, difficulty in publishing work by new or young scientists, and delay in publishing innovative work. Commoner stated that ''the real danger in the system is that it threatens to blunt the cutting edge of scientific progress'' (1). These criticisms have some validity and where studies of the system have been done, weaknesses have been found (2,3). Some journals such as *Lancet* and the *American Journal of Medicine* have at various times not used peer review and these publications flourished (4).

Review and discussion of the editorial process and of the system of peer review for the *Archives* may be helpful to the reader and writer, reviewer and editorial board member, expert and/or peer. This allows me the opportunity to thank the members of the editorial board for their efforts. For them, work with the journal is truly a labor of love and a contribution to our discipline. We also are grateful to the many surgeons and other physicians who have reviewed manuscripts for us as external reviewers. Their contributions are tremendously appreciated and their names are listed annually in the journal in recognition of their service for the *Archives*.

First, some facts

From 1979 to 1983, 3,576 manuscripts were submitted to the editor of the *Archives*. Of this number, 1,251 (35%) were accepted and 2,325 (65%) could not be accepted. These manuscripts were all reviewed by the editor and assistant editor and initial decisions were made as to whether the manuscripts should be sent to reviewers, accepted for publication without further review, or rejected. Few manuscripts are accepted by the editor without review by members of the editorial board and/or outside reviewers.

There are societies affiliated with the *Archives* in which the papers presented at the

From *Archives of Surgery*, 1985, 120 (August), 885–888. Copyright 1985, American Medical Association.

society's annual meeting are published in the *Archives*. These affiliation agreements do not provide for automatic acceptance of all papers. However, such papers have been considered by each program committee, which constitutes an initial review. Editorial board members are members of the society, attend the meeting, and hear the papers presented. The recording secretary is a member of the editorial board, and in some societies the manuscripts submitted after presentation at the meeting are again reviewed by the program committee. As many more abstracts are submitted to the program committee than can be accepted for the program, this constitutes a selective peer review process on a competitive basis. Finally, the editor reviews each of the society's manuscripts in detail. Approximately 90% of such manuscripts are accepted as presented. Ten percent or more may be sent for review by the editorial board. Approximately 5% of the manuscripts are eventually rejected because the manuscript and presentation do not adequately represent the claims or information of the initial abstract. There were 520 such manuscripts in this category.

Some manuscripts are rejected by the editor's office without further review. These are usually case reports, which may describe the 45th case of a disease process no longer requiring reports in the literature. Case reports are published in the *Archives* only if they provide new information, a new diagnosis, a new treatment, a new perspective, or a valuable lesson. Case reports are useful in hospital conferences as an educational device. Such presentations, however, are their own reward and usually need not be published. There were 1,087 in this category (54% of the rejected manuscripts). The manuscripts were returned to the author with such comments as "The *Archives* receives many more case reports than it is able to publish." Other materials rejected by the editor without review include intemperate manuscripts or letters or editorials lacking the intent to educate or attempts to set the record straight. Attacks, accusations, unkind remarks, or claims of priority are not acceptable. The *Archives* does not exist to verify or substantiate priorities in word or deed.

Most manuscripts for peer review were sent to a member of the editorial board with related expertise and to one outside reviewer with special knowledge or capability in the area of the submitted work. Of this group, 548 (44%) were accepted without revision and 698 (56%) were returned to the authors with detailed recommendations for revision in 1984. Approximately 1,000 manuscripts were rejected after review and, in most cases, detailed critiques were sent to the author. Most of the accepted manuscripts are returned to authors with requests for clarification of results, conclusions, or details of experiments. Approximately 8% of the manuscripts returned to authors for revision are not resubmitted. In my experience, with my own manuscripts submitted to other journals, I have benefited from and appreciated a careful and thoughtful review. My manuscripts were improved by the recommendations of unnamed colleagues. Most authors for the *Archives* appreciate the detailed and thorough reviews given to their work, and positive suggestions for improving the clarity of their messages.

The rights of authors and readers

The purpose of a journal is to promote scientific communication and to publish the original work of clinicians, investigators, and observers for the educational and informational benefit of readers, surgeons, and physicians (and ultimately for their patients). The journal has responsibilities to all constituencies.

A. The author(s) should expect:

1. Respect for his or her submission as a contribution to the field of surgery. The author is trying to communicate and his or her efforts should be encouraged, regardless of the impression of a reviewer. Thus, we are grateful to authors for sending their material to the *Archives*. Without them, there would be no journal. Disparaging comments are never transmitted to an author. Criticisms of content, of scientific design and statistical evaluation must be included, but overall indictments or subjective comments are not necessary.

2. A prompt reply. Once mailed, a manuscript will not arrive on the editor's desk for about a week. The initial review takes several more days. If a manuscript is sent to a reviewer, we ask that it be returned within two weeks. However, the process of mailing, reviewing, and returning usually takes about a month. Thus, an author should expect a reply in four to six weeks. We strive to be faster, but sometimes there are delays – for example, a manuscript may be on the bottom of a stack of work of a busy reviewer. Perpetually slow reviewers so declare their lack of interest in participating in the activities of the journal.

3. Confidentiality of the report. Anyone participating in peer review must be far above the use of a privileged communication for his or her own work or a quick report on similar works. Although every reviewer knows that a manuscript for review is a privileged communication, they may not be rigorous in maintaining this confidence. The problem for surgeons, as I see it, is not in direct use of someone else's information, but rather in the subtle forgetfulness of where an idea came from. Sharing a manuscript being reviewed with one's laboratory colleagues could lead to a flurry of activity in that laboratory to catch up or get ahead. Such activity never results in scientific progress but only in "me-too-ism."

4. A reply from the journal that provides clear information about the review process. If the author's manuscript is accepted, then the response is clear and definitive. If the recommendation is for acceptance if certain revisions are made, then these should be clearly stated. The author then has a clear message. He or she may decide to revise the manuscript according to the recommendations and resubmit it. If that is done as recommended, then acceptance should be virtually assured. I have always insisted that once recommendations are made to an author and he or she complies with the suggested revisions, no further considerations of new ideas or revisions can be recommended. In other words, include it the first time.

5. The right of rebuttal. If the author disagrees with the reviewers, we expect to hear from him or her and usually do. Neither I, Dr Wright, or our reviewers are sacred. We have been known to reconsider. I enjoy hearing from an author who believes that a review was not accurate, complete, or even fair. A debate between author and reviewer, moderated by the editor, can be healthy and productive, and I encourage it. If an author resubmits a manuscript and counterattacks the reviewer, this is fine, if such a debate will improve the journal and the manuscript. Such a debate may continue between reviewer and author until resolution is brought about or other referees may be brought in. We recognize that reviewers and editors are as fallible as are authors. Thus the initial review need not be a final decision, but rather a takeoff point for further adjudication, discussions, and review. This process has been very well described by Alfred Soffer, MD, in his editorial "The Open Editorial Office"(5).

If a manuscript is rejected, the author deserves to be given a reason for the decision.

Editors, editorial boards, and referees have been likened to gatekeepers letting in only the select few, or traffic officers directing the flow of manuscripts away from one journal and to others. A note about how sorry the journal or the editor is does not suffice. The author learns nothing from this treatment, and may submit the manuscript to another journal only to repeat the same process.

Reasons for a rejection may include the following: (*a*) the wrong journal for the message provided (ie, basic research submitted to a clinical journal); (*b*) a message with limited interest or importance; (*c*) a well-known message or conclusion; (*d*) information that is not new, or has been published previously by the same or other authors; (*e*) conclusions that are not substantiated by the data; (*f*) inadequately tested or verified recommendations to promulgate use by surgeons; and (*g*) recommendations that may be dangerous if used generally.

6. An acceptable article may be rejected if there is a backlog of material to be published and the delay is long. In the *Archives,* material accepted is usually published within six months. Authors also have a responsibility to follow the rules or directions of the journal to authors, to provide a synopsis-abstract, and to use good English, proper syntax, and clear journalism, avoiding slang and jargon. The author must assure the editor and readers that this is an original manuscript and unpublished work. Repeated publication of the same information is considered fraudulent. An author has the right to contest a rejected manuscript. Such a rebuttal will fall on receptive ears, but may not reverse the verdict. The author may not recognize flaws in his work, or we and the reviewers may not recognize potential scientific progress. We all make mistakes – errors of judgment – but we will consider and reconsider and re-review.

B. The reader should expect:

1. A journal that provides important new information related to his or her professional activities.

2. Articles that are accurate, easy to read, contain all necessary information, do not require referral to prior publications to understand the present study, and have concise discussions, clear well-substantiated conclusions, and complete and accurate (but not overwhelming) bibliographies.

3. Information that does not mislead, suggest dangerous or untried procedures, or speculate beyond the data.

4. A balanced editorial fare or menu that is not repetitious or redundant, covers a broad spectrum of the field, and provides information about new and exciting developments.

5. An opportunity to disagree with authors and editors and to debate issues or provide new insights from their experiences that are helpful for readers.

Reviewers

The responsibility of reviewers is great, but their pay is small (nonexistent). For almost all reviewers, their work is a labor of love to provide the best in the surgical literature. They work anonymously to allow free and honest critiques. Most reviewers are members of the editorial board and their names are printed each month in the *Archives.* The names of all external reviewers are published yearly. This general anonymity does not excuse invective, put-downs, or personal attacks, which our reviewers assiduously avoid. They work to improve the literature and to stimulate authors to better scholarship and contributions to the literature. These unsung heroes provide an immense contribution, particularly when they write a detailed critique of the good and/or flawed features of a manuscript. These can be returned to the author whether the manuscript is accepted with revision or rejected. Thus, there is an educational experience provided for authors. It is not helpful to an author when a reviewer puts an "X" in squares labeled "Accept" or "Reject" without explanation. Nor is it helpful to the editor. The editor does not know if the decision was based on personal beliefs or scientific acumen. It has been suggested that reviewers should sign their reviews and be identified. I disagree. Few of us would be as direct and critical as is necessary. It is the editor's responsibility to be sure that reviews are fair and balanced. Some have suggested that the authors and institutions should not be known to the reviewers. This idea has some merit.

The biggest hazard for a reviewer is to react favorably to work that confirms his or her thoughts and to reject work that disagrees with his or her theories. Here is where a real expert can become an enemy to scientific progress, because he or she may be very close to what is happening and hence unwilling to recognize a new lead or a new direction. Our job is to encourage scientific curiosity. Perhaps a new idea, incompletely worked out, should be published as a challenge, not as a fait accompli. It is easier to criticize than it is to encourage.

The hazards then for the expert reviewer are to:

1. Be too close to the work to recognize a totally new idea.
2. Be unable to recognize work in conflict with his or her own.
3. Insist on his or her own criteria and prejudices rather than considering those of others.
4. Use the Matthew effect ("to him that hath shall be given") and more readily publish the work of established authorities.

The opposite of this, of course, would be a reviewer with little knowledge of the problem who might recommend acceptance of a marginal contribution. I am pleased that most reviewers for the *Archives* provide detailed reviews and critiques and do not simply check the Accept-Reject boxes. A detailed critique not only helps the journal but contributes to scientific writing in general. Again, we salute our reviewers.

The editors

Editors have an immense responsibility. Some might call it power (6). If there is power, it must be used humbly. First of all, the author's rights and privileges must be protected. Authors must recognize and believe that the editor can be trusted with their prized possession – the product of their pen. Authors must believe that their manuscript will be reviewed honestly, fairly, and carefully, with confidence, concern, and positive – albeit honest – feedback.

1. The contribution of reviewers and editorial board members must be recognized. They must know that their efforts are important and contribute to the course of the journal. There may be differences of opinion between reviewers and editors, but the bottom line must be the editor's opinion based on the best information and recommendations he or she can get. We have published manuscripts that our reviewers have recommended not be published because we believed that surgeons should read them and decide for themselves. I have published manuscripts that I would have rejected but that the reviewers

felt should be published. The final decision is always that of the chief editor. If the two or three reviewers all recommend acceptance, we will generally go with that. If all reviewers recommend rejection, that decision is also usually but not always final. Split decisions are adjudicated. There is no right or wrong. Only so many manuscripts can be published and these should be the best possible. There is a hazard in not publishing an exciting development because its time has not yet come.

2. Selection of reviewers. The fate of a manuscript may be determined by the reviewers selected by the editor. There are tough reviewers, hatchet men who are judgmental rather than instructive. Others recommend that most everything be published if there is room in the journal: "let the readers decide." The editor must know the reviewers and work to assure fairness in the review process. Freedom from all biases is sought but seldom achieved. All of us have some biases and prejudices. Failure to recognize them is the error. Disagreement among reviewers is cited as a weakness of the peer review process. I believe, rather, it is a strength, for reviewers should be selected because of different viewpoints. Not all reviewers have detailed scientific knowledge, literary skill, and discrimination in all areas of surgery.

3. Passing the buck. Reviewers are consultants to the editor. Therefore, the editor should not pass the buck or hide behind his editorial board. At one time I wrote to authors, "I am extremely sorry to tell you that the reviewers did not recommend or give your manuscript a high enough priority for publication." This was hiding behind the reviewers, as if the editor were wonderful and the reviewers were villains. Rejection is not easy, and none of us wants to receive such a notice. Authors best will accept rejection if there is an honest, direct reason given for the decision.

4. Clinical experiences vs research reports. An editor and reviewers must be aware of a potential double standard in the surgical literature. It is easier to write, review, and publish clinical experiences – 100 patients with carcinoma of the pancreas, for example – than it is to carry out, report, review, and publish a research paper. I find that a reviewer may recommend for publication the report of a small series of cases of an unknown entity, but will have substantial criticism of a clinical research report in which all the variables could not be controlled. A tremendous amount of effort may have gone into a detailed basic or clinical research effort, only to be rejected by zealous reviewers. It is much easier to be critical of a scientific effort than it is of a clinical experience, which is actually a collection of anecdotes based on the variations of a disease process.

On the other side of the coin is the possibility of publishing something that may lead surgeons astray – where readers may say "The *Archives of Surgery* says we should do this" – but the recommendation is ill-considered.

The balance between intellectual stimulation, encouragement, and practical substantiation is the crux of the editorial process. Thus we have reviews – in most cases peer, in some cases peerless. Both are needed. The editor has final responsibility to his board, to the authors, and to the readers. The balance of forces is important, and hopefully out of this balance comes a healthy publication, which includes:

—Excellent authors and reviewers –
—A careful peer and/or peerless review process – and
—Concern for progress in surgery and contributions to betterment of the care of patients.

On the balance, careful, considerate, and concerned peer review assures the quality publication of archival journals such as the *Archives*. The process provides a collegial educational process for author, reader, reviewer, and editor. Imperfections do not negate the benefits of a journal that is stronger and better because of its editorial board and reviewers. Readers, authors, and the editor applaud their efforts, which promote and stimulate, rather than stifle, science in surgery.

References

1. Commoner B: Peering at peer review. *Hosp Pract* 1978;13:25–29.
2. Ingelfinger FJ: Peer review in biomedical publication. *Am J Med* 1974;56:686–692.
3. Lock S: Peer review weighed in the balance. *Br Med J* 1982;285:1224–1226.
4. Douglas-Wilson I: Editorial review: Peerless pronouncements. *N Engl J Med* 1977;296:877.
5. Soffer A: The open editorial office. *Chest* 1978;73:125.
6. Warren R: Power and prejudice. *Arch Surg* 1978;113:13.

14

Irresponsible authorship and wasteful publication

Edward J. Huth

Fraud in scientific publication is a dramatic abuse and it readily catches the eye of the popular press and the public. But there are abuses that because of their frequency and ubiquity should concern us more than the extreme of fraud. These are abuses of two kinds: irresponsible authorship and wasteful publication.

Public evidence of these abuses is scanty and largely anecdotal, although they have been discussed in the literature (1,2). Aside from May's study (3) of duplicate papers in one small corner of mathematics, however, I do not know of any thorough and quantitative studies of the extent and frequency of these problems.

Irresponsible authorship

I take authorship to mean that an author who is the sole author of a paper has been solely responsible for the work it reports and that all coauthors in a multiauthor paper have been sufficiently involved in the reported work and in the writing of the paper to be able to take public responsibility for its contents (4).

The first species of irresponsible authorship is *unjustified authorship*. There are the authors who simply made technical suggestions and did not take part in the research, did not help write the paper, and did not see the final version submitted to the journal. There is the departmental chairman who did not take part in the research. There is the laboratory technician who did routine work that would have been done regardless of the study and who could not defend the paper's content. There is the principal author's spouse listed as second author on a paper about bowel disease who has a degree in library science and gathered numbers from clinical records.

Unjustified authorship is not simply a problem of numbers. Growing numbers of authors per paper may be justified by growing complexity of research, but editors are seeing numbers that seem disproportionately large for the work the papers seem to represent.

Incomplete authorship, the second species of irresponsible authorship, is probably rare. This abuse is a failure to include as authors persons who had responsibility (5) for critical content of a paper.

Wasteful publication

Abuses of authorship rarely seem to damage the efficiency of science or seriously sap its resources. But they do undermine the ethic of honesty. Abuses that may be doing more damage involve wasting the resources of scientific publication.

From *Annals of Internal Medicine*, 1986, 104, pp. 257–259. Reproduced with permission.

The abuse of *divided publication* is the breaking down of findings in a single piece of research into a string of papers, each of which is what Broad (1) has tagged as the ''LPU'' or ''Least Publishable Unit.'' The research could probably have been reported in a single paper. But why should the investigators confine themselves to one paper when they can slice up data and interpretations into two, three, four, five, or more papers that will better serve their needs when they face promotion or tenure committees? ''Salami science'' does not always equal baloney, but such divided publication is often an abuse of scientific publication.

When five papers report findings that could have been reported in one, the editorial process, including peer review, has been turned on five times instead of once. Peer review is expensive in time and in money, for journal offices and for reviewers. Divided publication produces unnecessary press and postage costs for journals and the costs of multiple indexing and abstracting for what should have been represented once. Should we squander the resources of science in such multiplied costs?

Repetitive publication – republishing essentially the same content in successive papers or in chapters, reviews, and papers – also wastes resources. In one episode involving this journal about 2 years ago, we published a paper about a serious adverse pulmonary effect due to a new cardiovascular drug. A paper published in a radiological journal five months later described the same effect in apparently the same patients. The authors of the two papers were different but the papers came from the same medical school. Case details strongly suggested that the same cases had been reported twice. At least one author of the second paper must have been aware of the first paper because that author had been acknowledged for reviewing it. An excuse for this duplication might have been to get the message to two audiences unlikely to see each other's journals. But is the cost of duplicating the message for two audiences justified? For some decades the cost for searching through secondary services for information in a journal not usually seen by the searcher might have justified such duplicative publication. Now, the ease, speed, and relatively low cost of searching scientific literature through online bibliographic services discredit this excuse. One good reason to object to the repetition in this episode is that the re-reporting of the four cases misrepresents the incidence of the reported adverse drug effect. A literature search would turn up eight cases instead of four. A closely related abuse is producing the papers I call ''meat extenders,'' papers that add data to the authors' previously reported data, without reaching new conclusions.

None of these abuses is dramatically unethical in the sense that fakery and fraud are. The scientific community might not even agree on whether repetitive and duplicative publication are unethical. Wasteful publication might be seen as justified by needs to compete for institutional and financial support to ensure academic survival. Scientists do not realize that they help pay the excessive costs for peer reviewers, editors, professional societies, bibliographers, and libraries if they subscribe to journals or use any of these services.

Possible remedies

These abuses arise from the value publishing brings to individuals and particularly to their institutions. Publications are accomplishments that lead to income and power. I am skeptical that enunciating standards for scientific publication, no matter how rational, will readily influence what is in essence an economic problem. Science involves big money and attracts highly competitive career seekers. Short of a basic change in how science is rewarded and rewards itself, what might be done about abuses of authorship and wastes in publication? Dr. Angell proposes in her paper (6) what might be the best remedy; let me suggest some others.

A first major step could be wide and public acceptance among all scientific disciplines of clearly defined and specific criteria for authorship. Very few disciplines appear to have such criteria. The American Psychological Association has developed criteria (7); the Council of Biology Editors has published a short statement, not full criteria, on authorship (8); and the American Chemical Society has published a statement (9) on ethics of publication that covers authorship. The International Committee of Medical Journal Editors has recently issued several short statements defining authorship (10–12).

A second step could be specific requirements on authorship by scientific journals: an acknowledgment or footnote in every co-authored paper could state the exact contribution by each author that has justified authorship. Alternatively, the statement might be required in an accompanying letter. This procedure might reduce the number of abuses by at least forcing application of some kind of criteria.

A third step, one *Annals* took a few years ago, could cut back the abuse of naming persons as authors who have not seen the final version of the paper. We require that each author sign a "Conditions of Publication" form before we publish the paper. Each author thus affirms having seen the final version and agrees to its publication. Such a form could also require authors to indicate their particular contributions to the paper, such as study design, analysis of data, writing the first draft. Even if such required forms did not eliminate all abuses, they might at least raise awareness that authorship implies having taken on responsibilities and not just willingness to accept credit.

Divided publication may be more difficult for editors to deal with. When a piece of work has been chopped up for two or more papers, they are usually submitted to different journals at about the same time. Unless the authors are honest enough to cite the other papers, the peer reviewers and editors are not likely to be aware of the divided pieces. Editors who become aware of the multiple papers may face problems in asking the authors to withdraw one or more papers from the other journals and to combine them.

Editors can probably do more about repetitive publication. Editors can ask peer reviewers to call attention to any prior publication of the content of the paper under review. Many reviewers do this now, some even checking through online bibliographic searchers, but more might do so if asked specifically.

Editors can require authors to affirm by signature on an appropriate form that the present paper or the essence of its content has not been accepted for publication or already published elsewhere. This procedure could raise authors' awareness that editors are alert to such abuses.

Editorial offices could search bibliographic databases to see whether a similar if not identical paper has already been published. A few years ago this procedure would have been too costly in time and money for most journals when the search had to be carried out with paper indexes that often were not current. Now that we have relatively cheap and up-to-date online services, most journals could probably afford to use such searches for papers to be accepted.

All of us in science have ethical obligations to maintain honest authorship and to prevent wasting space in the expensive vehicles that are scientific journals. Our resources are not unlimited and must be shared.

References

1. Broad WJ. The publishing game; getting more for less. *Science.* 1981;**211:**1137–9.
2. Kronick DA. *The Literature of the Life Sciences: Reading, Writing, Research.* Philadelphia: ISI Press; 1985:67.
3. May KO. Growth and quality of the mathematical literature. *Isis.* 1968;**59:**363–71.
4. [Huth EJ]. Authorship from the reader's side [Editorial]. *Ann Intern Med.* 1982;**97:**613–4.
5. Relman AS. Responsibilities of authorship: where does the buck stop? *N Engl J Med.* 1984;**310:**1048–9.
6. Angell M. Publish or perish: a proposal. *Ann Intern Med.* 1986;**104:**261–2.
7. *Publication Manual of the American Psychological Association.* Washington, D.C.: American Psychological Association; 1983:20–1.
8. Ethical conduct in authorship and publication. In: CBE Style Manual Committee. *CBE Style Manual: A Guide for Authors, Editors, and Publishers in the Biological Sciences.* 5th ed. Bethesda, Maryland: Council of Biology Editors; 1983:1–6.
9. American Chemical Society. ACS ethical guidelines to publication of chemical research. In: *The ACS Style Guide.* Washington, D.C.: American Chemical Society; 1986:217–22.
10. Editorial consensus on authorship and other matters. *Lancet.* 1985;**2:**595.
11. International Committee of Medical Journal Editors. Guidelines on authorship. *Br Med J.* 1985;**291:**722.
12. Huth EJ. Standards on authors' responsibilities [Editorial]. *Ann Intern Med.* 1985;**103:**797.

15

Reporting provocative results:
Can we publish "hot" papers without
getting burned?

James L. Mills

In April 1981, *JAMA* published an article reporting an association between spermicide use around conception and congenital disorders (1). The authors were careful to note that "the results should be considered tentative until confirmed by other data." Nevertheless, their findings were taken up by the media and lawyers and treated as if they were established facts. Pregnant women who had used spermicides around conception became alarmed, and spermicide manufacturers were sued by former users who had had malformed infants.

Some journals publish exciting positive findings but are loath to publish subsequent negative investigations that contradict them. *JAMA,* to its credit, published an editorial the following year explaining why the association should be considered tentative or preliminary (2), along with several studies (3,4) that did not find any association between spermicides and birth defects. Subsequently, a number of negative studies appeared in other journals (5), and Food and Drug Administration hearings determined that there was insufficient evidence for an association between spermicides and birth defects to warrant a warning label (6).

However, the damage was done. Ortho Pharmaceutical Corp (Raritan, NJ), a major spermicide manufacturer, lost a $4.7 million suit brought by a spermicide user whose child was born with limb anomalies (7). The *Wall Street Journal* (May 20, 1986, p 5) reported that Ortho was considering removing spermicides from the market, a claim other company spokesmen later denied (*Wall Street Journal,* May 21, 1986, p 5). Today, spermicide manufacturers face numerous lawsuits despite a Food and Drug Administration statement that spermicides do not cause birth defects (8) and a statement from a distinguished teratologist and coauthor of the original paper that condemned the use of their data to prove that spermicides cause birth defects (9). This sad story demonstrates what can happen when a provocative or "hot" paper is published in a major journal, despite the best efforts of the authors and editors to present the data in proper perspective.

What makes a paper provocative? Provocative papers present exciting new ideas or results. Provocative papers have a major impact on the public or the scientific community. Sometimes they are preliminary or tentative, but not always. When they are correct, such as the report identifying the molecular structure of nucleic acids (10), they can dramatically accelerate the progress of medical research. When they are incorrect, they can lead investigators down blind alleys, as happened when nickel poisoning was suggested as

From *Journal of the American Medical Association,* 1987, 258(23), pp. 3428–3429. The author wishes to thank Mark Klebanoff, M.D., and George Rhoads, M.D., for reviewing the manuscript and Diane Wetherill for technical assistance.

138

the cause of legionnaires' disease (11,12). In the extreme case, they can cause great damage. The study demonstrating that diethylstilbestrol prevented toxemia, fetal death, and other bad pregnancy outcomes (13) led to several million women being placed at increased risk for vaginal cancer for no real benefit (14). Today, we face the same challenge of determining which provocative findings will lead to great advances in our understanding of disease and which will lead to disaster. For example, will lymphokine-activated killer cells and interleukin 2 (15) join the ranks of the great advances in cancer therapy or will they be a false alarm?

In our current litigious and socially volatile climate, it is increasingly difficult for authors and editors to know what to do with hot findings. Can major medical journals afford to publish such papers? Certainly, if the study results are correct, they need to be disseminated as quickly as possible. If incorrect, the studies need to be repeated, and the evidence that they are not reproducible also needs to be reported as quickly as possible, preferably in the same journal. In either case, it seems desirable to have provocative findings appear in high-visibility journals.

How, then, can hot studies be handled? The primary responsibility must fall on the authors. They have four options: A finding may be (1) discarded, (2) "buried" in a small-circulation journal, (3) reported as a letter to the editor, or (4) published by a major journal. First, the authors must decide whether or not the findings are reasonable. I once uncovered an association between a very popular analgesic and malformations. Even after using a second data set to confirm the findings, I was not certain that the malformations were not the result of the infections for which the analgesics were taken. I put this study into the trash. Discarding data has its disadvantages, however. It can result in important findings being withheld from the scientific community, and it can damage the career of a young investigator. Despite these dangers, investigators must be encouraged to do it when they do not have complete confidence in their findings. The analgesic issue, incidentally, has never been resolved.

A colleague asked me to review a paper that reported an association between birth defects and a controversial contraceptive. I asked what he planned to do with it. "We're not sure if it's true," he replied. "We're going to bury it." "Burial" is researchers' slang for publication in a journal that is read by only a small group of specialists in the field. This makes it possible to present data to a select group of colleagues without attracting undue public attention. Unfortunately, burial can be too effective a method of concealing data. Fetal alcohol syndrome was actually reported five years before its discovery by Jones et al (16). The data were published in a little known French journal (17) and would probably never have reached the public had it not been for the independent observations of the US investigators. With the increasing popularity of computer literature searches, burial may not be as safe an option in the future.

Letters to the editor serve to disseminate information quickly and provide a forum for raising questions. They are viewed as less than definitive by the media. Unfortunately, they are usually not peer reviewed, leave little room for describing study design, and earn their authors little credit in the academic world.

Finally, there is the major medical journal. When the authors choose this option, the hot paper becomes the editor's responsibility. The traditional review process provides several methods for evaluating provocative papers. A rigorous review will identify many flawed studies; however, unpaid volunteer reviewers will not always provide high-quality reviews. As a reviewer, I can attest to the fact that papers with novel or unexpected results are the most difficult to assess. One looks for flaws, but frequently none are evident even in studies one knows from other sources to be of poor quality. Errors in study design may be concealed or may simply not be mentioned in the methods section. Where no problems in design or analysis are evident and no additional information is available, the reviewer is forced to base the decision to accept or reject on intuition: do the results make sense?

Next comes the editorial board's review. The editors may abdicate their responsibilities and take the reviewers' suggestions without question. More properly, they can add their own wisdom to the reviewers'. Where doubts remain about the validity of a paper, the conservative approach calls for rejection. This approach can have embarrassing consequences for the editor. I recall Dr Rosalyn Yalow's address to the Endocrine Society after she won the Nobel Prize. She announced with obvious glee that she still had the rejection letter from a well-known journal (which she mentioned by name), turning down the research that was to win her the prize. The editor's other option is to publish the article with a cautionary editorial, but there are limits to this approach. Each paper requires a skilled editorial writer and space in the journal.

One would hope that the best efforts of authors, reviewers, and editors would result in provocative papers being published in the appropriate journals, but far too often these traditional methods are proving ineffective. New approaches are needed in a society where the paper published today will be the six o'clock news tonight and the basis for a lawsuit in the morning.

It has been suggested (9) that hot findings not be published until they have been reported at meetings and other investigators have had the opportunity to review the results. This suggestion has the major advantage of not putting questionable results before the public. It would also permit other investigators with similar data sets to try to confirm the findings. Yet, it could prove impractical in a system in which rewards come with publication and where there is the risk that others will duplicate the work and publish first.

Journals could create a separate category for provocative results that require confirmation. Authors might object, but such studies would be more clearly identified. Epidemiologists identify studies that test for a variety of possible associations by the term *hypothesis-generating*. Positive results from hypothesis-generating studies are not automatically assumed to be causal. It may be hard to identify speculative papers, but some rules of thumb are helpful. Studies without a clear a priori hypothesis, those where positive results appear to be due to multiple comparisons, and those reporting chance observations are strong candidates for the speculative category.

Often the tentative nature of a study is obvious to the expert but not to the general scientific or lay reader. The expert's knowledge could be passed along without making the review and publication process too cumbersome by adding a section to the reviewer's comments designated for publication immediately following the study. These commentaries could be published anonymously (encouraging candor) or with the reviewer's name (encouraging quality) at the editor's discretion. When the editor deems it appropriate, this approach could be expanded into a formal discussion among reviewers.

The final and, perhaps, the most difficult step toward publishing hot papers without courting disaster is education. The academic community, the legal profession, and the media must recognize their responsibilities. Universities should place less emphasis on number of publications when deciding on promotions. This would eliminate some marginal papers and allow investigators the luxury to "sit on" questionable results until they can be confirmed. Lawyers must recognize that one paper rarely provides a final, definitive answer. The concept that consistency of findings across studies is needed to prove causality should make its way into the courtroom. Journalists must restrain their natural desire for an exciting story. It does the public no service to report that spermicides are related to birth defects without also noting that the investigators consider their results tentative. Journalists, like lawyers, should be given a better appreciation of the process of scientific investigation.

The spermicide experience demonstrates the risks that we take when we publish provocative findings in America today. Nonetheless, provocative studies should be published. Authors, editors, those who report medical findings to the public, and those who use them in courts of law must recognize the potential danger inherent in reporting tentative results and must accept new responsibilities to minimize that danger. As never before, hot findings must be handled with care.

References

1. Jick H, Walker AM, Rothman KJ, et al: Vaginal spermicides and congenital disorders. *JAMA* 1981;245:1329–1332.
2. Oakley GP: Spermicides and birth defects. *JAMA* 1982;247:2405.
3. Shapiro S, Slone D, Heinonen O, et al: Birth defects and vaginal spermicides. *JAMA* 1982;247:2381–2384.
4. Mills JL, Harley EE, Reed GF, et al: Are spermicides teratogenic? *JAMA* 1982;248:2148–2151.
5. Bracken MB: Spermicidal contraceptives and poor reproductive outcomes: The epidemiologic evidence against an association. *Am J Obstet Gynecol* 1985;151:552–556.
6. National Center for Drug and Biologics: *Minutes of the Fertility and Maternal Health Drugs Advisory Committee Meeting.* Bethesda, Md, Food and Drug Administration, 1983.
7. *Wells v Ortho Pharmaceutical Corp,* 788 F2d 741 (11 Cir 1986).
8. Data do not support association between spermicides, birth defects. *FDA Drug Bull* 1986;16:21.
9. Holmes L: Vaginal spermicides and congenital disorders: The validity of a study. *JAMA* 1986;256:3095.
10. Watson JD, Crick FHC: Molecular structure of nucleic acids: A structure of deoxyribose nucleic acid. *Nature* 1953;171:737–738.
11. Chen JR, Francisco RB, Miller TE: Legionnaires' disease: Nickel levels. *Science* 1977;196:906–908.
12. Sunderman FW: Perspectives on Legionnaires' disease in relation to acute nickel carbonyl poisoning. *Ann Clin Lab Sci* 1977;7:187–200.
13. Smith OW, Smith G van S: The influence of diethylstilbestrol on progress and outcome of pregnancy as based on a comparison of treated with untreated primagravidas. *Am J Obstet Gynecol* 1949;58:994–1009.
14. Brackbill Y, Berendes HW: Dangers of diethylstilbestrol: Review of a 1953 paper. *Lancet* 1978;2:520.
15. Rosenberg SA, Lotze MT, Muul LM, et al: Observations on the systemic administration of autologous lymphokine-activated killer cells and recombinant interleukin–2 to patients with metastatic cancer. *N Engl J Med* 1985;313:1485–1492.
16. Jones KL, Smith DW, Ulleland CN, et al: Patterns of malformations in offspring of chronic alcoholic mothers. *Lancet* 1973;1:1267–1271.
17. Lemoine P, Harousseau H, Borteyru JP, et al: Les enfants de parents alcooliques: Anomalies observees a propos de 127 cas. *Ouest Med* 1968;21:476–482.

QUESTIONS FOR DISCUSSION

1. When a multicenter study involves twenty or more researchers whose significant contributions warrant formal recognition, what is an appropriate way to determine who receives authorship credit? In what order should those who qualify as authors be listed? How should the others' work be acknowledged?
2. Can news organizations report "ground-breaking" scientific findings from professional journals without misleading the public about their significance? If so, how? If not, why not?
3. In a highly competitive area of research, is it better to be the first to publish an important but incomplete finding, or to have a later paper that is complete and accurate?

RECOMMENDED SUPPLEMENTAL READING

"Guarding the Guardians: A Conference on Editorial Peer Review (Editorial)," Drummond Reenie, *Journal of the American Medical Association*, 1986, 256, pp. 2391–2392.
"Ensuring Integrity in Biomedical Publication," Patricia K. Woolf, *Journal of the American Medical Association*, 1987, 258, pp. 3424–3427.
"Problems with Peer Review and Alternatives," Richard Smith, *British Medical Journal*, 1988, 296, pp. 774–777.

PART VI

Research with Human Subjects

INTRODUCTION

One of the most sensitive and difficult aspects of scientific work occurs when human beings are used as subjects of experimentation. In working to advance knowledge that may benefit humanity, researchers may place individual subjects at risk of harm. In all such research, investigators must respect their human subjects as voluntary participants in a collaborative effort. Investigators who are also responsible for their subjects' medical care must further balance these efforts with their professional duty to seek their patients' benefit.

Modern consideration of these tensions began with the trials of Nazi physicians and scientists after World War II for their unethical research on Jews, Gypsies, prisoners, and the physically and mentally disabled. The tribunal composed the Nuremberg Code, guidelines on human research, which established a moral framework for the conduct of future investigations on humans. It focuses on subjects' voluntary consent to participate and researchers' duty to protect their subjects from related harm. Together with the World Medical Association's Declaration of Helsinki, the Nuremberg Code remains the fundamental comprehensive statement of research ethics worldwide.

Two decades after Nuremberg, however, many researchers still gave inadequate thought to their subjects' consent. In 1966, the U.S. Public Health Service (PHS) mandated that institutions receiving PHS research and training grants review all research involving human subjects to ensure that the subjects' rights and welfare were protected, and that appropriate procedures were used to obtain their consent. Protecting subjects from the risks of research and documenting their free and informed consent to participate has since become a significant aspect of every research protocol conducted in government-funded institutions.

Protecting subjects from risk itself poses ethical dilemmas. Clinician-researchers have observed that even a thorough disclosure of risks may be completely misunderstood by subjects who hope to benefit from a study. Recently, the practice of excluding women subjects of childbearing age, in an effort to protect their future children from unknown risks, has been criticized sharply. Critics claim that such exclusion gives an incomplete clinical picture of the effects of drugs and other treatments, and ultimately harms more women and children than it protects. The full ethical demands of consent and the protection of human subjects remain to be worked out.

16
The Nuremberg Code

The proof as to war crimes and crimes against humanity

Judged by any standard of proof the record clearly shows the commission of war crimes and crimes against humanity substantially as alleged in counts two and three of the indictment. Beginning with the outbreak of World War II criminal medical experiments on non-German nationals, both prisoners of war and civilians, including Jews and "asocial" persons, were carried out on a large scale in Germany and the occupied countries. These experiments were not the isolated and casual acts of individual doctors and scientists working solely on their own responsibility, but were the product of coordinated policy-making and planning at high governmental, military, and Nazi Party levels, conducted as an integral part of the total war effort. They were ordered, sanctioned, permitted, or approved by persons in positions of authority who under all principles of law were under the duty to know about these things and to take steps to terminate or prevent them.

Permissible medical experiments

The great weight of evidence before us is to the effect that certain types of medical experiments on human beings, when kept within reasonably well-defined bounds, conform to the ethics of the medical profession generally. The protagonists of the practice of human experimentation justify their views on the basis that such experiments yield results for the good of society that are unprocurable by other methods or means of study. All agree, however, that certain basic principles must be observed in order to satisfy moral, ethical and legal concepts:

    1. The voluntary consent of the human subject is absolutely essential.

    This means that the person involved should have legal capacity to give consent; should be so situated as to be able to exercise free power of choice, without the intervention of any element of force, fraud, deceit, duress, over-reaching, or other ulterior form of constraint or coercion; and should have sufficient knowledge and comprehension of the elements of the subject matter involved as to enable him to make an understanding and enlightened decision. This latter element requires that before the acceptance of an affirmative decision by the experimental subject there should be made known to him the nature, duration, and purpose of the experiment; the method and means by which it is to be conducted; all inconveniences and hazards reasonably to be expected; and the effects

From *Trials of War Criminals before the Nuernberg Military Tribunals under Control Council Law No. 10*, vol. 2 (Washington, D.C.: U.S. Government Printing Office, 1949), pp. 181–182.

upon his health or person which may possibly come from his participation in the experiment.

The duty and responsibility for ascertaining the quality of the consent rests upon each individual who initiates, directs or engages in the experiment. It is a personal duty and responsibility which may not be delegated to another with impunity.

2. The experiment should be such as to yield fruitful results for the good of society, unprocurable by other methods or means of study, and not random and unnecessary in nature.

3. The experiment should be so designed and based on the results of animal experimentation and a knowledge of the natural history of the disease or other problem under study that the anticipated results will justify the performance of the experiment.

4. The experiment should be so conducted as to avoid all unnecessary physical and mental suffering and injury.

5. No experiment should be conducted where there is an *a priori* reason to believe that death or disabling injury will occur; except, perhaps, in those experiments where the experimental physicians also serve as subjects.

6. The degree of risk to be taken should never exceed that determined by the humanitarian importance of the problem to be solved by the experiment.

7. Proper preparations should be made and adequate facilities provided to protect the experimental subject against even remote possibilities of injury, disability, or death.

8. The experiment should be conducted only by scientifically qualified persons. The highest degree of skill and care should be required through all stages of the experiment of those who conduct or engage in the experiment.

9. During the course of the experiment the human subject should be at liberty to bring the experiment to an end if he has reached the physical or mental state where continuation of the experiment seems to him to be impossible.

10. During the course of the experiment the scientist in charge must be prepared to terminate the experiment at any stage, if he has probable cause to believe, in the exercise of the good faith, superior skill and careful judgment required of him that a continuation of the experiment is likely to result in injury, disability, or death to the experimental subject.

17
Clinical investigations using human subjects

U.S. Public Health Service, Division of Research Grants

Subject

Clinical Investigations Using Human Subjects

Applicability

All PHS Research and Research Training Grants in Support of Such Clinical Investigations (including General Research Support Grants)

Effective date

Immediately

Background

The National Advisory Health Council on December 3, 1965, recommended to the Surgeon General as follows:

Be it resolved that the National Advisory Health Council believes that Public Health Service support of clinical research and investigation involving human beings should be provided only if the judgment of the investigator is subject to prior review by his institutional associates to assure an independent determination of the protection of the rights and welfare of the individual or individuals involved, of the appropriateness of the methods used to secure informed consent, and of the risks and potential medical benefits of the investigation.

The Surgeon General accepted the recommendation of the Council and instructed the Grants Policy Officer to develop implementing procedures for research and research training grants.

Statement of policy

No new, renewal, or continuation research or research training grant in support of clinical research and investigation involving human beings shall be awarded by the Public Health Service unless the grantee has indicated in the application the manner in which the grantee

U.S. Public Health Service, Division of Research Grants, memo PPO #129, February 8, 1966, and supplement, April 7, 1966.

institution will provide prior review of the judgment of the principal investigator or program director by a committee of his institutional associates. This review should assure an independent determination: (1) of the rights and welfare of the individual or individuals involved, (2) of the appropriateness of the methods used to secure informed consent, and (3) of the risks and potential medical benefits of the investigation. A description of the committee of associates who will provide the review shall be included in the application.

Procedure

The above policy becomes effective immediately and will be incorporated in all PHS research and research training grant regulations and research and research training policy statements as soon as possible. In the meantime, the attached memorandum from the Surgeon General explains the policy to grantee institutions.

The PHS staff who administer the initial review of applications for clinical research and investigation involving human beings (including the administrative review for continuation applications) shall ascertain that each application includes the information required by this policy and shall obtain this information, if necessary, in a document signed by both the principal investigator or program director and the official authorized to sign for the institution.

Originating office

The Surgeon General, Public Health Service

Approved by

Grants Policy Officer, OSG

Subject

Clinical Investigations Using Human Subjects

Applicability

1. All Supplemental Research and Research Training Grants, including General Research Support Grants
2. All Training (including RCP) Awards

Effective date

Immediately

Statement of policy

The requirements stated in PPO #129, dated February 8, 1966, are applicable to all new, renewal and continuation research and research training grants (including general research support grants). These requirements are extended (1) to include supplemental awards to the above grants and (2) to all new, renewal, supplemental and continuation research fellowships, training grants, research career program awards and direct traineeships.

Originating office

Office of the Chief, Division of Research Grants

Approved by

Grants Policy Officer, OSG

18

False hopes and best data: Consent to research and the therapeutic misconception

Paul S. Appelbaum, Loren H. Roth, Charles W. Lidz,
Paul Benson, and William Winslade

Following a suicide attempt, a young man with a long history of tumultuous relationships and difficulty controlling his impulses is admitted to a psychiatric hospital. After a number of days, a psychiatrist approaches the patient, explaining that he is conducting a research project to determine if medications may help in the treatment of the patient's condition. Is the patient interested, the psychiatrist asks? The answer: "Yes, I'm willing to do anything that might help me."

The psychiatrist returns over the next several days to explain the project further. He tells the patient that two medications are being used, along with a placebo; medications and placebo are assigned randomly. The trial is double-blinded; that is, neither physician nor patient will know what the patient is receiving until after the trial has been completed. The patient listens to the explanation and reads and signs the consent form. Since the process of providing information and obtaining consent seems, on the surface, exemplary, there appears to be little reason to question the validity of the consent.

Yet when the patient is asked why he agreed to be in the study, he offers some disquieting information. The medication that he will receive, he believes, will be the one most likely to help him. He ruled out the possibility that he might receive a placebo, because that would not be likely to do him much good. In short, this man, now both a patient and a subject, has interpreted, even distorted, the information he received to maintain the view – obviously based on his wishes – that every aspect of the research project to which he had consented was designed to benefit him directly. This belief, which is far from uncommon, we call the "therapeutic misconception." To maintain a therapeutic misconception is to deny the possibility that there may be major disadvantages to participating in clinical research that stem from the nature of the research process itself.

Research risks and the scientific method

The unique aspects of clinical research include the goal of creating generalizable knowledge; the techniques of randomization; and the use of a study protocol, control groups, and double-blind procedures. Do these elements create a body of risks or disadvantages for research subjects? The answer lies in understanding how the scientific method is often incompatible with one of the first principles of clinical treatment – the value that the legal philosopher Charles Fried calls "personal care."[1]

According to the principle of personal care, a physician's first obligation is solely to

From *Hastings Center Report*, 1987, 17, (April) pp. 20–24. © The Hastings Center. The authors acknowledge the invaluable assistance of Paul Soloff, M.D., in the collection of the data described in this paper.

the patient's well-being. A corollary is that the physician will take whatever measures are available to maximize the chances of a successful outcome. A failure to adhere to this principle creates at least a potential disadvantage for the clinical research subject: there is always a chance that the subject's interests may become secondary to other demands on the physician-researcher's loyalties.[2] And the methods of science inhibit the application of personal care.

Randomization, an important element of many clinical trials, demonstrates the problem. The argument is often made that comparisons of multiple treatment methods are legitimately undertaken only when the superiority of one over the other is unknown; thus the physician treating a patient in one of these trials does not abandon the patient's personal care, but merely allows chance to determine the assignment of treatments, each of which is likely to meet the patient's needs.[3]

But as Fried and others have noted, it is very unlikely that two treatments in a clinical trial will be identically desirable *for a particular patient*. The physician may have reason to suspect, for example, that a given treatment is more likely to be efficacious for a particular patient, even if overall evidence of greater efficacy is lacking. This suspicion may be based on the physician's previous experience with a subgroup of patients, the patient's own past treatment experience, the family history of responsiveness to treatment, or idiosyncratic elements in the patient's case. Subjects may have had previous unsatisfactory responses to one of the medications in a clinical trial, or may display clinical characteristics that suggest that one class of medications is more likely to benefit them than another.

Ordinarily, these factors would guide the therapeutic approach. But in a randomized study physicians cannot allow these factors to influence the treatment decision, and efforts to control for such factors in the selection of subjects, while theoretically possible, are cumbersome, expensive, and may bias the sample. Thus reliance on randomization represents an inevitable compromise of personal care in the service of attaining valid research results. There are at least two reports in the literature of physicians' reluctance to refer patients to randomized trials because of the possible decrement in the level of personal care.[4]

The use of a study protocol to regulate the course of treatment – essential to careful clinical research – also impedes the delivery of personal care. Protocols often indicate the pattern and dosages of medication to be administered or the blood levels to be attained. Even if they allow some individualization of medication, changes in time or magnitude may be limited. Thus patients who do not respond initially to a low dose of medication may not receive a higher dose, as they would if they were being treated without a protocol; on the other hand, patients experiencing side effects, which could be controlled by lowering their dosage, yet which are not so severe as to require withdrawal from the study, cannot receive the relief they would get in a therapeutic setting.

Analogously, adjunctive medications or forms of therapy, which may interfere with measurement of the primary treatment effect, are often prohibited. The exclusion of adjunctive medications, such as sleeping medications or decongestants, may increase a patient's discomfort. The requirement for a "wash-out" period, during which subjects are kept drug-free, may place previously stable patients at risk of relapse even before the experimental part of the project begins. And alternating placebo and active treatment periods may mean that a patient who responds well to a medication must be taken off that drug for the purposes of the study; conversely, patients who improve on placebo must be subject to the risks of active medication. In sum, the necessary rigidities of an experimental protocol often lead investigators to forgo individualized treatment decisions.

The need for control groups or placebos and double-blind procedures can produce similar effects. In the therapeutic setting patients will rarely receive medications that are deliberately designed to be pharmacologically ineffective; the ethics of those occasional situations when placebos are employed clinically are hotly disputed.[5] Yet, placebos are routinely employed in clinical investigations, without the intent of benefiting the individual subject.

Similarly, clinicians in a nonresearch setting will never allow themselves to remain ignorant of the treatment patients are receiving. Double-blind procedures, however, are necessary to ensure the integrity of a research study, even if they delay recognition of side effects or drug interactions, or have other adverse consequences.

Are these disadvantages so important that they should routinely be called to the attention of research subjects? That issue raises an empirical question: how prevalent is the therapeutic misconception?

Studies on consent

Our findings suggest that research subjects systematically misinterpret the risk/benefit ratio of participating in research because they fail to understand the underlying scientific methodology.[6]

This conclusion is based on our observations of consent transactions in four research studies on the treatment of psychiatric illness, and our interviews with the subjects immediately after consent was obtained. The studies varied in the extent of the information they provided to subjects. Two of the studies compared the effects of two medications on a psychiatric disorder (one used, in addition, a placebo control group). A third study examined the relative efficacy of two dosage ranges of the same medication. And a fourth examined two different social interventions in chronic psychiatric illness, compared with a control group.

The populations in these studies ranged from actively psychotic schizophrenic patients to nonpsychotic, and in some cases, minimally symptomatic, borderline, and depressed patients. Our questions were based on information included on the consent form with regard to the understanding of randomized or chance assignment; and the use of control groups, formal protocols, and double-blind techniques. Eighty-eight patients comprised the final data pool, but since all of the issues addressed here were not relevant to each project the sample size varied for each question.

We found that fifty-five of eighty subjects (69 percent) had no comprehension of the actual basis for their random assignment to treatment groups, while only twenty-two of eighty (28 percent) had a complete understanding of the randomization process. Thirty-two subjects stated their explicit belief that assignment would be made on the basis of their therapeutic needs. Interestingly, many of these subjects constructed elaborate but entirely fictional means by which an assignment would be made that was in their best interests. This was particularly evident when information about group assignment was limited to the written consent forms and not covered in the oral disclosure; subjects filled vacuums of knowledge with assumptions that decisions would be made in their best interests.

Similar findings were evident concerning other aspects of scientific design. With regard to nontreatment control groups and placebos, fourteen of thirty-three (44 percent) subjects failed to recognize that some patients who desired treatment would not receive it. Concerning use of a double-blind, twenty-six of sixty-seven subjects (39 percent) did not understand that their physician would not know which medication they would receive; an additional sixteen of sixty-seven subjects (24 percent) had only partially understood this. Most striking of all, only six of sixty-eight subjects (9 percent) were able to recognize a single way in which joining a protocol would restrict the treatment they could receive. In the two drug studies in which adjustment of medication dosage was tightly restricted, twenty-two of forty-four subjects (50 percent) said explicitly that they thought their dosage would be adjusted according to their individual needs.

Two cases illustrate how these flaws in understanding affect the patient's ability to assess the benefits of the research. The first demonstrates the effect of a complete failure to recognize that scientific methodology has other than a therapeutic purpose. The second demonstrates a more subtle influence of a therapeutic orientation on a subject who understands the overall methodology but has certain blindspots.

In the first case, a twenty-five-year-old married woman with a high-school education was a subject in a randomized, double-blind study that compared the use of two medications and a placebo in the treatment of a nonpsychotic psychiatric disorder. When interviewed, she was unsure how it would be decided which medication she would receive, but thought that the placebo would be given only to those subjects who "might not need medication." The subject understood that a double-blind procedure would be used, but did not see that the protocol placed any constraints on her treatment. She said that she considered this project not an "experiment," a term that implied using drugs whose effects were unknown. Rather, she considered this to be "research," a process whereby doctors "were trying to find out more about you in depth." She decided to participate because, "I needed help and the doctor said that other people who had been in it had been helped." Her strong conviction that the project would benefit her carried through to the end of the study. Although the investigators rated her a nonresponder, she was convinced that she had improved on the medication. She attributed her improvement in large part to the double-blind procedures, which kept her in the dark as to which medication she was receiving, thereby preventing her from persuading herself that the medication was doing no good. She was quite pleased about having participated in the study.

In the same study, another subject was a twenty-five-year-old woman with three years of college. At the time of the interview, she had minimal psychiatric symptoms and her understanding of the research was generally excellent. She recognized that the purpose of the project was to find out which treatment worked best for her group of patients. She spontaneously described the three groups, including the placebo group, and indicated that assignment would be at random. She understood that dosages would be adjusted according to blood levels and that a double-blind would be used. When asked directly, however, how *her* medication would be selected, she said she had no idea. She then added, "I hope it isn't by chance," and suggested that each subject would probably receive the medication she needed. Given the discrepancy between her earlier use of the word "random" and her current explanation, she was then asked what her understanding was of "random." Her definition was entirely appropriate: "by lottery, by chance, one patient who comes in gets one thing and the next patient gets the next thing." She then began to wonder out loud if this procedure was being used in the current study. Ultimately, she concluded that it was not.

In this case, despite a cognitive understanding of randomization, and a momentary recognition that random assignment would be used, the subject's conviction that the investigators would be acting in her best interests led to a distortion of an important element of the experimental procedure and therefore of the risk/benefit analysis.

The comments of colleagues and reports by other researchers have persuaded us that this phenomenon extends to all clinical research. Bradford Gray, for example, found that a number of subjects in a project comparing two drugs for the induction of labor believed, incorrectly, that their needs would determine which drug they would receive.[7] A survey of patients in research projects at four Veterans Administration hospitals showed that 75 percent decided to participate because they expected the research to benefit their health.[8] Another survey of attitudes toward research in a combined sample of patients and the general public revealed the thinking behind this hope: when asked why people in general should participate in research, 69 percent cited benefit to society at large and only 5 percent cited benefit to the subjects; however, when asked why *they* might participate in a research project, 52 percent said they would do it to get the best medical care, while only 23 percent responded that they would want to contribute to scientific knowledge.[9] Back in the psychiatric setting, Lee Park and Lino Covi found that a substantial percentage of patients who were told they were being given a placebo would not believe that they received inactive medication,[10] and Vincenta Leigh reported that the most common fantasy on a psychiatric research ward was that the research was actually designed to benefit the subjects.[11]

Responding to the problem

Should we do anything about the therapeutic misconception? It could be argued that as long as the research project has been peer-reviewed for scientific merit and approved for ethical acceptability by an institutional review board (IRB), the problem of the therapeutic misconception is not significant enough to warrant intervention. In this view, some minor distortion of the risk/benefit ratio has to be weighed against the costs of attempting to alter subjects' appreciation of the scientific methods. Such costs include time expended and the delay in completing research that will result when some subjects decide that they would rather not participate.

Whether we accept this view depends on the value that we place on the principle of autonomy that underlies the practice of informed consent. Autonomy can be overvalued when it limits necessary treatment, as it may, for example, in the controversy over the right to refuse psychotropic medications. There, we believe, patients' interests would best be served by giving claims to autonomy lesser weight.[12] But when we enter the research setting, limiting subjects' autonomy becomes a tool not for promoting their own interests, but for promoting the interests of others, including the researcher and society as a whole. We are not willing to accept such limitations for the benefit of others, particularly when, as described below, there may exist an effective mechanism for mitigating the problem.

Assuming that one agrees that distortions of the type we have described in subjects' reasoning are troublesome and worthy of correction, is such an effort likely to be effective? One might point to the data just presented to argue that little can be done to ameliorate the problem. The investigator in one of the projects we studied offered his subjects detailed and extensive information in a process that often extended over several days and included one session in which the entire project was reviewed. Despite this, half the subjects failed to grasp that treatment would be assigned on a random basis, four of twenty misunderstood how placebos would be used, five of twenty were not aware of the use of a double-blind, and eight of twenty believed that medications would be adjusted according to their individual needs. Is it not futile, then, to attempt to disabuse subjects of the belief that they will receive personal care?

Various theoretical explanations of our findings could support this view. Most people have been socialized to believe that physicians (at least ethical ones) always provide personal care.[13] It may therefore be very difficult, perhaps nearly impossible, to persuade subjects that *this* encounter is different, particularly if the researcher is also the treating physician, who has previously satisfied the subject's expectations of personal care. Further, insofar as much clinical research involves persons who are acutely ill and in some distress, the well-known tendency of patients to regress and entrust their well-being to an authority figure would undercut any effort to dispel the therapeutic misconception.

In response, more of our data must be explored. In each of the studies we observed, one cell of subjects was the target of an augmented informational process, which supplemented the investigator's disclosures to subjects with a "preconsent discussion." This discussion was led by a member of our research team who was trained to teach potential subjects about such things as the key methodologic aspects of the research project, especially methods that might conflict with the principle of personal care.

By introducing a neutral discloser, distinct from the patient's treatment team, we shifted the emphasis of the disclosure to focus on the ways in which research differs from treatment. Of the subjects who received this special education, eight of sixteen (50 percent) recognized that randomization would be used, as opposed to thirteen of the fifty-one (25 percent) remaining subjects; five of five (100 percent) understood how placebos would be employed in the single study that used them, compared with eleven of the fifteen (73 percent) remaining subjects; nine of sixteen (56 percent) comprehended the use of a double blind while only fifteen of fifty-one (31 percent) remaining subjects did so; and five of seventeen (29 percent) initially recognized other limits on their treatment as a result of constraints in the protocol, compared with one of the fifty-one (2 percent) other subjects.

Our data suggest that many subjects can be taught that research *is* markedly different from ordinary treatment. Other efforts to educate subjects about the use of scientific methodology offer comparably encouraging results.[14] There is no reason to believe that subjects will refuse to hear clear-cut efforts to dispel the therapeutic misconception.

Novel approaches such as we employed may be one thing, of course, while routine procedures are something else. Perhaps our data derive from an unusually gifted group of patient-subjects. Will the complexity of explaining the principle of the scientific method defy understanding by most research subjects?

Undercutting the therapeutic misconception, thereby laying out some of the major disadvantages of any clinical research project, is probably much simpler than it seems. About the goals of research, subjects could be told: "Because this is a research project, we will be doing some things differently than we would if we were simply treating you for your condition. Not all the things we do are designed to tell us the best way to treat *you*, but they should help us to understand how people with your condition *in general* can best be treated." About randomization: "The treatment you receive of the three possibilities will be selected by chance, not because we believe that one or the other will be better for you." About placebos: "Some subjects will be selected at random to receive sugar pills that are not known to help the condition you have; this is so we can tell whether the medications that the other patients get are really effective, or if everyone with your condition would have gotten better anyway."

One can quibble about the wording of specific sections, and complexities can arise with particular projects, but the concepts underlying scientific methodology are in reality quite simple. And as long as subjects understand the key principles of how the study is being conducted, investigators can probably omit some of the detail that currently clogs consent forms and confuses subjects about the minor risks that accompany the experimental procedures, such as blood drawing. Overall, then, we may end up with a much simpler consent process when we focus on the issue of personal care.

Who should have the task of explaining the therapeutic misconception to subjects? Clearly, investigators should be encouraged to discuss such issues with subjects and to include them on consent forms, but several problems arise here. First, it is decidedly *not* in investigators' self-interest for them to disabuse potential subjects of the therapeutic misconception. Experienced investigators, as we have reported elsewhere,[15] view the recruitment of research subjects as an intricate and extended effort to win the potential subject's trust. One of our subjects in this study described the process in these words: "It was almost as if they were courting me. . . . everything was presented in the best possible light." One could argue that it is unrealistic to expect investigators to raise additional doubts about the benefits that subjects can expect; any effort in that regard will result in resistance by investigators, particularly those who have yet to internalize the justifications for informed consent in general.

Second, even investigators who recognize the desirability of subjects making informed decisions may have great trouble conveying this particular information. When a researcher tells subjects that he or she is not selecting the treatment that will be given or that the medications being used may be no more effective than a placebo, the researcher is confessing uncertainty over the best approach to treatment, as well as the likely outcome. Harold Bursztajn and colleagues have argued that the essential uncertainty of all medical practice is precisely what physicians need to convey in *both* research and treatment settings.[16] Yet, as Jay Katz points out, physicians have been systematically socialized to underplay or ignore uncertainty in their discussions with patients.[17] In a recent report of physicians' reluctance to enter patients in a multicenter breast cancer study, 22 percent of the principal investigators cited as a major obstacle to enrolling subjects difficulty in telling patients that they did not know which treatment was best.[18]

Third, few researchers who are also clinicians feel comfortable acknowledging, even to themselves, that the course of treatment may not be optimally therapeutic for the patient. Thus, there appear such statements as the following, which recently was published in *The Lancet:* "A doctor who contributes to randomized treatment trials should not be thought of as a research worker, but simply as a clinician with an ethical duty to his patients not to go on giving them treatments without doing everything possible to assess their true worth."[19] The author concludes that since randomized trials are not really research, there is no need to obtain *any* informed consent from research subjects. Although this conclusion may be extreme, the example emphasizes the difficulties of getting investigators to admit to themselves, much less to their patient-subjects, the limits they have accepted on the delivery of personal care.

If there is concern with particular protocols, IRBs might consider supplementing the investigators' disclosure and the "courtship" process with a session in which the potential subject reviews risks and benefits with someone who is not a member of the research team. (John Robertson has proposed a similar approach, albeit out of other concerns.[20]) The neutral explainer would be responsible to the IRB and would be trained to emphasize those aspects of the research situation about which the IRB has the greatest concern. This approach might be especially appropriate when the investigator is also the subject's treating physician and the methodology used is likely to be interpreted as therapeutic in intent. The model we employed of using a trained educator (nurses are natural candidates for the job) worked well. It is certainly more manageable and less disruptive than the oft-heard suggestions that patient advocates or consent monitors sit in on every interaction between subject and investigator.

There may be advantages to using a trained, neutral educator, apart from aiding subjects' decision-making. Subjects' perceptions of the research team as willing to "level with them," even to the point of explaining why it might not be in subjects' interests to participate in the study, may increase their trust and cooperation. On the other hand, failure to deal with the therapeutic misconception during the consent process could increase distrust of researchers and the health care system in general, if subjects later come to feel they were "deceived," as a few did in the studies we observed. Enough experiences of this sort could further heighten public antipathy to medical research, particularly if they are publicized as some have been.[21] The scientific method is a powerful tool for advancing knowledge, but like most potent clinical procedures it has side effects that must be attended to, lest the benefits sought be overwhelmed by the disadvantages that accrue. With careful planning, the therapeutic misconception can be dispelled, leaving the subjects with a much clearer picture of the relative risks and benefits of participation in research.

Notes

1. Charles Fried, *Medical Experimentation: Personal Integrity and Social Policy* (New York: American Elsevier Publishing Co., 1974).
2. Arthur Schafer, "The Ethics of the Randomized Clinical Trial," *New England Journal of Medicine* 307 (Sept. 16, 1982), 719–24.
3. "Consent: How Informed?" *The Lancet* I (June 30, 1984), 1445–47.
4. Kathryn M. Taylor, Richard G. Margolese, and Colin L Soskolne, "Physicians' Reasons for Not Entering Eligible Patients in a Randomized Clinical Trial of Surgery for Breast Cancer," *New England Journal of Medicine* 310 (May 24, 1984), 1363–67; Mortimer J. Lacher, "Physicians and Patients as Obstacles to Randomized Trial," *Clinical Research* 26 (December 1978), 375–79.
5. Sissela Bok, "The Ethics of Giving Placebos," *Scientific American* 231:5 (May 1974), 17–23.
6. Paul S. Appelbaum, Loren H. Roth, and Charles W. Lidz, "The Therapeutic Misconception: Informed Consent in Psychiatric Research," *International Journal of Law and Psychiatry* 5 (1982), 319–29; Paul Benson, Loren H. Roth, and William J. Winslade, "Informed Consent in Psychiatric Research: Preliminary Findings from an Ongoing Investigation," *Social Science and Medicine* 20 (1985), 1331–41.
7. Bradford H. Gray, *Human Subjects in Medical Experimentation: A Sociological Study of the Conduct and Regulation of Clinical Research* (New York: John Wiley & Sons, 1975).
8. Henry W. Riecken and Ruth Ravich, "Informed Consent to Biomedical Research in Veterans

Administration Hospitals,'' *Journal of the American Medical Association* 248 (July 16, 1982), 344–48.

9. Barrie R. Cassileth, Edward J. Lusk, David S. Miller, and Shelley Hurwitz, ''Attitudes Toward Clinical Trials Among Patients and Public,'' *Journal of the American Medical Association* 248 (August 27, 1982), 968–70.

10. Lee C. Park and Lino Covi, ''Nonblind Placebo Trial: An Exploration of Neurotic Patients' Responses to Placebo When Its Inert Content is Disclosed,'' *Archives of General Psychiatry* 12 (April 1965), 336–45.

11. Vincenta Leigh, ''Attitudes and Fantasy Themes of Patients on a Psychiatric Research Unit,'' *Archives of General Psychiatry* 32 (May 1975), 598–601.

12. Paul S. Appelbaum and Thomas G. Gutheil, ''The Right to Refuse Treatment: The Real Issue is Quality of Care,'' *Bulletin of the American Academy of Psychiatry and the Law* 9 (1982), 199–202.

13. Cassileth et al., *op cit.*

14. Jan M. Howard, David DeMets, and the BHAT Research Group, ''How Informed Is Informed Consent? The BHAT Experience,'' *Controlled Clinical Trials* 2 (1981), 287–303.

15. Paul S. Appelbaum and Loren H. Roth, ''The Structure of Informed Consent in Psychiatric Research,'' *Behavioral Sciences and the Law* 1:3 (Autumn 1983), 9–19.

16. Harold Bursztajn, Richard I. Feinbloom, Robert M. Hamm, and Archie Brodsky, *Medical Choices, Medical Chances: How Patients, Families, and Physicians Can Cope with Uncertainty* (New York: Free Press, 1984).

17. Jay Katz, *The Silent World of Doctor and Patient* (New York: Free Press, 1984).

18. Taylor, et al., *op cit.*

19. Thurston B. Brewin, ''Consent to Randomized Treatment,'' *The Lancet* II (Oct. 23, 1982), 919–21.

20. John A. Robertson, ''Taking Consent Seriously: IRB Intervention in The Consent Process,'' *IRB: A Review of Human Subjects Research* 4:5 (September-October 1982), 1–5.

21. Dava Sobel, ''Sleep Study Leaves Subject Feeling Angry and Confused,'' *New York Times* (July 15, 1980), p. C–1.

19

Declaration of Helsinki: Recommendations guiding physicians in biomedical research involving human subjects

World Medical Association

Introduction

It is the mission of the physician to safeguard the health of the people. His or her knowledge and conscience are dedicated to the fulfillment of this mission.

The Declaration of Geneva of the World Medical Association binds the physician with the words, ''The health of my patient will be my first consideration,'' and the International Code of Medical Ethics declares that, ''A physician shall act only in the patient's interest when providing medical care which might have the effect of weakening the physical and mental condition of the patient.''

The purpose of biomedical research involving human subjects must be to improve diagnostic, therapeutic and prophylactic procedures and the understanding of the aetiology and pathogenesis of disease.

In current medical practice most diagnostic, therapeutic or prophylactic procedures involve hazards. This applies especially to biomedical research.

Medical progress is based on research which ultimately must rest in part on experimentation involving human subjects.

In the field of biomedical research a fundamental distinction must be recognized between medical research in which the aim is essentially diagnostic or therapeutic for a patient, and medical research, the essential object of which is purely scientific and without implying direct diagnostic or therapeutic value to the person subjected to the research.

Special caution must be exercised in the conduct of research which may affect the environment, and the welfare of animals used for research must be respected.

Because it is essential that the results of laboratory experiments be applied to human beings to further scientific knowledge and to help suffering humanity, the World Medical Association has prepared the following recommendations as a guide to every physician in biomedical research involving human subjects. They should be kept under review in the future. It must be stressed that the standards as drafted are only a guide to physicians all over the world. Physicians are not relieved from criminal, civil and ethical responsibilities under the laws of their own countries.

Adopted by the 18th World Medical Assembly, Helsinki, Finland, June 1964, and amended by the 29th World Medical Assembly, Tokyo, Japan, October 1975; 35th World Medical Assembly, Venice, Italy, October 1983; and the 41st World Medical Assembly, Hong Kong, September 1989. © World Medical Association

I. Basic Principles

1. Biomedical research involving human subjects must conform to generally accepted scientific principles and should be based on adequately performed laboratory and animal experimentation and on a thorough knowledge of the scientific literature.

2. The design and performance of each experimental procedure involving human subjects should be clearly formulated in an experimental protocol which should be transmitted for consideration, comment and guidance to a specially appointed committee independent of the investigator and the sponsor provided that this independent committee is in conformity with the laws and regulations of the country in which the research experiment is performed.

3. Biomedical research involving human subjects should be conducted only by scientifically qualified persons and under the supervision of a clinically competent medical person. The responsibility for the human subject must always rest with a medically qualified person and never rest on the subject of the research, even though the subject has given his or her consent.

4. Biomedical research involving human subjects cannot legitimately be carried out unless the importance of the objective is in proportion to the inherent risk to the subject.

5. Every biomedical research project involving human subjects should be preceded by careful assessment of predictable risks in comparison with foreseeable benefits to the subject or to others. Concern for the interests of the subject must always prevail over the interests of science and society.

6. The right of the research subject to safeguard his or her integrity must always be respected. Every precaution should be taken to respect the privacy of the subject and to minimize the impact of the study on the subject's physical and mental integrity and on the personality of the subject.

7. Physicians should abstain from engaging in research projects involving human subjects unless they are satisfied that the hazards involved are believed to be predictable. Physicians should cease any investigation if the hazards are found to outweigh the potential benefits.

8. In publication of the results of his or her research, the physician is obliged to preserve the accuracy of the results. Reports of experimentation not in accordance with the principles laid down in this Declaration should not be accepted for publication.

9. In any research on human beings, each potential subject must be adequately informed of the aims, methods, anticipated benefits and potential hazards of the study and the discomfort it may entail. He or she should be informed that he or she is at liberty to abstain from participation in the study and that he or she is free to withdraw his or her consent to participation at any time. The physician should then obtain the subject's freely-given informed consent, preferably in writing.

10. When obtaining informed consent for the research project the physician should be particularly cautious if the subject is in a dependent relationship to him or her or may consent under duress. In that case the informed consent should be obtained by a physician who is not engaged in the investigation and who is completely independent of this official relationship.

11. In case of legal incompetence, informed consent should be obtained from the legal guardian in accordance with national legislation. Where physical or mental incapacity makes it impossible to obtain informed consent, or when the subject is a minor, permission

from the responsible relative replaces that of the subject in accordance with national legislation.

Whenever the minor child is in fact able to give a consent, the minor's consent must be obtained in addition to the consent of the minor's legal guardian.

12. The research protocol should always contain a statement of the ethical considerations involved and should indicate that the principles enunciated in the present Declaration are complied with.

II. Medical research combined with professional care (Clinical research)

1. In the treatment of the sick person, the physician must be free to use a new diagnostic and therapeutic measure, if in his or her judgement it offers hope of saving life, reestablishing health or alleviating suffering.

2. The potential benefits, hazards and discomfort of a new method should be weighed against the advantages of the best current diagnostic and therapeutic methods.

3. In any medical study, every patient – including those of a control group, if any – should be assured of the best proven diagnostic and therapeutic method.

4. The refusal of the patient to participate in a study must never interfere with the physician-patient relationship.

5. If the physician considers it essential not to obtain informed consent, the specific reasons for this proposal should be stated in the experimental protocol for transmission to the independent committee (I, 2).

6. The physician can combine medical research with professional care, the objective being the acquisition of new medical knowledge, only to the extent that medical research is justified by its potential diagnostic or therapeutic value for the patient.

III. Non-therapeutic biomedical research involving human subjects (Non-clinical biomedical research)

1. In the purely scientific application of medical research carried out on a human being, it is the duty of the physician to remain the protector of the life and health of that person on whom biomedical research is being carried out.

2. The subjects should be volunteers – either healthy persons or patients for whom the experimental design is not related to the patient's illness.

3. The investigator or the investigating team should discontinue the research if in his/her or their judgement it may, if continued, be harmful to the individual.

4. In research on man, the interest of science and society should never take precedence over considerations related to the well-being of the subject.

20
Wanted:
Single, white male for medical research

Rebecca Dresser

In June 1990, congressional investigators issued a startling report. The General Accounting Office revealed that despite a 1986 federal policy to the contrary, women continued to be seriously underrepresented in biomedical research study populations. According to the National Institutes of Health, this practice "has resulted in significant gaps in [our] knowledge" of diseases that affect both men and women.[1] In short, many of the important human health data generated by the modern biomedical research revolution are data about men.

The failure to include women in research populations is ubiquitous. An NIH-sponsored study showing that heart attacks were reduced when subjects took one aspirin every other day was conducted on men, and the relationship between low cholesterol diets and cardiovascular disease has been almost exclusively studied in men. Yet coronary heart disease is the leading cause of death in women. Similarly, the first twenty years of a major federal study on health and aging included only men. Yet two-thirds of the elderly population are women. The recent announcement that aspirin can help prevent migraine headaches is based on data from males only, even though women suffer from migraines up to three times as often as men.[2]

The list goes on: studies on AIDS treatment frequently omit women, the fastest growing infected population. An investigation of the possible relationship between caffeine and heart disease involved 45,589 male research subjects. Most amazing is the pilot project on the impact of obesity on breast and uterine cancer conducted – you guessed it – solely on men. Moreover, the customary research subject not only is male, but is a white male. African-Americans, Latinos, and other racial and ethnic groups have typically been excluded from studies, again in spite of a formal NIH guideline encouraging the inclusion of such groups in study populations. Children and elderly persons also have received short shrift, particularly in the testing of new drugs. And in basic research, even female rats are frequently excluded as research subjects![3]

The physiology of women and men differs in ways that can affect how disease and treatment manifest themselves. Beyond the obviously sex-linked diseases such as uterine and prostate cancer, there is evidence that heart disease, AIDS, depression, and numerous other ostensibly "gender-neutral" conditions are expressed differently in women and men. A similar situation exists among different racial and ethnic groups. Lupus, for example, reportedly affects one in 750 women generally, but its incidence is one in 245

From *Hastings Center Report*, 1992, 22 (January-February), pp. 24–29. © The Hastings Center. The author would like to thank Dena Davis and Mike Grodin for their comments on an earlier draft of this article, and Laura Chisholm for encouraging her to write on this topic.

among African-American women and one in 500 among Latinas.[4] Such differences make it inappropriate simply to generalize findings based on one gender or racial group to all human beings. As a result of the past over-representation of white men in research populations, physicians now frequently lack adequate evidence on whether women and people of color will be helped, harmed, or not affected at all by numerous therapies now endorsed as promoting "human health."

NIH officials have admitted that the agency's policy on expanding study populations was inadequately publicized as well as substantively feeble, simply recommending that investigators proposing studies "consider" the inclusion of women and minority groups. In the four years that elapsed between the policy's announcement and the GAO report, NIH continued to review numerous proposals that either gave no information on the gender of their study populations, or proposed all-male studies without a rationale for doing so. The GAO report also notes that the NIH itself had no policy to ensure the inclusion of women in its intramural research program. Indeed, according to *Science* correspondent Joseph Palca, Acting Director William Raub said that a small group of NIH staff still had "disdain" for the policy encouraging inclusion.

After the GAO report was released, NIH officials did attempt to mend fences. In December 1990 they issued special instructions to grant applicants providing that clinical research grants "will be *required* to include minorities and women in study populations." Omission or inadequate representation of these groups must be accompanied by "a clear compelling rationale."[5] Raub also established an office of research on women's health, which will coordinate a new women's health study involving several thousand women.[6]

Time will tell whether these actions reduce reliance on the white male subject. But disturbing questions remain. In a country that prides itself on its progress in promoting gender and racial equality, how could the federal government sanction such a nakedly discriminatory practice? Why wasn't the original NIH policy more strongly worded and more effectively implemented? Moreover, why was a special NIH policy necessary at all? Why didn't the researchers themselves adopt a more inclusive practice? And finally, why didn't the institutional review boards charged with research oversight demand a more inclusive approach? During the twenty-plus years of intense analysis and debate on the ethics of research on human subjects, how did this glaring moral mistake elude our scrutiny? In this paper, I examine some of the possible sources of this national ethical blindspot.

Alleged justifications for the exclusionary practice

Some scientists and officials have explained that there often is "scientific" justification for studying only white males. Clean, simple data are needed for studies; the more alike the subjects, the more any variation can be attributed to the experimental intervention. Including women would "complicate" a study due to the hormone changes of the menstrual cycle. I have two responses to this claim. First, even if it is scientifically justifiable to study humans who have a similar physiology, why study white men? Perhaps the choice of racial group can be supported by its dominant proportion in the U.S. population, but not so for the choice of gender. In this country, women are numerically in the majority. Why then the choice of the minority white male? Why is it female, but not male, hormones that "complicate" research? Second, focusing on one type of human physiology reduces the generalizability of the experimental data. Although there is probably a place for such narrowly focused projects, why have they so rarely been conducted on anyone but white men? Again, what accounts for the relative infrequency of studies on homogeneous populations of other kinds of people?

One can also challenge the notion that a study conducted on physiologically close subjects is usually the "best" scientific approach. Such a judgment divorces the concept of scientific merit from its broader context. A project may be designed with the greatest of scientific elegance, but if the data it produces have little value to society, it is not necessarily a meritorious project. Merit, at least in the context of government funding decisions, is tied to a proposal's promise of benefit to society.[7] If NIH's goal is to award support to the projects most likely to advance our knowledge of important human health concerns, it would seem that white-male-only clinical investigations of widespread conditions such as coronary artery disease and aging would have less merit than studies that provided data with broader applicability. In fact, the latest NIH directive explicitly instructs its scientific reviewers to consider inclusion of women and minorities in study populations when they evaluate a proposal's scientific merit.

Two other explanations have been offered for the practice of excluding women from study populations. One is concern for the condition of women who could become pregnant while enrolled as research subjects. Threats of miscarriage, birth defects, and so forth are cited as justifications for omitting women. Exclusion is appropriate, it is alleged, to protect potentially pregnant women and their potential children. The Department of Health and Human Services regulations governing human subjects research sets special conditions on research involving fetuses and pregnant women, and the Food and Drug Administration guidelines for clinical evaluation of drugs restricts but does not ban participation of "women of childbearing potential" in clinical trials.[8] Certainly caution is warranted here. But is maternal-fetal protection always a valid reason for failing to include female subjects?

Our nation has a long history of excluding women from various activities on grounds that participation would harm the "weaker sex," and thus often denying women the significant benefits of participation. Likewise, the failure to conduct biomedical research on women denies them the benefits of research. The vast majority of women who are not pregnant cannot with sufficient confidence take advantage of numerous health recommendations that have emerged from men-only research studies. In the name of *potential* protection for *potentially* pregnant women and their fetuses, all women have lost opportunities to improve and extend their lives.

Complete exclusion of women subjects is an unnecessarily blunt instrument to accomplish the goal of maternal-fetal protection. The exclusionary approach, as Carol Levine notes, "assumes that all women are alike, that all women are sexually active, and that all are unreliable in their contraceptive practices."[9] To the contrary, as one physician pointed out, "Most female cardiac patients are not planning to get pregnant."[10] Neither are the women likely to be subjects in an aging study!

If a study poses a legitimate threat to the potential offspring of women participants, two options come to mind. One is simply to exclude fertile women of reproductive age. Again, however, this seems overbroad; indeed, this is the approach the Supreme Court recently struck down in *Johnson Controls* as violating federal law prohibiting sex discrimination in the workplace.[11] It would be better to adopt a more nuanced approach. In her recent article on the underrepresentation of women in HIV/AIDS research, for example, Levine endorses a three-tiered categorization system to address the problem. Many, perhaps most, human studies fail to pose a foreseeable risk to future children. The unknown and unforeseeable teratogenic risk that accompanies practically any physiological intervention fails to justify excluding fertile women from studies in this category. Similarly, women should have the opportunity to enroll in studies that present known risks to future children, but also have the potential for significantly benefiting the research participants. In these two categories of research, adequate disclosure of the risks and potential benefits of research participation, together with the availability of highly reliable contraceptives and abortion, would give women a reasonable choice regarding whether to accept the risks of participating. The possibility that a few women might become pregnant, might choose against abortion, and might have a child who is harmed by exposure to an experimental intervention is too small to justify the current exclusionary practices. The risk of tort liability in such cases is also small. Women who consent to the risk of harm to potential offspring and who decide against abortion when they become unexpectedly pregnant would be unlikely to recover damages. Any injured children might themselves have a claim, however. Perhaps some form of legislative immunity is needed here. But it should be recognized that the current approach also fails to protect health professionals and drug manufacturers against liability. The present practice merely moves the source of the claims to the damaged future children of women patients who receive drugs and other treatments in the clinical setting.

A third research category is more complicated, however. Levine argues that sexually active fertile women should be excluded from studies that present both a known significant risk to potential offspring and minimal or unknown benefit to women subjects, because parents have a moral responsibility to make reasonable efforts to protect their future children's health and the knowledge sought from such studies is obtainable through other means. Given the ever-present danger of contraceptive failure, the misunderstandings "informed" subjects may have about a protocol's risks and potential benefits, and the possibility that subjects' awareness or appreciation of their exposure to risk could decline over time, it is better to conduct such studies on other groups, Levine contends. If early results reveal a possible substantial benefit for women participants, she suggests that the intervention could be made available to individual women off-protocol.

This would be appropriate, in my view, as long as the same approach is applied to sexually active fertile men. Researchers have been extremely concerned about reproductive risks to women, while largely neglecting the reproductive risks research participation may pose to men. There is growing evidence that many substances may be damaging to sperm, thereby creating the possibility of birth defects in offspring.[12] The emphasis on reproductive hazards to women thus is an unjustifiably narrow means of protecting children's health. If society deems the health of potential future children to justify the blanket exclusion of fertile women from certain research protocols, the exclusion should cover *all* fertile subjects whose offspring could be endangered, not just female ones. Furthermore, men's lengthier reproductive capacity could lead to their exclusion from risky studies for many more years than women.

The final rationale for women's exclusion from study populations involves alleged recruitment difficulties. For example, researchers in the aspirin and heart disease study claimed that they wanted to include women, but were unable to find enough potential subjects to do so. Their study population was physicians over age forty, they explained, and women comprised only 10 percent of this group.[13] Moreover, according to one NIH official, it was doubtful that a sufficient number of women would be "interested in participating and be content to go through the hassle of taking a placebo."[14] In other heart disease studies, researchers have asserted that they could not locate enough women with the condition. Although this is partly due to the lower overall incidence and later development of this disease among women, it turns out that another factor is the medical community's failure to recognize serious heart disease in women.[15]

Blaming the scarcity of potential women subjects for the exclusionary practice is unacceptable. In effect, this adds insult to injury by building on past bias to justify its perpetuation in a different realm. The traditional exclusion of women from the medical profession is the source of the small number of middle-aged women physicians. Health stereotypes about women – "women just don't get heart disease"; "women somaticize their emotional problems" – are one source of physicians' failure to recognize heart disease in women. As one physician put it,

If a fifty-year-old man goes to the doctor complaining of chest pains, the next day he will be on a treadmill taking a stress test. If a fifty-year-old woman goes to the doctor and complains of chest pains, she will be told to go home and rest.[16]

When heart disease studies exclude women, they only reinforce physicians' misplaced assumptions. And why was it assumed that women would be less interested than men in "go[ing] through the hassle of taking a placebo"? Women who were adequately informed of their risk of heart disease would have as much incentive as men to participate in the study.

Biomedical research studies should be designed to surmount the alleged difficulties in recruiting women. If enough female physicians are not available, why not study female nurses, or some other reasonably accessible group of women? (A recent observational study suggesting that low-dose aspirin could reduce cardiovascular disease in women was conducted on female nurses, but the authors emphasize the need for a randomized, controlled clinical trial to verify that a benefit exists, rule out serious risks, and determine an appropriate dose for women.)[17] If scientists conducting heart disease research are afraid that physicians will not refer enough women patients, then extra recruiting measures should be taken to ensure that they do. Research costs may go up, but the benefits of including women subjects are worth the expense.

What's wrong with exclusion

The current disparity between the health information we have about white males and the information we have about women and people of color contravenes basic ethical principles governing human experimentation. Most clearly violated is the principle of beneficence, which holds that biomedical research should be designed to maximize benefit and minimize harm. Proposals promising to advance knowledge of important human health and welfare concerns should receive funding priority. Awarding support to studies on white males withholds research benefits from other groups of people and possibly exposes such people to risk when they and their physicians follow recommendations based on data from white male subjects. When diseases disproportionately affecting women and people of color are given low funding priority, knowledge that could alter current ineffective or detrimental routine medical care is never produced.

The harm produced by the exclusionary practices is not easily dismissed. Simple extrapolation from white males to everyone else can be dangerous. One study, for example, found that due to physiological differences, African-Americans given the ''normal'' dose of lithium (established in trials on white men) frequently experienced toxic reactions, heightening their already high risk of renal failure. Similarly, the male-only studies of heart disease and cholesterol led the American Heart Association to recommend a diet that could actually exacerbate the risk of heart disease for women. Oral contraceptives can cause excessive cholesterol levels, yet it has not been systematically demonstrated that the cholesterol-lowering medication proven effective in men works when taken in conjunction with oral contraceptives.[18] The current lack of knowledge on the connection between diet and breast cancer denies women a potential opportunity to protect themselves against a frequently lethal disease that strikes one in nine women. Antiseizure and antidepressant drugs may require different doses over the menstrual cycle to achieve their desired effect, and the failure to calibrate asthma medication to this cycle may contribute to the existing premenstrual rise in asthma deaths.

Scientists and policymakers must recognize that the choice is not whether to protect women and people of color from research risks. Instead, the choice is whether to expose some consenting members of these groups to risk in the closely monitored research setting, or to expose many more of them to risk in the clinical setting without these safeguards, which is the result of the current approach.

The present situation also is unjust. The justice principle mandates fair distribution of the benefits and burdens of biomedical research. But instead, taxpayers excluded from study populations have been charged for research without the assurance that they will share in any health benefits it might produce. Historically disadvantaged groups have subsidized health benefits for the more privileged, while being denied similar benefits for themselves.

The modern response to past injustice in the selection of human subjects may have contributed to the current imbalance in study populations. Ethical codes governing experimentation on human subjects arose primarily in reaction to the horrors of the Nazi experiments, the Tuskegee syphilis study, and other research on vulnerable populations that exposed uninformed and unconsenting persons to extreme harm for the benefit of the better off. Hence, the overall reform goal was to eliminate such practices. This may have led to the notion that white middle- and upper-class men were the best people to bear the burdens of research participation. But these burdens have now been substantially reduced, while participation offers significant benefit to the members of other racial and ethnic groups. A move perhaps designed to protect disadvantaged groups has simply shifted potential harm away from research subjects and imposed it on people in the community who may be receiving inappropriate health information and medical treatment.

''Tuskegee fallout'' probably has contributed in an additional way to the present underrepresentation of people of color in study populations. In light of past scandals, some members of disadvantaged communities are justifiably suspicious of the research establishment's motivation in seeking their participation as subjects. But this product of past abuses ought not excuse the current underrepresentation. People of color also continue to experience a disproportionate share of economic, health care, and other deprivation that creates barriers to their research participation. Today's researchers face the task of educating these communities on the positive dimensions of research participation. Special support services may be necessary to facilitate the participation of those who wish to serve as subjects, including child care and transportation assistance. Furthermore, society has an obligation to ensure that members of these communities actually have access to any health care benefits produced by the research in which they participate.

The hidden roots of exclusion

How did white males come to be the prototype of the human research subject? Like the pronoun "he," it was taken for granted that the white male subject stood for all of us. In her examination of how the law treats differences among people, Martha Minow suggests some reasons for this. As individuals, she points out, we are all different from everyone else in countless ways. In society, however, certain differences are deemed relevant to how people are regarded. The choice of which differences "matter" inevitably reflects and reinforces existing social structures, and normality and abnormality are determined by the most powerful social group's (usually unstated) point of reference. Accordingly, "women are different in relation to the unstated male norm. Blacks, Mormons, Jews, and Arabs are different in relation to the unstated white Christian norm."[19] Members of the dominant group making decisions in reliance on this norm may discount or be oblivious to the influence of their particular perspective. To the contrary, they see themselves as "objective," and the existing social structure as "natural."

It is easy to see this process at work in the research setting. NIH officials and biomedical researchers have, consciously or unconsciously, defined the white male as the normal, representative human being. From this perspective, the goal of advancing human health can be achieved by studying the white male human model. Physical differences between males and females, or between whites and people of color, are unacknowledged or irrelevant in this world view. Including women and people of color would simply complicate the work, thus making it more difficult and costly, which would detract from the researchers' mission of improving human health and welfare. According to this world view, "special money" must be raised to study women and people of color, so that the "regular money" can be reserved for "normal" research.[20]

Perhaps there was also a more insidious influence on the decisions about study populations. At least some scientists and government officials might have believed it was not important even to find out whether data from studies on white males applied to women and people of color. We cannot dismiss the possibility that the exclusionary practice reflected implicit social worth judgments on who ought to have priority in obtaining the fruits of biomedical research. An emphasis on the economic costs of human disease could also have inadvertently contributed to the view that research should focus on the "normal" economic contributor, that is, the young or middle-aged white male.[21]

In attempting to trace the origins of the exclusionary practice, we must consider as well the identity of the major players in the research establishment. Science has been and to some extent still is largely populated by white males. The same is true of NIH officialdom, although the agency's new director is Bernadine Healy, who has initiated a new program focusing on the specific health needs of women. A white male-dominated group will assess the nation's biomedical research priorities from a particular vantage point. Decisions by such a group could intentionally or inadvertently undervalue the health concerns of "outsiders." When one researcher asked investigators about the exclusion of African-Americans from clinical trials, many responded that they simply had "never thought about" the matter.[22] Congresswoman Olympia Snow put it succinctly in her comment on the choice to study men to assess obesity's impact on breast and uterine cancer: "Somehow, I find it hard to believe that the male-dominated medical community would tolerate a study of prostate cancer that used only women as research subjects."[23]

An overly simplistic concept of equality might also have helped to create homogeneous study populations. In many social contexts, advancing the ideal of equality requires decision-makers to disregard gender, racial, and ethnic differences among people. If all human beings have equal moral value, then in some sense they are identical and inter-changeable. If all people are identical, then it might appear that any human subject could adequately represent the general human population. In this framework, it would be unnecessary to recruit research subjects according to their gender, race, or ethnicity; the white male subject could stand for everyone. Gender, racial, and ethnic differences that affect health and disease must, however, be recognized if women and people of color are to have truly equal access to the health benefits of biomedical research.

Remedying the situation: The downside

Even though there are compelling reasons to conduct research on the possible health effects of gender, race, and ethnicity, one must also acknowledge that adverse conse-quences could flow from such research. Studies of women and particular racial and ethnic groups could indicate that these populations are more susceptible to conditions that reinforce group stereotypes. Thus, for example, research suggesting that monthly hormone fluctuations make women more prone than men to depression and other emotional dis-turbances could become potent ammunition for those seeking to exclude women from important policy positions. Certain evidence indicating significant physiological differ-ences between men and women could trigger controversy similar to that surrounding Carol Gilligan's work on gender differences in psychological and moral development, which some feminists see as strengthening the traditional picture of women as nurturing, sacrificing, and passive. When gender, racial, and ethnic differences are characterized as "natural," they may be deemed impervious to change. The role of environment in shaping human physiology and behavior can be ignored, thus reducing the pressure to minimize the environmental sources of difference.

Moreover, as Gilligan reminds us, our culture "hasn't been able to represent difference without hierarchy."[24] There is a danger that studies finding gender, racial, and ethnic health differences will be used to support unjust discrimination against historically ex-cluded groups. The employment and other discrimination experienced by African-Americans carrying sickle-cell trait is just one example of this pattern. Meanwhile, the potential value of certain health differences found in these groups could be ignored. For instance, women's relative physical endurance and longevity are differences that could justify a female-dominated workforce in at least some settings. Yet this biological ad-vantage has had virtually no influence on employment policy; instead, policies tend to focus on pregnancy- and family-related "problems" of employing women.

The lessons of exclusion

The revelations of gender and other biases in the study of human health reminds us of how far we are from fully escaping the discriminatory legacies of the past. Much of our current social structure still embodies, albeit often inadvertently, the idea that the white man is the best to represent all people. Yet in many significant respects, he is not. Biomedical research must respond to this reality.

The immediate task for scientists and government officials involves revamping study design and reordering funding priorities to remedy past exclusionary practices. The NIH and other funding agencies should back up their paper policies with concrete implementation measures, including the added financial expenditures that may be necessary to ensure more representative study populations. There is also a need for more carefully reasoned policies governing the inclusion of women – and men – of reproductive potential in clinical research. Institutional review boards ought to consider explicitly the composition of proposed study populations in determining whether the selection of subjects is equitable. But the remedies also extend beyond this realm. One task is to continue and to redouble the effort to reduce the disproportionate representation of white men in important scientific and policy positions. Diversity among powerful decisionmakers is one of the best methods to guard against conscious as well as unconscious discriminatory practices.

Second is the challenge to use the emerging knowledge about biological differences for the benefit of historically disadvantaged groups. Perhaps we have come far enough to recognize such differences without transforming them into tools for maintaining the traditional social hierarchy. Particular biological characteristics of women and members of nonwhite racial and ethnic groups must not be viewed through the narrow prism of the status quo, which too frequently labels "difference" as "problem." From a wider perspective, the contributions of people who are "different" can in some cases be "better." Moreover, sometimes, as Martha Minow has noted, it is the system that should adjust to embrace the difference. The goal is to move beyond the restrictive traditional patterns of labeling difference toward a richer, more expansive view.

Last is a message for bioethicists. The discovery of bias in selecting human subjects hints at the existence of other as yet unrevealed forms of bias in medicine and biomedical research. In this vein, a recent analysis of court decisions suggests that judges give less weight to incompetent women's prior statements on life-sustaining treatment than they do to men's. According to the authors, judges characterized men's remarks as mature, rational choices; in contrast, women's statements were deemed unreflective and emotional.[25]

Many of us in bioethics have been surprised by the recent disclosures of bias in clinical studies and practice. They serve notice that unjust discrimination in medicine and science can be more subtle than many of the issues on which we have focused our attention. Dramatic issues like surrogate motherhood and sex-selection indisputably raise serious ethical questions about the position of women in our society. The lesson of the recent revelations about research subject populations, however, is that we must also keep our eyes open to the subtler gender and other biases still plaguing contemporary medicine and science.

Notes

1. U.S. General Accounting Office, Statement of Mark Nadel, "National Institutes of Health: Problems in Implementing Policy on Women in Study Populations," 18 June 1990.
2. Andrew Purvis, "A Perilous Gap," *Time,* Special Issue on Women (Fall 1990), pp. 66–67; Joseph Palca, "Women Left Out at NIH," *Science* 248 (29 June 1990): 1601; Judy Grande,

"Gender Gap Plagues U.S. Health Studies," *Cleveland Plain Dealer,* 30 July 1990; "Aspirin Every Two Days Found to Reduce Migraines," *New York Times,* 3 October 1990. According to one NIH official, the study of breast and uterine cancer was considering the effects of particular nutrients on estrogen metabolism, and researchers chose male subjects in the belief that estrogen metabolism is similar in men and women.

3. Bruce Nussbaum, "Under-the-Counter Drug Testing," *New York Times,* 19 February 1991; Paul Cotton, "Is There Still Too Much Extrapolation from Data on Middle-Aged White Men?" *JAMA* 263 (23 February 1990): 1049–50; Kathleen Nolan, "AIDS and Pediatric Research," *Evaluation Review* 14 (October 1990): 464–81; Greg Sachs and Christine Cassel, "Biomedical Research Involving Older Human Subjects," *Law, Medicine and Health Care* 18 (Fall 1990): 234–43.

4. Warren Leary, "Uneasy Doctors Add Race-Consciousness to Diagnostic Tools," *New York Times,* 25 September 1990.

5. National Institutes of Health, Priority Announcement, "Special Instructions to Applicants Using Form PHS 398 Regarding Implementation of the NIH/ADAMHA Policy Concerning Inclusion of Women and Minorities in Clinical Research Study Populations," 1 December 1990.

6. Bernadine Healy, "Women's Health, Public Welfare," *JAMA* 226 (24 July 1991): 566–68.

7. Rebecca Dresser, "Measuring Merit in Animal Research," *Theoretical Medicine* 10 (1990): 21–34.

8. Food and Drug Administration, *General Considerations for the Clinical Evaluation of Drugs* (Washington, D.C.: U.S. Government Printing Office, 1977); Carol Levine, "Women and HIV/AIDS Research: The Barriers to Equity," *IRB: A Review of Human Subjects Research* 13, no. 1–2 (1991): 18–22.

9. Levine, "Women and HIV/AIDS Research."

10. Purvis, "A Perilous Gap."

11. *Automobile Workers v. Johnson Controls,* III S. Ct. 1196, 1991.

12. Mary Becker, "Can Employers Exclude Women to Protect Children?" *JAMA* (24 October 1990): 2113–17.

13. Palca, "Women Left Out."

14. Paul Cotton, "Examples Abound of Gaps in Medical Knowledge," *JAMA* 263 (23 February 1990): 1051–55.

15. Purvis, "A Perilous Gap"; "Sex Bias in Treatment of CAD Reported in SAVE Trial Review," *The Newspaper of Cardiology,* June 1990, p. 11; Richard Steingart, Milton Packer, Peggy Hamm, et al., "Sex Differences in the Management of Coronary Artery Disease," *NEJM* 325 (25 July 1991): 226–30.

16. Judy Grande, "Cleveland Clinic Struggles to Find Women for Heart Study," *Cleveland Plain Dealer,* 5 August 1990.

17. JoAnn Manson, Meir Stampfer, Graham Colditz, et al., "A Prospective Study of Aspirin Use and Primary Prevention of Cardiovascular Disease in Women," *JAMA* 266 (24 July 1991): 521–27.

18. Cotton, "Examples Abound."

19. Martha Minow, *Making All the Difference: Inclusion, Exclusion, and American Law* (Ithaca, N.Y.: Cornell University Press, 1990), pp. 49–74.

20. Cotton, "Examples Abound."

21. Council on Ethical and Judicial Affairs, American Medical Association, "Gender Disparities in Clinical Decision Making," *JAMA* 226 (24 July 1991): 559–62.

22. Cotton, "Is There Still Too Much Extrapolation?"

23. Grande, "Gender Gap."

24. Anastasia Toufexis, "Coming from a Different Place," *Time,* Special Issue on Women (Fall 1990), pp. 64–66.

25. Steven Miles and Allison August, "Courts, Gender and the 'Right to Die,'" *Law, Medicine and Health Care* 18 (Spring/Summer 1990): 85–95.

QUESTIONS FOR DISCUSSION

1. Identify several groups of people who are often recruited for medical research, but who may not be completely free to refuse to participate. What conditions might coerce them into becoming subjects? Should such groups automatically be excluded from research?

2. Is the Nuremberg Code's statement on the subject's freedom to withdraw from a research project adequate protection from the risks of unanticipated events? How do the researcher's responsibilities to stop a study complement this safeguard?

3. What are some of the difficulties inherent in relying on written consent documents to provide information on a research protocol? Who should obtain the subject's consent, and how?

RECOMMENDED SUPPLEMENTAL READING

"Ethics and Clinical Research," Henry K. Beecher, *New England Journal of Medicine,* 1966, 274, pp. 1354–1360.

Proceed with Caution. Predicting Genetic Risks in the Recombinant DNA Era, Neil A. Holtzman, Baltimore, MD: Johns Hopkins University Press, 1989.

"Gender Disparities in Clinical Decision Making," American Medical Association Council on Ethical and Judicial Affairs, *Journal of the American Medical Association,* 1991, 266, pp. 559–562.

"Research on Human Populations: National and International Guidelines," Bernard M. Dickens, Larry Gostin, & Robert J. Levine (eds.), *Law, Medicine & Health Care,* 1991, 19, pp. 157–266.

PART VII

The Use of Animals in Biological Research

INTRODUCTION

The use of animals in biomedical research is a topic of considerable public debate. Due to the controversial nature of experimentation with animal subjects, and its importance to biomedical research, it is vital for researchers to know and understand the differing views of others.

Many critics of research with animals believe that simply having the capacity to suffer, known as sentience, gives nonhuman animals the right to be treated as ends in themselves, rather than simply as means to human ends. Arthur Caplan claims that the burden of proof for justifying the use of animals rests with investigators. Since many animals are both sentient and purposive, he finds that they have a *prima facie* right to be left alone. For Caplan, the use of animals in research is tragic even where justified; at the least, researchers must recognize their moral responsibilities to animal subjects, eliminating waste and duplication and minimizing their suffering.

Among members of the scientific establishment there is increasing concern about the proper use and care of animals, and there are efforts worldwide to refine, reduce, replace, review, and regulate animal research. As society will be involved in determining whether and how animals will be used in science, it is essential that scientists engage in a constructive dialogue with their critics, and educate the public about the medical advances made possible by animal use.

21

Beastly conduct:
Ethical issues in animal experimentation

Arthur L. Caplan

The legitimacy of means and the legitimacy of ends in animal experimentation

There has been a great deal of argument in recent years over the subject of animal experimentation. Few topics are able to elicit the degree of moral vehemence and passion that this topic does. Accusations of moral blindness fly back and forth between vivisectionists and antivivisectionists. Bills are submitted almost willy-nilly at both the federal and state level, lobbying efforts on both sides of the issue are best described as fierce, and the disputants seem to delight in holding meetings and conferences at which their opponents are persona non grata – on both sides opponents are rarely invited, and, if they somehow manage to appear, they are made the object of calumny usually reserved only for criminals or even politicians (12).

Despite the political and sociological vortex surrounding the issue of animal experimentation, it would be wrong for those on either side to underestimate the sincerity and thoughtfulness that can underlie much of the noise and rhetoric characteristic of current public debates over the issue. In recent years a rather rich philosophical literature (10,11) has developed on the subject of the moral responsibilities of human beings toward animals, and this literature surely must be reckoned with by all parties to the debate. Just as it is wrong to suppose that all vivisectionists are callous brutes, unconcerned about the effects of their work on their animal subjects, it is also wrong to assume that all antivivisectionists are misanthropic kooks who are too emotionally unstable to recognize the benefits that derive from research involving animals.

Before considering some of the moral questions that arise in the context of the practice of experimentation involving animals, it is important to make a distinction between two issues that are often conflated by parties on both sides of the issue. Oftentimes scientists go to great lengths to demonstrate to each other and the general public that they take every possible precaution to assure the humane treatment of any animals that may be used for experimental purposes. Scientists often note with pride that they have, through their own voluntary efforts, established clear codes of conduct about the care and handling of laboratory animals. Moreover, most reputable scientists in America and other nations

From *Annals of the New York Academy of Science*, 1983, 406, pp. 159–169. The author wishes to acknowledge De Anti-Vivisectie Stichting of The Netherlands for the opportunity to present some of the material in this paper in a series of lectures at the Universities of Leiden, Groningen, Wachningen, Nijmegen, and the Free University of Amsterdam; Corrie Smid, Eleanor Seiling, Janet Caplan, and Peter Singer for helpful conversations regarding many of the ideas presented in this paper; and the support of the Marilyn M. Simpson Charitable Income Trust in preparing this paper. Reproduced with permission.

go to great lengths to minimize, through the use of anesthetics, anesthesia, and other means, the pain or suffering that animals endure as a result of the process of experimentation.

The many efforts now made to reduce animal suffering and to ensure the proper care and handling of animals used for research purposes are often brought forward in response to criticisms leveled by antivivisectionists concerning the enterprise of animal research. Unfortunately, persons who question the moral legitimacy of animal experimentation are not likely to be dissuaded from their view by demonstrations of the care and concern shown by those engaged in the practice.

There are really two issues involved in thinking about research involving animals and questions of humane care are pertinent only to one of them – (1) is it morally legitimate to conduct research upon animals?; (2) if it is morally permissible to utilize animals for research purposes, what moral responsibilities must be discharged by those engaged in such research? Questions on what conduct constitutes humane care, guidelines on the handling and transport of animal subjects, and efforts to teach students and professionals techniques that will minimize animal suffering and pain consequent to research interventions are all only relevant to the question of professional duty within the research context. However, before these issues can be usefully discussed, it is necessary to examine the prior question of whether it is morally justifiable to conduct any research on animals. For if the answer to this question is no, then no amount of guidelines, restraint, educational effort, or codified standards will suffice in response to criticisms of the activity.

The major areas of contention concerning the moral legitimacy of animal research

If one reviews the various public pronouncements (1,3,6,7,10,12) made about the issue of animal experimentation by parties on both sides of the issue, it quickly becomes evident that there exist three major areas of dispute. First, there is a good deal of disagreement about the need to conduct any research upon animals. Second, there is much disagreement about the moral value to be assigned to animals. Much of the attention to issues of animal sentience and consciousness in debates about the ethics of animal research are spin-offs from this issue since the more animals are felt to possess mental powers equivalent to or closely resembling those possessed by humans, the more various people feel disposed to assign moral worth to such creatures. Third, there is a good deal of tacit or between-the-lines argument about the moral priority that ought be accorded the whole issue of the ethics of animal experimentation. Many persons admit that the question of the legitimacy of animal experimentation is a vexing one, but there is no agreement over whether the topic is one that ought to command wide public attention and legislative concern. Other issues, such as human starvation, malnutrition, war, crime, poverty and the like are felt, oftentimes, to deserve precedence over the fates of animals in research laboratories (12).

It is interesting to compare and contrast the positions taken by the 'pro' and 'anti' vivisection camps on these three major issues. To some degree some of the stereotyping and caterwauling so characteristic of disputes over this issue can be defused by a little reflection over the stances adopted by the parties to the debate on the major question surrounding the legitimacy of the research enterprise.

The provivisection point of view

Need

Provivisectionists argue that it is ludicrous to talk at the present time about the complete replacement or elimination of animals from the context of experimentation. If human health and well-being are to be improved, if human safety is to be assured in both medical and non-medical contexts, and if human knowledge is to advance, then some amount of animal experimentation must be conducted. It is simply not possible, given our present knowledge, to utilize alternatives to animals and simultaneously maintain publicly acceptable levels of human health and well-being. In part, this is due to the fact that testing chemicals or pharmaceutical substances on cells or other limited organic systems fails to capture the complexities involved in the processing of such substances by whole organisms. The pursuit of such universally recognized human goods, as health, safety, and knowledge, requires that some animals be utilized in research contexts.

Moral equality

Most provivisectionists do not accept the equation of animals and humans as entities deserving of equal moral consideration and concern. Some believe that animals do not suffer or feel pain in ways analogous to that experienced by human beings, and, thus, do not deserve the same sort of protections and considerations as human beings do in experimental settings. Others favoring vivisection simply see human beings and their goals and purposes as more worthy of moral respect than the goals and purposes of members of the animal kingdom. Thus, the general health of human beings or the welfare of any specific individual human being counts for far more, in their view, than the well-being or health of any single animal or groups of animals. This view is reflected in the fact that scientists will often comment to each other in private that they have actually heard some antivivisectionists say that they would rather one baby be used for experimental purposes than one thousand rats. Such statements are held up as exemplifying the moral blindness of those who would equate animal welfare with human welfare.

Priority

Many persons involved with or supportive of the use of animals in experimental studies find it hard to believe that so much energy, money, and time is devoted to this issue by opponents of such practices. They note that there is plenty of misery about in both the human and animal kingdoms and that antivivisectionists might better devote their frenetic energies to obviating the many other clear injustices that exist in the world. Why, it is sometimes asked, don't antivivisectionists attempt to stop such practices as pet abuse, hunting, or meat-eating rather than focus as they do on animal research? The numbers of animals who suffer at the hands of humans are surely greater in these other contexts, and these would therefore seem to be more appropriate places for political and legislative intervention by those concerned with animal welfare.

The antivivisectionist point of view

Need

Antivivisectionists believe that while it may be true that not all animal experimentation can be abolished (some believe that all could), it is nevertheless true that far more could be eliminated than is presently the case. They argue that there exist many techniques for replacing animals in experiments, including cellular studies, computer simulations, and careful field studies upon animals in natural settings. Moreover, they argue, even more could be done in the way of replacement and reduction in the number of animals used in scientific research but for the pernicious influence of the animal breeding industry, which has no obvious interest in seeing animal experimentation curbed or in developing suitable substitutes for whole live animals. Antivivisectionists see the continued and ongoing reliance of scientists upon animal studies as the natural outcome of an economic and political situation in which various parties have powerful vested interests in assuring the continuance of the status quo with regard to animal research.

It should also be noted that while most opponents of animal research do not challenge the legitimacy of such goals as the assurance of human health and safety or the advancement of human knowledge, they find defenses of animal research couched in terms of these broad social goals inadequate. First, they argue, it is not clear that human knowledge is likely to be advanced by the kinds of studies and experiments to which animals are currently put by scientists. There is simply too much waste, replication, and redundancy in scientific experimentation to justify the toll imposed on animals in the name of advancing scientific knowledge. Second, it is not clear that human health is always advanced by animal research since ultimately all drugs and procedures must be tried on humans anyway.

More importantly, they note, a good deal of animal experimentation is conducted in order to assure the American consumer a suitable range of cosmetics, toiletries, and other aesthetic paraphernalia. These are hardly indispensable aspects of human existence, and the antivivisectionists have been quick to note that safety with regard to perfumes and underarm deodorants is hardly an awe-inspiring moral imperative when assessing the legitimacy of the animal sacrifices involved in order to attain safety with regard to these frivolous ends.

Moral equality

Sophisticated critics of the entire enterprise of animal research argue that science itself is in many ways responsible for skepticism about the acceptability of animal research. While there have existed strong traditions within both science and religion committed to the view that animals are nothing more than dumb brutes or automata, the fact is that scientific research has, over the years, revealed essential similarities between humans and animals with respect to many physical and mental properties. Surely, such critics note, we know enough about the physiology, neurology and behavioral capacities of higher vertebrates to make us realize that these creatures can feel pain, can suffer, and that they ought not be treated any differently than we would treat any human being endowed with such capacities and traits. There is an implicit demand for consistency behind much of the antivivisectionist opposition to research on animals – what we would not dream of doing to a child, a fetus, a newborn, a demented person, a retarded person, a senile person, a comatose person, or a dead person, we ought not dream of doing to a sentient animal.

The argument from consistency does not commit the antivivisectionist to the equation of animals and humans in terms of their moral worth. Rather, the view held by most antivivisectionists is that animals have the minimal properties capable of conferring moral standing upon an entity – sentience, consciousness, or the capacity to feel pain. These properties, or some one of them, seem sufficient for according moral status to animals. Animals and humans both possess, on this view, minimally sufficient attributes for becoming the objects of moral concern. Both kinds of organisms satisfy minimal requirements for being valued, and in this sense they ought be viewed as of equal moral worth.

Priority

While antivivisectionists argue that animals and humans are equal in terms of their both possessing capacities that qualify them for moral concern and respect, antivivisectionists give a higher priority to the need to attend to animal suffering than do many proponents of research. The primary reason that seems to motivate the view that animal suffering deserves our legislative and regulatory attention is that animals are not in a position to avoid the types of suffering they encounter in the laboratory. While it is true that animals cause each other harm in nature, the fact remains that the sorts of suffering they often encounter in research settings is entirely due to the activities of human beings. Human beings, thus, are responsible for inflicting an additional measure of pain and suffering upon creatures who are unable to protect themselves against these evils. While human beings can, assumedly, avoid at least some of the pain and misery they inflict on their fellows in various situations, animals in laboratories cannot and thus possess a special claim to human moral attention because they are so utterly dependent on humans for alleviating the suffering they encounter.

The issue of moral equality

Having presented the basic outlines of the dispute about animal experimentation, the rest of this essay will focus on the thorny question of the moral worth of animals and humans. For, if it is true that at least some partisans on both sides of the issue are in basic agreement that human health, well-being, and safety are desirable goods, and, that the production of human knowledge that promotes these ends is also good, then it would seem that the real issue dividing 'pro' and 'anti' vivisectionists is the degree to which sacrifices and concessions have to be made with regard to these goods in order to promote animal wellbeing and decrease animal suffering. Both the level of priority accorded the enterprise of animal experimentation as a moral question and the zeal with which alternatives to animal use are pursued pivot around the degree to which animals are seen as worthy of moral concern. The moral equality of animals and humans is thus the crucial issue dividing the two sides in current disputes, and it is this question which merits close, critical scrutiny if any progress is to be made toward settling the issue.

Much of the basis for the belief that animals and humans have an equal claim to moral consideration arises from an awareness of recent history in the discipline of ethics (11). During the past two hundred years or so, many human beings have come to realize that differences in sex, race, ethnic group, or sexual preference are not relevant properties for excluding individuals from the moral realm. The recent popularity of the story of the Elephant Man in the movies and on Broadway derives in part from the message conveyed by the leading character of the play, John Merrick, that despite his deformed and even ghastly appearance, he is still a person worthy of moral concern and respect. Physical form and appearance are not in themselves reasons for excluding someone or even something from the sphere of our moral concern. Thus, while animals are certainly different in their shape, form, and physical appearance from human beings, these differences are not in themselves sufficient for establishing a relevant moral difference between animals and humans any more than are the various shapes, colors, and sizes of human beings.

Some persons have turned to other criteria besides physical differences for distinguishing between the moral worth of animals and humans. Reason, language, intentionality, self-awareness, and a sense of personal identity have all been suggested as properties possessed by humans which distinguish them from animals with respect to their moral worth (2). But there are problems in using these properties as a basis for distinguishing animals from humans concerning moral worth. Many human beings lack some or all of the aforementioned properties. Certainly fetuses, comatose persons, and dead persons can be said to lack all of them. Yet, we do not feel free to do as we please with individuals who are in one of these categories of humanhood. It is also the case that the mental powers of many humans are, at various times, often severely impaired or entirely absent, i.e. when they are asleep, under the influence of drugs, etc., and yet we do not believe that the moral worth of such persons evaporates with the temporary disappearance of their mental powers.

Nor is it evident that animals lack the capacities and abilities to manifest some or all of the mental properties often held to distinguish man and beast. There is a voluminous literature in ethology and comparative psychology that indicates that at least some animals are capable of primitive forms of reasoning, intentionality, language, and self-awareness (1,3,5). Certainly enough evidence has accumulated in the behavioral and biological sciences to cast suspicions on claims for the complete absence of higher mental states and abilities in the animal world. Given the uncertainty surrounding the question of animal awareness, it seems reasonable, in light of what we know about other similarities and commonalities between humans and animals, to err in the direction of commonality when in doubt until definitive evidence can be produced – that what has proven true with regard to genetic, morphological, physiological, biochemical, and anatomical properties is not true with respect to mental properties.

Given the fact that not all humans always possess fully developed mental powers and the likely circumstance that at least some animals do, there would appear to be no basis for drawing a hard and fast line between animals and humans in terms of physical or mental properties. What is important about this claim is that the moral worth of entities does seem linked in important ways to abilities and capacities to suffer, feel pain, or have their goals and purposes frustrated. While it is evident that bodily form or physical appearance are unimportant in deciding whether one ought to be concerned about the welfare of another creature, it is true that certain properties must be presumed if talk about welfare is to make any sense. The ability to feel pain, to suffer anxiety or stress, and the capacity to have one's desires, purposes, or intentions frustrated, all seem to be grounds for speaking meaningfully about the welfare of something. If a creature can experience pain, then, other things being equal, it certainly seems wrong to inflict pain on that creature. Similarly, if an organism, be it human or animal, seeks to fulfill some purpose or end – to drink some water, return home, to rest—it seems wrong (again, other things being equal) to frustrate such desires or purposes.

Sentience and purposiveness seem to be the kinds of properties that confer moral worth on creatures. Any entity, human or non-human, terrestrial or nonterrestrial, that could reasonably be said to possess sentience or purpose seems to be the sort of thing to which it is reasonable to attribute moral worth (4,6). Unless some reason can be given for interfering with or hindering a creature so endowed, it seems inherently wrong to inflict pain on a sentient entity or to frustrate the purposes and goals of such a creature.

It is with respect to the properties of sentience or purposiveness that humans and animals can be said to be of equal moral worth. Most humans and many animals seem to possess some degree of sentience. They are alert to stimuli and will seek those they find pleasant and attempt to avoid those they find noxious. Many animals and most humans seem to harbor any number of desires, aspirations, intentions, and purposes as can be inferred from the efforts they will make to attain certain goals or to overcome certain obstacles that may stand between them and the objects of their desires. While the issue of sentience and purposiveness is in part a scientific question, at least with regard to the distribution and degree of such properties in the biological world, there would seem to be good reasons for thinking that these properties represent excellent candidates for conferring moral worth upon entities (4).

It should be noted that in arguing that sentience and purposiveness are sufficient properties for attributing moral worth to an entity, this does not mean that both or either property is necessary for having moral worth. Creatures may someday be found on this or other planets that lack these traits, but possess still others that might make them objects of our moral respect. Moreover, the fact that an entity possesses sentience or purposiveness only satisfies the minimal conditions requisite for having moral worth. It may be possible to distinguish further among various creatures as to which ones have more or higher degrees of these salient features. It would surely be a logical error to infer from the fact that animals meet minimal conditions for having moral worth that there are no relevant differences with respect to these properties that distinguish humans and animals – for example, few animals will modify their behavior toward other animals as a result of reading this paper, while it is possible that some human beings may do so.

If it is true that the existence of sentience and/or purposiveness are sufficient traits for imputing moral worth to someone/something, then it would seem there exists what philosophers term *prima facie* duties (2,9) that ought be exercised toward such creatures. Unless one can justify the behavior by an appeal to some higher moral reason or purpose, it would be wrong to harm or frustrate any creature, including an animal, for no reason. Perhaps the cruelest or meanest activity that humans can engage in is the harming or frustrating of others, human and animal, for no reason other than simple meanness of spirit. In some ways human beings are actually in a better position than minimally endowed animals to cope with the frustration and pain of being deceived, fooled, hindered, tricked, or duped since humans are at least bright enough to occasionally figure out what is going on and take steps to avoid or end their suffering. Animals, confronted with malevolent owners or mischievous children, are competent enough to serve as the objects of malevolent intentions (as the pet owners or children know all too well), but are not competent enough to avoid or evade their plight.

It is important to distinguish between an entity's having moral worth, a status I have argued derives from the properties of sentience and purposiveness, and an entity's being a moral agent. Or, in other words, to distinguish between being a moral object and a moral agent. It is true that many animals and some humans lack all of the properties of mentation we commonly associate with *Homo sapiens*. It would be ludicrous to think that we could hold all animals and humans morally responsible for their actions or that we should expect moral reciprocity from any creature capable of sentience and purpose. What is sufficient in terms of properties that concern moral worth or standing is hardly sufficient in terms of properties that confer moral agency and moral responsibility. We need not determine the nature of the properties that would be sufficient for establishing moral competence among creatures (although it is interesting to note that historically not a few animals have been punished by their owners and even by courts as liable for the untoward outcomes of their behavior!) in this paper. All that need be noted is that the class of moral agents is far smaller than the class of moral objects, and that arguments about the moral equality of animals and humans concern the latter status and not the former.

Sentience and purposiveness as criteria of moral worth

I have argued thus far that both sentience and purposiveness seem to me to be properties sufficient for conferring moral worth on entities who possess them. However, I have not faced the question of whether these properties must both be present, or whether either one of them is sufficient by itself for establishing moral worth. Since moral considerableness entails a number of responsibilities on human agents in terms of their not harming or interfering with creatures that have moral worth, it is important to look carefully at these two properties to see whether they are independent and individually adequate for conferring moral worth.

In recent arguments about the ethics of animal experimentation, some philosophers (10,11), notably and most vocally Peter Singer in his book *Animal Liberation,* have argued for the sufficiency of sentience as a property for conferring moral worth upon entities. Singer presents a four-part argument in this book that runs as follows: (1) Any creature that is sentient has an interest in not suffering and not feeling pain; (2) all interests must be taken into account in deciding how we ought to behave; (3) equal interests in not suffering or experiencing pain must be counted equally; (4) we should act to bring about the greatest amount of good and to minimize suffering and pain. Thus, if animals can suffer and feel pain as a result of being sentient, Singer argues we must treat them impartially in assessing the practice of animal experimentation. What counts is not only the degree to which human safety is assured and human health promoted, but the degree to which animal suffering is exacerbated by experimental procedures. We should not engage in any particular experiment where the degree of suffering or pain produced in sentient creatures is not outweighed by the amount of benefit to be produced for other sentient creatures, animal and human.

Singer's position is one of classical utilitarianism – the costs and benefits of every action must be computed as best as can be done and decisions about the acceptability or non-acceptability of any action or practice turn on the beliefs we have about the overall effects of the action or practice in terms of goods versus suffering produced. In most cases, Singer argues (11), animal experiments fail to be justifiable since, given animal sentience, the degree of suffering involved cannot, with certainty, be predicted to be outweighed by the goods to be obtained by engaging in any given case of animal experimentation. Since we should be impartial as to the source of suffering when it occurs, animals and humans being equally deserving of moral consideration when they are capable of suffering or feeling pain, we ought to modify our current experimental practices accordingly and drastically decrease the use of animals in research.

The difficulties confronting Singer's criterion of sentience and his four-part argument are many (9,10). For example, it is not clear that most scientists would disagree with the claim that human benefit ought outweigh animal suffering if animal experimentation is to be morally legitimated (12). Indeed, as critics of Singer's view point out, the issue of how much suffering is caused by animal experiments is an empirical question and it is not clear that the benefits do outweigh the harms in assessing most cases of animal research.

More seriously, Singer's argument against animal experiment founders on two other issues. First, his position would seem to permit experimentation on any creatures which cannot, for whatever reason, suffer or feel pain. Thus, if we can make animal experimentation, or human experimentation for that matter, pain-free, we would appear to be justified in conducting research that would produce benefits in terms of health, well-being, safety, or knowledge. Also, if we could produce vast benefits to animals or humans by utilizing only a few animals or humans in painful experiments, this practice would also escape moral condemnation since, on Singer's construction of the argument, it is only the net outcome of experimentation that legitimates the activity.

I suspect that sentience and the corresponding ability it confers upon animals to suffer or feel pain is a bit too lofty a standard to invoke in thinking about the question of moral worth. It seems wrong to treat humans or animals who are incapable of suffering or feeling pain as undeserving of moral respect and consideration. For example, even if a human being were rendered unable to feel pain or to suffer by surgical intervention or through the use of drugs, I doubt whether members of our society would want to say that such persons could then be used in any way scientists deemed useful in the process of research.

It is interesting to note that Singer's view, while popular in antivivisectionist circles these days, does not lead to the view that all animal experimentation is wrong. Nor does it lead to the view that animals have rights – a concept that is antithetical to a utilitarian analysis of moral worth. However, if we look to purposiveness and intentionality rather than sentience and the ability to suffer as the standard of moral worth, I think we come closer to locating the kind of criterion that motivates much of the moral concern about animal experimentation.

If animals and humans are so organized as to be purposive creatures with various desires, drives, intentions, and aspirations, it seems wrong to cavalierly frustrate these purposes. It might be argued that if animals and humans are biologically constituted so as to pursue their own existence, which is a fact quite consistent with current thinking in evolutionary theory, then it is morally wrong to interfere with or deprive animals of the opportunity to fulfill this basic drive. In other words, animals and humans, endowed by nature with a will to survive, have a right to survive – rights being consequent upon the purposiveness and teleological orientation of living things (9). If all creatures who possess purposiveness have a right to be left alone to pursue their ends, then the basic moral repugnance felt by many people about animal experimentation can be easily under-stood – most experimentation deprives animals of the right to exist, or, at minimum, frustrates certain basic drives and intentions they manifest. While human beings are under no moral obligation to aid their fellows or animals in the pursuit of their basic purposes, they do appear to be under some constraint not to uncaringly interfere with other organisms.

I believe that purposiveness rather than sentience is a property that suffices for conferring moral worth upon entities. When organisms have sufficient organization to have basic drives, desires, and intentions, be they amoebas, bees, birds, or retarded humans, it is wrong to interfere with their efforts to fulfill these desires. It needs to be quickly added that such interference is wrong unless there exists some other reason or justification for doing so. The fact is that, as is the case with the abortion debate, most persons erroneously believe that once animal rights are established, the issue of animal experimentation is settled (2). If it is wrong to interfere with purposive creatures, then no animal research could ever be morally legitimate. But such a view confuses the question of how moral worth and moral rights arise with the question of what to do when rights conflict – a common, ordinary, and unavoidable consequence of the nature of the world we live in.

No animals or humans capable of purposiveness should be interfered with by others, other things being equal. But other things are rarely equal. If humans are to survive, they must eat, and animals may have to suffer the consequences. If human beings are to fulfill their desires to have medicines, then some creatures will have to suffer in the course of discovering whether different substances have therapeutic value. While it is true that we ought not interfere with or hinder the bringing to fruition of the desires and purposes of others, animals and humans, in a world of limited resources and conflicting purposes, some creatures will, of necessity, have their basic rights overridden.

The legitimacy of animal experimentation reconsidered

It should be evident from the preceding discussion that science has no one to blame but itself for the existence of worries about the ethics of animal experimentation. Science has shown the degree to which sentience and purposiveness permeate the animal kingdom, and thus has raised doubts about the validity of causing harm to or interfering with creatures who may not differ all that much from human beings in the properties that count from a moral point of view. If sentience or, minimally, purposiveness are sufficient for conferring moral worth on things, and if we are to be consistent in our moral practices and beliefs, then we may have to rethink our ordinary attitudes about the legitimacy of animal experimentation.

Perhaps the strongest caveat to emerge from an analysis of the morality of animal research is that the burden of proof always rests upon the experimenter to justify the use of animals in experimental contexts. The antivivisectionist has nothing to prove; many animals used in experiments are sentient and purposive, and thus have *prima facie* rights to live and be left alone. Those who would override or abrogate these rights must provide compelling reasons for doing so. Humility and sensitivity, not arrogance and hubris, must be the hallmarks of animal research since it is only out of ignorance and expediency that we put members of the animal kingdom to our purposes rather than theirs.

The other conclusion that follows from the analysis of the moral legitimacy of animal experimentation is that such activity is always morally tragic. No matter what goods are promoted by the process, some creatures who are unable to alter their circumstances will have their basic rights of life and fulfillment infringed. Since this is so, it would seem imperative that steps be taken to reduce waste and duplication in the use of animals for research purposes, put more funds toward the development of alternatives to animal testing, and make the public aware of the moral trade-offs that must be faced in deciding how best to achieve human well-being, health, safety, and knowledge at the expense of animal suffering. Ultimately, the public will have to decide what sorts of trade-offs are morally acceptable when animal and human interests conflict.

References

1. Bowd, A. D. 1980. Ethical reservations about psychological research with animals. Psychol. Rec. **30**(Spring): 201–210.
2. Caplan, A. L. 1978. Rights language and the ethical treatment of animals. *In* Implications of History and Ethics to Medicine – Veterinary and Human. L. McCullough & J. P. Morris, Eds.: 126–135. Texas A&M University Press. College Station, Tex.
3. Fox, M. S. 1981. Experimental psychology, animal rights, welfare and ethics. Psychopharm. Bull. **17**(2): 80–84.
4. Goodpaster, K. E. 1978. On being morally considerable. J. Phil. **76**(6): 308–324.
5. Griffin, D. R. 1976. The Question of Animal Awareness. Rockefeller University Press. New York.
6. Hoff, C. 1980. Immoral and moral uses of animals. N. Eng. J. Med. **302**(2): 115–118.
7. Morris, R. K. & M. W. Fox, Eds. 1978. On the Fifth Day: Animal Rights and Human Ethics. Acropolis Books. Washington, D.C.
8. Passmore, J. 1976. Man's Responsibility For Nature. Scribner's. New York.
9. Regan, T. 1980. Animal rights, human wrongs. Environ. Ethics **2**(2): 99–120.
10. Regan, T. & P. Singer, Eds. 1976. Animal Rights and Human Obligations. Prentice-Hall. Englewood Cliffs, N.J.
11. Singer, P. 1975. Animal Liberation. Avon Books. New York.
12. Visscher, M. B. 1979. Animal rights and alternative methods. The Pharos (Fall): 11–19.

22
Use of animals in experimental research: A scientist's perspective

Ruth Ellen Bulger

Modern science has made great strides toward understanding basic biological processes and toward improving the health and safety of humankind and of certain animal species. The discoveries of antibiotics, vaccines, and other treatment modalities, and technologies such as transplantation surgery, are only a few of the remarkable advances made possible partly by the use of experimental animals in research. But what have been the costs of these advances with respect to animals sacrificed during the process of discovery? The Office of Technology Assessment (1986) estimates that 17–22 million vertebrates are used each year. Other estimates are considerably higher. A.N. Rowan (1984) estimated that a total of 70 million animals are utilized yearly, 40% being used for research, 20% for toxicology testing, 26% for drug development, 8% for teaching, and 6% for other purposes. Can this use and destruction of animals be justified in moral terms by the counterbalancing of the good accomplished in improving the health and safety of human beings and animals?

This paper will look briefly at the thoughts of certain philosophers about the use (or misuse) of animals for the explicit purposes of human beings. The concerns of philosophers, and subsequently of bioethicists, have intensified recently as the latter group has tried to assess moral rights of humans (including infants, those comatosed, or those severely retarded) and then to relate these rights to those of animals. The concerns related to animal use were crystalized into a movement called "animal liberation" by the appearance of a book by Peter Singer (1975) called *Animal Liberation: A New Ethic for Our Treatment of Animals* pertaining to how moral standing can be attributed to a person or object (Caplan, 1984). Singer says that we not only practice sexism and racism, but we practice "speciesism." Society maintains that human beings are better than animals, but Singer believes that all animals are equal and, therefore, human suffering is morally the same as animal suffering. This present paper will therefore review some basic premises of individuals and groups who wish to accord to animals rights that are equivalent to those normally afforded to humans, and to consider what the implications of this position are to research based on animal experimentation.

The concerns of animal rights groups have stimulated both laws and other regulatory activities by the legislative, executive, and judicial branches of our government, resulting in considerable tightening of standards by which animals can be utilized for research purposes. Such actions have profound effects on research and therefore necessitate that individual scientists and their professional societies understand the positions of animal rights groups, define their own positions, and interpret their use of animals to the rest of

From *Anatomical Record,* 1987, 219, pp. 215–220. Reprinted by permission of Wiley-Liss, a division of John Wiley and Sons, Inc.

society (if warranted). It also makes mandatory that scientists, who wish to continue their use of animal models, establish meaningful codes of behavior to regulate their own practices with respect to animal experimentation before their actions are entirely mandated by others; these codes must be such as to encourage maximal benefit from the use of these valuable animals in research and the minimization of pain experienced by the animals.

Philosophers and animal use

Then God said, "Let Us make man in Our image, according to Our likeness; and let them rule over the fish of the sea and over the birds of the sky and over the cattle and over all the earth, and over every creeping thing that creeps on the earth." Genesis 1:26

Although Aristotle (384–322 BC) made anatomic dissections of animals for scientific study and teaching, the first recorded experiments on living animals were performed by Erasistratus of Alexandria (304–258 BC), who studied the function of the airways and heart in a pig (Fox, M.A., 1986; Shapiro, 1986). Since that time, animal experimentation has been an integral part of the process of accumulation of knowledge about anatomy and physiology. Philosophers had little problem justifying such use, since animals were not generally thought to be the moral equivalent of human beings. Augustine (354–430 AD) recognized that animals suffered pain but did not find them related to us by a common nature, since they lacked a rational soul (Rowan, 1984). Since God had given human beings rule over animals, St. Thomas Aquinas (1225–1274) felt their treatment was a matter of indifference, except that individuals were encouraged to pity animals in pain as a matter of human compassion (Rowan, 1984). Descartes (1596–1650) had no objections to use of animals in experiments, since he denied that they could feel pain. He viewed animals only as complex machines (Levine, 1984). Human bodies, he said, were distinguished from animal bodies because of the presence of an immortal human soul. Ensoulment for Descartes was distinguished by the capacity to use language and ensouled beings included all and only human beings (Benjamin, 1987).

Locke (1632–1704) and Hume (1711–1776), on the basis of empirical observations, did not find animals to be like machines. Locke found causing pain and death to animals to be morally wrong, and Hume argued that the minds of animals and humans worked in the same way (Rowan, 1984). Animals were not seen as self-conscious by Kant (1724–1804) and hence were only a means to an end – the end being man. He found cruelty to animals to be wrong, since a person predisposed to being cruel to animals might "become hard also in his dealings with" human beings (Lloyd, 1986; Benjamin, 1987). A utilitarian thesis was proposed by Jeremy Bentham (1748–1831) in which pain and pleasure governed behavior. He likewise proposed a system to achieve the greatest happiness for the greatest number. Since the ability to experience pain or pleasure determines whether a being qualifies for moral consideration, both human beings and animals qualify equally according to these ideas (Benjamin, 1987; Rowan, 1984). This capacity to experience pain is called sentience.

Claude Bernard (1813–1878) was one of the most respected scientists of the nineteenth century. He recognized that experiments must be done on either human beings or animals, and as too many dangerous experiments were already undertaken on human beings, it was essentially moral to experiment on animals, even though the experiments might be painful or dangerous to the animal, if the results were useful to human beings (Bernard, in Reisen, 1977). The thought that human beings were different qualitatively from other animals was challenged by the theory of evolution proposed by Darwin, according to Bates and Humphrey (1956), who recognized the relationships among the species. "I have now recapitulated the facts and considerations which have thoroughly convinced one that species have been modified, during the long course of descent. This has been effected chiefly through the natural selection of numerous successive, slight, favourable variations" (Bates and Humphrey, 1956, p. 251). Darwin's work proposed that differences between human beings and animals were only those of degree, not of kind.

Two other groups of individuals became part of the debate on the moral status of animals, the antivivisectionists and the bioethicists. Bioethics is a systematic study of questions of value that arise in biomedical and behavioral fields (Walters and Kahn, 1986). Major moral principles in bioethics are the same as those debated in ethics more generally such as nonmaleficence, beneficence, justice, equality, veracity, and autonomy (Bok, 1977). In considering such acts as euthanasia bioethicists have become involved in considering the relevance of various abilities possessed by human fetuses, handicapped newborns, and severely demented and permanently comatosed individuals to their moral status. Since certain nonhuman animals have similar or even more developed capabilities than some groups of human beings, certain bioethicists have questioned our moral values with respect to these animals (Dresser, 1986).

Antivivisectionism began as a major movement in Victorian England in the mid-nineteenth century. The group was a diverse one that expressed concern about animal suffering, advocated abolition of animal experiments, and campaigned for passage of corrective legislation (Levine, 1984). This group also served as a mostly reactionary outlet for anxieties stemming from changes in society and its values relating to such areas as the idea that experimental medicine was a threat to the religious and moral foundations of society (Fox, M.A., 1984).

More recently, organizations that are active in attempting to ban animal research call themselves "animal liberation," "animal rights," or "moral rights" movements. These groups have been influenced by the concerns of bioethicists. Many of them build their case on the platform of the equal status of animals and human beings (Levine, 1984). Tannenbaum lists various views to which these moral rights groups often subscribe, including the belief that the majority of animals (including companion, farm, and laboratory mammals) not only have moral rights, but have the same rights as human beings. They are held to have these rights at least in part because they have many of the same mental capabilities and activities as people. Animals' moral rights are violated when they are used as food or in research without their consent. Laws should enforce their moral rights including the ability to have lawsuits brought forth on their behalf. Groups that subscribe to some or all of these doctrines include the Animal Legal Defense Fund, the Animal Liberation Front, The Coalition to End Animal Suffering in Experiments, The International Society for Animal Rights, The People for the Ethical Treatment of Animals, and The United Action for Animals (Tannenbaum, 1986).

Shapiro (1986) named 80 bills introduced in state legislatures aimed at curbing or banning the use of animals in research. He also noted the complacency of research scientists in countering these groups. Trull and Kalikow (1984) have called attention to the fact that animal rights groups are now dominated by experienced activist social reformers who are transforming the movement into sophisticated and effective organizations.

The two lines of social reform represented by the antivivisectionists and bioethicists became partially confluent in 1975 with Peter Singer's *Animal Liberation* (Singer, 1975), in which Singer maintained that animals can experience pain and suffering and that this property of sentience alone is sufficient to confer moral worth upon them. In his view, our society is guilty of "speciesism," the biased contention that human beings are superior to other animals. Singer posits that any creature that is sentient has an interest in not suffering; that the interests of all species must be taken into account in deciding any action or policy; that the interests of all species including human beings and other animals should count equally; that we should always act to maximize good and to minimize the suffering, animals' interests being weighted equally with those of humans. He takes the utilitarian view, believing that experiments are justifiable only when they give rise to more good than suffering. Most animal experiments do not pass this test according to his evaluation. Animal experiments are justifiable, in his view, only when we would consider using a human, "even a retarded human," for this same experiment (Caplan, 1984).

Since the publication of *Animal Liberation* in 1975, a variety of other ethicists and animal welfare proponents have taken stands on whether animals have moral rights, moral worth, moral value, natural rights, or intrinsic worth. They have then tried to weigh these rights with respect to the rights of human beings, using a variety of criteria to determine whether animal rights exist. The most frequently used criterion has been the possession of sentience. In assigning this criterion, various individuals have stressed behavioral and neurophysiological similarities between human beings and other animals (Benjamin, 1987; Dubner, 1983; Fox, M.A., 1984). Since pain can be caused by both doing and not doing experiments, and the pain responses of animals are largely unknown, more research into animal pain and its prevention is warranted (Kitchell, 1983; Overcast and Sales, 1985).

Others have attempted to use the distinction between simple consciousness and self-reflective consciousness as a criterion for differentiation between animals and human beings and their respective rights, finding human beings more highly developed with respect to self-reflective consciousness and claiming therefore greater moral worth for human beings (Benjamin, 1987). The conclusion that a definite line can be drawn between species on the basis of these criteria can be challenged by the findings of Darwin, from which a gradual evolution of self-consciousness might be deduced (Bates and Humphrey, 1956; Overcast and Sales, 1985). The use of language and cognition has also been used in support of the greater moral worth of humans (Ristau, 1983). However, research into animal behavior indicates that chimpanzees have both problem-solving and analytical ability (Fox, M.A., 1984) and that a variety of species have some degree of awareness, cognition, and language (1986).

There is no consensus on the existence of animal rights; and in instances where agreement on animal rights does exist, there is no agreement regarding the underlying derivation of these rights. The conclusions drawn from the presence or absence of rights also vary among the individuals who propose them. It seems that there are about as many views on the subject as there are viewers. Paton (1984) finds no basis for the claim of natural rights for animals, but agrees that they do have inherent worth; humans can accept duties to animals because of this natural worth. M.A. Fox (1984) sees animal experimentation as ethically sound because it is morally neutral. He says that animals have value only from benefits derived by human use, but he argues that they should not be mistreated since the mistreatment of animals diminishes human moral character. Hoff (1980) finds human beings unique but claims that animals do have moral standing. It is therefore wrong to use animals in research unless some major benefit for human beings or other animals results. Tannenbaum (1986) holds that animals have moral rights and inherent moral value independent of humans. Caplan (1984) maintains that animals are sentient and possess purposiveness; he therefore recognizes their prima facie rights to live and be left alone; the burden of proof of the necessity to use animals in research rests upon the scientist in each experimental context. Caplan asserts it is imperative that steps be taken to reduce waste and duplication in animal research and that more funding be used for developing alternatives. M.W. Fox (1986) maintains that animals have natural rights, intrinsic worth, and interests, and possibly souls. These animal rights pose moral injunctions that constitute a humane and ecologically sound ethic. He argues that it is imperative for humankind to develop moral laws and codes to protect plant and animal species (Fox, 1981).

It is noteworthy that the arguments of these observers (all males) revolve around the concerns of justice and rights. One of the most profound recent observations made about the moral development of human beings is that not only justice and rights are important (Kohlberg, 1970), but also the capacity for caring relationships (Gilligan, 1982). The fact that certain animals have a well-developed ability to set up meaningful relationships with each other and with human beings in the past has never been mentioned as being of any worth. Some of the opinions of animal rights advocates that are dismissed as sentimentality by scientists may have a basis in their unstated recognition of this ability in animals, which is, in fact, now considered to be of moral significance for human beings (Gilligan, 1982).

Dresser (Dresser, 1986) divides these contemporary positions in respect to animal treatment into three categories:

1. The "humane treatment" view concentrates on improving the quality of the life of laboratory animals without compromising the benefits that can be derived from their use in research. The animal's interests in avoiding pain, suffering, and distress are of enough moral significance to require that the research must advance the welfare of others.

2. The utilitarian view determines the morality of specific research projects according to the balance between the harm to the experimental animals and the anticipated benefits to human beings. The exact weighing is problematic because of the uncertainty in assessing the positive and negative experiences of animals in relation to those of human beings and in assessing the ultimate benefit of the knowledge to be gained.

3. The deontological, or rights-based, position argues that all animals have specific rights that should almost always have priority over the general rights of others. This is held to be true even though animals are dependent on others to assert their rights. The proper extent of this protection is, however, disputed by various individuals.

Scientific progress and regulation

Animals have been used in research to provide a variety of kinds of information. Research in the basic sciences increases our scientific understanding of biology but does not always relate immediately to solving a known health problem. Much of this information subsequently becomes important to the understanding and treatment of disease, but the lag time between discovery and clinical use can be long and unpredictable; and some of this information is more purely of intellectual worth. Other research is more directly clinical and its use in promoting better health is more rapidly obvious with a shorter lag period.

Another major area of animal use involves the testing of the short- and long-term safety of human exposure to various chemicals and drugs. The development of new chemotherapeutic agents and other treatment modalities constitutes a fourth area of animal experimentation. Bioassays that utilize animals, and animal sources of biological products such as antibodies or hormones also consume animals. Finally, animals are used in education at all levels. The work of Archibald et al. (1985), Lloyd (1986), Dukelow (1983), Fox, M.A. (1984) and Fox, M.W. (1986) document some of the information gained through the use of animals.

There has been increasing interest in alternatives to the use of animals in research, testing, and education (Office of Technology Assessment, 1986). Alternatives will not eliminate animal use, since animals will still be needed to study problems that involve various organ systems acting in concert or studies of recovery after injury, but alternative methods can be used for studies of processes occurring on a less complex level. Changing the testing procedures for toxicity studies would make a substantial impact on the number of animals used. In fact, some changes have already taken place. One of the oldest, most criticized, and least sophisticated animal tests is the LD_{50} test (which determines the lethal dose for 50% of the test animals) used as a screen for short-term toxicity. Such tests have been modified to utilize three to ten times fewer animals (Holden, 1986; Fox, M.A., 1984). A second much-criticized test used for product testing is called the Draize eye irritancy test, in which substances to be tested are placed on the cornea of rabbits' eyes. This test is also being modified to use lower doses of less concentrated solutions. In vitro methods to test the irritancy of such substances are currently under development. One such method utilizes the chorioallantoic membrane of a chick embryo (Office of Technology Assessment, 1986).

Other replacement technologies being developed include the use of chemical tests to replace bioassays; the use of microbiological tests for carcinogenicity screening, such as the Ames test using *Salmonella* bacteria or a newer modification called the Hayes test, which uses *E. coli* (Rowan, 1984; Fox, M.A., 1984); cell or organ culture (which can even be done on tissues derived from human beings) for a variety of uses such as cell biology, toxicity testing, and carcinogenesis; the use of isolated perfused organs or tissues, or isolated single cells to study a variety of cell and organ functions; the exploitation of computers for data processing, drug predictions, molecular conformation studies, modeling of organ function, teaching of students, and improved literature searches to avoid duplication of experiments (Fox, 1984); the use of mannequins, mechanical models, or audiovisual aids for teaching; and, in certain specific cases, the use of human in place of animal experimentation. Human beings have been used in autoexperimentation and epidemiological studies, and as volunteers in well-controlled studies undertaken with proper oversight and informed consent. In this regard, however, it is important to point out that both the Nuremberg Code (1977) and the Helsinki Declaration (World Medical Association, 1977) do require that all protocols be based on results from adequately performed laboratory and animal experiments.

Although continued work to provide well-substantiated models using animal alternatives is important, Watkins (1986) has reported a decrease in funding provided by companies this year for support of the laboratories at the Rockefeller University that are involved with in vitro toxicological assay development. Some funding for development of alternate methods to animal testing procedures for investigators is being provided by the International Foundation for Ethical Research (Watkins, 1986).

A variety of federal and state laws, regulations, and policies now affect the use of animals in research by investigators. These include the following important documents.

1. The Animal Welfare Act (Public Law 99–198), revised in 1985, requires humane handling, care, treatment, and transportation of animals by dealers, research facilities, and exhibitors. Each institutional facility needs to provide assurances that professionally acceptable standards are followed in experiments, to describe procedures likely to produce animal pain or distress, to provide adequate veterinary care, and to ensure that alternatives to those painful procedures have been considered.

2. The Health Research Extension Act of 1985 (Public Law 99–158) mandates the establishment of animal care committees at all locations doing biomedical or behavioral research with Public Health Service funds. Applicants for National Institutes of Health funding must demonstrate compliance with the act. In addition, each facility must show that training in humane animal maintenance and care has been provided. This is a federal law enforcing part of the previously existing Public Health Service policy.

3. The Guide for the Care and Use of Laboratory Animals (Department of Health and Human Services, 1985) gives guidelines to which all institutions receiving Public Health Service funding must adhere for professional and humane care and use of laboratory animals.

4. The Public Health Service Policy on Humane Care and Use of Laboratory Animals by Awardee Institutions (NIH, 1986) is a policy that ensures professional use and care of vertebrate animals involved in Public Health Service-supported research, training, and testing. It includes provisions for the training and instruction of scientists, animal technicians, and others involved in animal care, treatment, or use. It specifies procedures for establishing institutional animal care and use committees.

In addition, most states have statutes that forbid cruelty to and neglect of animals. Some states regulate the use of pound animals for research purposes. Inglehart (1985) and Overcast and Sales (1985) have reviewed some of this legislation.

A scientist's statement

When it is deemed morally legitimate to conduct research on animals, one must consider which moral responsibilities must be discharged by those engaged in animal-based experimental research (Caplan, 1983, 1984). Scientists not only should be committed to the welfare of animals used in experimental procedures, but should ensure that society understands their concerns.

The statement of practice that is proposed in this paper relies heavily on the "humane treatment" view of animal experimentation (Dresser, 1986). Whether humane treatment of animals derives its moral sanction from the effects on other human beings or derives from the animals' inherent rights, it is morally relevant for scientists to treat animals humanely. The aspects of this statement that stem from humane animal treatment are now supported by federal laws and regulations as well. The statement that follows also derives partially from considerations of a utilitarian view of balancing pain and suffering of animals against ultimate benefits to be derived from the research for human beings and other animals.

In light of the views of many members of society, and owing to the suffering of animals that does occur as a result of scientific research, it is important for scientists to question their goals and methods as they devise research protocols. In my opinion, however, the balancing is better done by the individual scientists with review by the animal care and use committees of their institution than by some external force such as that of law, since the scientists are in the best position to evaluate all aspects of the experiments. The following statement is not derived from the deontological position. There is much disagreement in our pluralistic society about the morality of this deontological position. As a scientist, I personally do grant inherent worth to animals and have decided in my own studies to avoid certain types of experiments that I believe violate these animal rights. This is a conviction that ultimately is derived from personal beliefs that are not common to all of society; therefore, I see no compelling reason that it should be part of any general statement. The statement, as proposed, could be perceived as a statement of minimum principles. Investigators must use their own thoughtful and educated opinions on the moral relevance of the deontological view in designing their own studies.

The basic moral issues surrounding the use or prohibition of use of animals for experimental purposes currently are based on various presuppositions. The attainment of additional knowledge on sentience, self-consciousness, and language will help clarify the issues, but conflicting values will still exist. The scientific community, which believes in appropriate and sensitive use of animals, can still do so while shifting away from the traditional view of humankind as a ruler of nature toward the view of peoples as diverse as the ancient Greeks and Native Americans that sees humankind as meant to exist in harmony with the other animals and all of nature. It is my view that a shift in this direction is occurring. Issues that scientists need to consider when utilizing animals in experimental procedures can be grouped under the three R's originally proposed by Russell and Burch (1959): *refinement, reduction,* and *replacement.* They introduced the idea of a gradual replacement of animals by using alternative techniques. Silcock (1986) recently has suggested various means of *refinement* in modern experimental procedures. In the following paragraphs, there is an extension of the three R's to include factors that are pertinent in 1987 and should be considered by current biomedical investigators. In addition, a fourth R – that of *review* – is added.

1. Refinement of the experiments provides for a decrease in the incidence or severity of inhumane procedures. Experiments should be designed to avoid unnecessary physical and/or mental suffering or injury to the animals. Anesthetic and analgesic agents to decrease pain in procedures and/or tranquilizers to limit distress should be employed whenever possible. Acceptable means of euthanasia should be used prior to recovery, if at all possible. New instrumentation that would decrease pain and noninvasive imaging procedures should be used whenever possible. Scientifically qualified and trained investigators with a high degree of skill should conduct the experiments. The individuals involved should be able to identify signs of pain in their experimental animals. Some of these suggestions are now mandated by the laws and regulations referred to above.

Optimal physical facilities must be used with proper caging and handling procedures, as outlined in the Public Health Service's Guide for the Care and Use of Laboratory Animals (DHHS, 1985), under the supervision of trained veterinarians. The appropriate review of protocols and facilities must be undertaken by the Institutional Animal Care and Use Committees and be done in a timely manner. The mandated education of investigators must be efficient and useful, dealing with the appropriate information to help the investigator to understand the state-of-the-art animal handling procedures as well as alternatives, without becoming burdensome to their time or effort.

2. Reduction, or the decrease in the number of animals used within the experimental situation, can be expressed in a variety of ways. The objectives of each experiment should be well defined so that the importance of data gained can be weighed with respect to the worth of the animals. A clearly formulated experimental protocol should be developed, derived from an understanding of the course of the disease to be studied and from a thorough knowledge of the related scientific literature. Well-substantiated procedures should be used. Fruitful results should be anticipated that are not procurable by other methods and that should be of ultimate benefit to society. A goal of the research must be publication of the results so as to make subsequent repetition of the experiment unnecessary. Adequate record keeping is mandatory.

The number of animals used per experiment, the number of controls done, and the number of trials per experiment should be kept at a minimum; however, the number must be sufficient to provide adequate data to give significant experimental results. Improvements in methods of information retrieval, establishment of a computer-based registry of negative results, and prompt publication of experimental findings should minimize duplication and repetition of experiments. In certain situations, animals and animal tissue can be shared among investigators as long as such sharing is consistent with experimental design.

3. Replacement will not eliminate all animal use, but can partially decrease the use of animals in certain types of study. Replacement focuses attention on such alternative methods as use of chemical tests, computer models, tissue culture techniques, audiovisual aids in teaching, and microbiological agents in screening for carcinogens. It can also mean the replacement of animals higher on the evolutionary scale with those in a lower position. Investigators need to be cognizant of advances in the development of replacement technologies both as an area in which to focus their research interest and, once developed, in their optimum use within the experimental research laboratory.

4. One way to deal with the problem of the regulation of proper use of laboratory animals is to impose an adequate *review* process on the problem. Dresser (1985) provided details of a model that attempts to integrate competing ethical claims based on the existing system used to regulate research on human subjects. She develops potential standards and procedures for one method of regulation. Movement toward such a procedure is demonstrated by the recent Health Research Extension Act of 1985 (Public Law 99–158) and the subsequent Public Health Service Policy on Humane Care and Use of Laboratory Animals and by the Animal Welfare Act (Public Law 99–198).

Scientists should take a positive and active position in determining appropriate courses of action. They should consider the issues raised by the assignment of moral rights to animals and how these positions should best be balanced against the benefits gained in society by continued scientific progress and advances in health care for human beings and animals. They should not assume that the general public understands these issues. The decisions of scientists should be reflected in their actions in conducting animal experiments and also in their role in educating the public about the importance of the use of experimental animals in advancing knowledge and improving health care. It is the members of society at large who will ultimately decide upon the appropriate bounds for animal use in experimental research (Myers, 1984).

References

Archibald, J., J. Ditchfield, and H.C. Rowsell, eds. (1985) The Contribution of Laboratory Animal Science to the Welfare of Man and Animals: Past, Present, and Future. Eighth Symposium of the International Council for Laboratory Animal Science (ICLAS)/Canadian Association for Laboratory Animal Science (CALAS). Gustav Fisher Verlag, Stuttgart, pp. 1–522.

Bates, M., and P.S. Humphrey, eds. (1956) The Darwin Reader. Scribner's, New York, pp. 1–470.

Benjamin, M. (1987) Ethics and Animal Consciousness (1987) In: Social Ethics, Morality and Social Policy. 3rd Ed. T.A. Mappes and J.S. Zembaty, eds. McGraw-Hill, New York, pp. 476–484.

Bernard, C. (1865/1977) Vivisection. In: An Introduction to the Study of Experimental Medicine. Reprinted in Ethics in Medicine: Historical Perspectives and Contemporary Concerns. S.J. Reiser, A.J. Dyck, and W.J. Curran, eds. M.I.T. Press, Cambridge, MA, pp. 257–259.

Bok, S. (1977) The Tools of Bioethics. (Essay excerpted from an address delivered at the Eastern Sociological Society Meeting.) Reprinted in Ethics in Medicine. Historical Perspectives and Contemporary Concerns. S.J. Reiser, A.J. Dyck, and W.J. Curran, eds. M.I.T. Press, Cambridge, MA, pp. 137–141.

Caplan, A. L. (1983) Beastly conduct: Ethical issues in animal experimentation. Ann. N.Y. Acad. Sci., *406:*159–169.

Caplan, A. (1984) Moral stewardship and our ethical responsibility to animals. In: National Symposium on Imperatives in Research Animal Use: Scientific Needs and Animal Welfare. NIH, Washington, DC, pp. 99–109.

DHHS (Department of Health and Human Services) (1985) Guide for the Care and Use of Laboratory Animals (revised). NIH Publication #86–23. DHHS, Washington, DC.

Dresser, R. (1985) Research on animals: Values, politics and regulatory reform. Southern California Law Review, *58:*1147–1201.

Dresser, R. (1986) Animal experimentation. In: Biolaw: A Legal and Ethical Reporter on Medicine, Health Care, and Bioengineering. University Publications of America, pp. 253–271.

Dubner, R. (1983) Pain research in animals. Ann. N.Y. Acad. Sci., *406:*128–132.

Dukelow, W.R. (1983) Nonhuman Primate Models for Human Disease. CRC Press, Boca Raton, FL, pp. 1–201.

Fox, J.G. (1985) Laboratory animal medicine. Changes and challenges. Cornell Vet., *75:*159–170.

Fox, M.A. (1984) Animal experimentation: Avoiding unnecessary suffering. In: National Symposium on Imperatives in Research Animal Use: Scientific Needs and Animal Welfare. NIH Publication #85–2746. DHHS, Washington, DC, pp. 111–115.

Fox, M.A. (1986) The Case for Animal Experimentation. An Evolutionary and Ethical Perspective. University of California Press, Berkeley, pp. 1–262.

Fox, M.W. (1981) The question of animal rights. Vet. Rec., *109:*37–39.

Fox, M.W. (1984) Towards a philosophy of veterinary medicine. Vet. Rec., *115:*12–13.

Fox, M.W. (1986) Laboratory Animal Husbandry. Ethology, Welfare and Experimental Variables. State University of New York Press, Albany.

Gilligan, C. (1982) A Different Voice: Psychological Theory and Women's Development. Harvard University Press, Cambridge, MA.

Hoff, C. (1980) Immoral and moral uses of animals. N. Engl. J. Med., *302:*105–118.

Holden, C. (1986) A pivotal year for lab animal welfare. Science, *232:*147–150.

Inglehart, J.K. (1985) The use of animals in research. N. Engl. J. Med., *313:*395–400.

Kitchell, R.L. (1983) Animal Pain. Perception and Alleviation. R.L. Kitchell, H.H. Erickson, E. Carstern, and L.E. Davis, eds. American Physiology Society, Bethesda, MD.

Kohlberg, L. (1970) Education for justice: A modern statement of the Platonic view. In: Moral Education. Five Lectures. N.F. Sizer and T.R. Sizer, eds. Harvard University Press, Cambridge, MA, pp. 56–83.

Levine, C. (1984) Should animal experimentation be stopped? In: Taking Sides: Clashing Views on Controversial Bio-Ethical Issues. Levine, ed. Dushkin Publishing Group, Guilford, CT, pp. 222–223.

Lloyd, W.E. (1986) Safety Evaluation of Drugs and Chemicals. Hemisphere Publishing Corp., McGraw-Hill International, Washington, DC.

Myers, D. (1984) Animal rights, academic freedom, and progress in biomedical research. Cancer Invest., *2*:497–498.

NIH (National Institutes of Health) (1986) Public Health Service Policy on Humane Care and Use of Laboratory Animals. Office for Protection of Research Risks. NIH, Washington, DC.

Nuremberg Code (1977) Trials of War Criminals Before the Nuremberg Military Tribunals Under Control Council Law. No. 10, *2*:181–182. Reprinted in Ethics in Medicine. Historical Perspectives and Contemporary Concerns. S.J. Reiser, A.J. Dyck, and W.J. Curran, eds. M.I.T. Press, Cambridge, MA, pp. 272–273.

Office of Technology Assessment (1986) Alternatives to Animal Use in Research, Testing, and Education. (OTA-BA–274). Author, Washington, DC 20510.

Overcast, T.D., and B.D. Sales (1985) Regulation of animal experimentation. J. Am. Med. Assoc., *254*:1944–1949.

Paton, W. (1984) Man and Mouse. Animals in Medical Research. Oxford University Press, Oxford.

Resources: Fall 1986 Pamphlet from the Center for Information on Research with Animals. A Program of the Foundation for Biomedical Research.

Ristau, C.A. (1983) Language, cognition, and awareness in animals? Ann. N.Y. Acad. Sci., *406*:170–186.

Rowan, A.N. (1984) Of Mice, Models, and Men: A Critical Evaluation of Animal Research. State University of New York Press, Albany, pp. 1–323.

Russell, W.M.S., and R.L. Burch (1959) The Principles of Humane Experimental Technique. Charles C. Thomas, Springfield, IL. Quoted in A.N. Rowan, Of Mice, Models, and Men: A Critical Evaluation of Animal Research. State University of New York Press, Albany.

Shapiro, H.M. (1986) Animal rights and biomedical research: No place for complacency. Anesthesiology, *64*:142–146.

Silcock, S.R. (1986) Refinement of experimental procedures. Alternatives to Laboratory Animals, *14*:72–84.

Singer, P. (1975) Animal Liberation. A New Ethic for Our Treatment of Animals. Avon Books, New York.

Tannenbaum, J. (1986) Animal rights: Some guideposts for the veterinarian. J. Am. Vet. Med. Assoc., *188*:1258–1263.

Trull, F.L., and N.A. Kalikow (1984) Animal rights movement: A threat to biomedical research? Cancer Invest., *2*:479–482.

Walters, L., and T.J. Kahn (1986) Bibliography of Bioethics. Kennedy Institute of Ethics, Georgetown University, Washington, DC, Vol. 12.

Watkins, T. (1986) Search for animal alternatives faces rough road. The Scientist, Dec. 15, *1*:6.

World Medical Association (1977) Declaration of Helsinki: Recommendations Guiding Medical Doctors in Biomedical Research Involving Human Subjects. Quoted in Ethics in Medicine. Historical Perspectives and Contemporary Concerns. S.J. Reiser, A.J. Dyck, and W.J. Curran, eds., M.I.T. Press, Cambridge, MA, pp. 328–330.

QUESTIONS FOR DISCUSSION

1. Is the physical size or species of an animal used in research related to its perceived moral status; that is, does concern for primates differ from that for dogs, or mice, or fruit flies? If so, why? If not, why not?
2. How is the role of the Animal Review Committee (ARC) similar to that of the Institutional Review Board that oversees research with human subjects? Are the protective functions of the ARC of a more scientific or ethical nature?
3. How should researchers who use animals respond to the challenges raised by the wide range of animal rights groups?

RECOMMENDED SUPPLEMENTAL READING

Guide for the Care and Use of Laboratory Animals (revised). Department of Health and Human Services (DHHS), NIH Publication #86–23, Washington, DC: DHHS, 1986.

"Animal Research at Stanford University: Principles, Policies, and Practices," James A. Thomas, Thomas E. Hamm, Jr., Pamela L. Perkins, Thomas A. Raffin, & the Stanford University Medical Center Committee on Ethics, *New England Journal of Medicine,* 1988, 318, pp. 1630–1632.

Animal Liberation: A New Ethics for Our Treatment of Animals, 3rd ed., Peter Singer, New York: New York Review Press, 1990.

PART VIII

The Work of the Academic Scientist

INTRODUCTION

The academic scientist is expected to undertake several roles at once, combining teaching, research, and service to society. The mechanisms for combining these roles vary throughout academia, according to the value that individual institutions assign different functions. The National Institutes of Health (NIH) and a variety of universities recently have issued policies and procedural guidelines governing the work of academic scientists in such areas as the supervision of trainees, data management, publication of findings, authorship, and research with human and animal subjects. Perhaps the most controversial of these policies is a federal mandate that recipients of institutional training grants from the National Institutes of Health and the Alcohol, Drug Abuse, and Mental Health Administration (ADAMHA) provide training in "the principles of scientific integrity."

Although many both inside and outside of academia may believe that teaching is the fundamental commitment of the university, academic scientists often consider basic research to be their most essential scholarly pursuit. In this view, the training of younger scientists and the application of knowledge are dependent functions of the research itself. Ernest L. Boyer challenges the traditional perspective on academic life with a definition of scholarship that is more integrated than hierarchical. For Boyer the scholarship of *discovery* must be complemented by the scholarship of *integration,* which interprets and gives contextual meaning to isolated findings; the scholarship of *application,* which offers new intellectual understanding of scientific findings in the act of using them; and the scholarship of *teaching,* which transmits, transforms, and extends knowledge into the future. Particularly as science becomes more specialized, such integration of academic life is essential to preserving science's broader intellectual commitments.

The apparent need for formal policies, whether governmental or institutional, suggests that there is significant uncertainty and disagreement about the nature of academic science. Whatever the formal guidelines, however, the values that institutions express by the totality of their practices – including promotion and tenure, interdisciplinary collaboration and peer review, admissions, funding of student assistantships, grading, and advising – will shape the self-image and social role of academic researchers.

23
Guidelines for investigators in scientific research

Harvard University, Faculty of Medicine, February 16, 1988

I.   Introduction

These guidelines describe practices generally accepted by members of the Faculty of Medicine and already in effect in their laboratories. The primary intent of codifying them is to bring them to the attention of those beginning their careers in scientific research. These recommendations are not intended as rules, but rather as guidelines from which each group of investigators can formulate its own set of specific procedures to ensure the quality and integrity of its research.

II.   Supervision of research trainees

Careful supervision of new investigators by their preceptors is in the best interest of the institution, the preceptor, the trainee, and the scientific community. The complexity of scientific methods, the necessity for caution in interpreting possibly ambiguous data, and the need for advanced statistical analysis, all require an active role for the preceptor in the guidance of new investigators. This is particularly true in the not uncommon circumstance of a trainee who arrives in a research unit without substantial experience in laboratory science.

Recommendations

1. The responsibility for supervision of each junior investigator should be specifically assigned to some faculty member in each research unit.

2. The ratio of trainees to preceptors should be small enough that close interaction is possible for scientific interchange as well as oversight of the research at all stages.

3. The preceptor should supervise the design of experiments and the processes of acquiring, recording, examining, interpreting and storing data. (A preceptor who limits his/her role to the editing of manuscripts does not provide adequate supervision.)

4. Collegial discussions among all preceptors and trainees constituting a research unit should be held regularly both to contribute to the scientific efforts of the members of the group and to provide informal peer review.

5. The preceptor should provide each new investigator (whether student, postdoctoral fellow, or junior faculty) with applicable governmental and institutional requirements for conduct of studies involving healthy volunteers or patients, animals, radioactive or other hazardous substances, and recombinant DNA.

Reprinted with permission from the Harvard Medical School.

III.   Data gathering, storage, retention

A common denominator in most cases of alleged scientific misconduct has been the absence of a complete set of verifiable data. The retention of accurately recorded and retrievable results is of utmost importance for the progress of scientific inquiry. A scientist must have access to his/her original results in order to respond to questions including, but not limited to, those that may arise without any implication of impropriety. Moreover, errors may be mistaken for misconduct when the primary experimental results are unavailable. In addition, when statistical analysis is required in the interpretation of data, it should be used in the design of studies as well as in the evaluation of results.

Recommendations

1. Custody of all original primary laboratory data must be retained by the unit in which they are generated. An investigator may make copies of the primary data for his/her own use.
2. Original experimental results should be recorded, when possible, in bound books with numbered pages. An index should be maintained to facilitate access to data.
3. Machine print-outs should be affixed to, or referenced from, the laboratory notebook.
4. Primary data should remain in the laboratory at all times and should be preserved as long as there is any reasonable need to refer to them. The chief of each research unit must decide whether to preserve such primary data for a given number of years or for the life of the unit. In no instance, however, should primary data be destroyed while investigators, colleagues, or readers of published results may raise questions answerable only by reference to such data.

IV. Authorship

A gradual diffusion of responsibility for multi-authored or collaborative studies had led in recent years to the publication of papers for which no single author was prepared to take full responsibility. Two critical safeguards in the publication of accurate, scientific reports are the active participation of each co-author in verifying that part of a manuscript that falls within his/her specialty area and the designation of one author who is responsible for the validity of the entire manuscript.

Recommendations

1. Criteria for authorship of a manuscript should be determined and announced by each department or research unit. The Committee considers the only reasonable criterion to be that the co-author has made a significant intellectual or practical contribution. The concept of "honorary authorship" is deplorable.
2. The first author should assure the head of each research unit or department chairperson that s/he has reviewed all the primary data on which the report is based and provide a brief description of the role of each co-author. (In multi-institutional collaborations, the senior investigator in each institution should prepare such statements.)
3. Appended to the final draft of the manuscript should be a signed statement from

each co-author indicating that s/he has reviewed and approved the manuscript to the extent possible, given individual expertise.

V. Publication practices

The Committee has observed certain practices that make it difficult for reviewer and reader to follow a complete experimental sequence: the rapid publication of data without adequate tests of reproducibility or assessment of significance, the publication of fragments of a study, and the submission of multiple similar abstracts or manuscripts differing only slightly in content. In such circumstances, if any of the work is questioned, it is difficult to determine whether the research was done inaccurately, the methods were described imperfectly, the statistical analyses were flawed, or inappropriate conclusions were drawn. Investigators should review each proposed manuscript with these principles in mind.

Recommendations

1. The number of publications to be reviewed at time of faculty appointment or promotion should be limited in order to encourage and reward bibliographies containing fewer but more substantive publications rather than those including many insubstantial or fragmented reports. (It has been suggested, for example, that no more than 5 papers be reviewed for appointment as Assistant Professor, nor more than 7 for Associate Professor, and no more than 10 for Professor.)

2. Simultaneous submission of multiple similar abstracts or manuscripts to journals is improper.

VI. Laboratory guidelines

Because each research unit addresses different scientific problems with different methods, each unit should develop its own specific guidelines to identify practices that seem most likely to enhance the quality of research conducted by its members. Those guidelines should be provided to the new investigator upon starting work.

24
Guidelines for the conduct of research at the National Institutes of Health

Bethesda, Maryland, March 21, 1990

Preface

The Guidelines for the Conduct of Research at the National Institutes of Health were written to make explicit the canons of good science that have traditionally governed the conduct of research in the Intramural Program at the National Institutes of Health (NIH). In the past, at NIH as in other academic communities, it could be assumed that investigators shared a common understanding and set of expectations regarding the conduct of research. For this reason, an unwritten code of conduct seemed adequate.

Today, the increasing complexity of research and the entry of far larger numbers of trainees into the research community make appropriate a written set of guidelines. NIH and other academic research centers have accordingly begun to issue guidelines to help both new and experienced investigators manage their work so as to safeguard the integrity of the research process.

The Guidelines that follow were developed by the Scientific Directors of the NIH. The Guidelines state expectations regarding the research process and indicate the responsibilities of investigators and research managers in resolving the various types of conflicts that may arise in the process of conducting, publishing and defending research.

. . .

Introduction

Scientists in the Intramural Research Program of the National Institutes of Health generally are responsible for conducting original research consonant with the goals of their individual Institutes, Centers, and Divisions.

NIH scientists, as all scientists, should be committed to the responsible use of the process known as the scientific method to seek new knowledge. While the general principles of the scientific method – formulation and testing of hypotheses, controlled observations or experiments, analysis and interpretation of data, and oral and written presentation of all of these components to scientific colleagues for discussion and further conclusions – are universal, their detailed application may differ in different scientific disciplines and in varying circumstances. It is clear, however, that only by adherence to the highest standards of intellectual honesty in formulating, conducting and presenting

Originally published by the National Institutes of Health, Bethesda, Maryland, March 21, 1990.

research does science advance and do scientists fulfill their contract with the community at large.

These Guidelines state general principles that NIH scientists are expected to follow in their research activities with regard to supervision of trainees, data management, publication practices, authorship, peer review and use of privileged information, and clinical investigations in order to promote the uniform application of the highest ethical standards to the conduct of all scientific research. It is the responsibility of each Laboratory or Branch Chief, and successive levels of supervisory individuals (especially Institute, Center, and Division Intramural Research Directors), to insure that each NIH scientist is cognizant of these Guidelines and to resolve issues that may arise in their implementation.

These Guidelines supplement existing NIH policies on the conduct of research. In particular, those policies concerning Institutional Review Board oversight of clinical research protocols; animal use; radiation, chemical and other safety issues; and other aspects of the Standards of Conduct for all federal employees remain parts of the canon of conduct for each scientist.

The formulation of these Guidelines is not meant to codify a set of rules, but rather to make explicit patterns of scientific practice that have been developed over many years and are followed by the vast majority of scientists, and to provide benchmarks when problems arise. Although no set of guidelines, or even explicit rules, can prevent willful scientific misconduct, it is hoped that formulation of these Guidelines will contribute to the continued clarification of the application of the scientific method in changing circumstances.

The community will ultimately judge the NIH by its adherence to these intellectual and ethical standards, as well as by its development and application of important new knowledge through scientific creativity.

Supervision of trainees

Research training is a complex process, the central aspect of which is an extended period of research carried out under the supervision of an experienced scientific mentor. This supervised research experience represents not merely performance of tasks assigned by the supervisor but rather a process wherein the trainee takes on an increasingly independent role in the choice of research projects, development of hypotheses and the performance of the work. Indeed, if training is to prepare a young scientist for a successful career as a research investigator, it must be geared toward providing the trainee with the aforementioned skills and experiences. It is particularly critical that the mentor recognize that the trainee is not simply an additional laboratory worker.

Each trainee should have a designated primary scientific mentor. It is the responsibility of this mentor to provide a training environment in which the trainee has the opportunity to acquire both the conceptual and technical skills of the field. In this setting, the trainee should undertake a significant piece of research, chosen usually as the result of discussions between the mentor and the trainee, which has the potential to yield new knowledge of importance in that field. The mentor has the responsibility to supervise the trainee's progress closely and to interact personally with the trainee on a regular basis in such a way as to make the training experience a meaningful one. Styles of research differ, both among fields and among investigators in a given field, so that no specific rules should be made about the number of trainees that is appropriate for a single mentor to supervise.

Nonetheless, mentors should limit the number of trainees in their laboratory to the number for whom they can provide an appropriate research experience.

There are certain specific aspects of the mentor-trainee relationship that deserve emphasis. First, mentors must be particularly diligent in avoiding the involvement of trainees in research activities that do not provide meaningful training experiences but which are designed mainly to further research or development activities in which the mentor has a potential monetary or other compelling interest. Second, training must impart to the trainee appropriate standards of scientific conduct. The mentor conveys these standards by instruction and by example. Third, mentors have a responsibility to provide trainees with realistic appraisals of their performance and with advice about career development and opportunities.

Data management

Research data, including detailed experimental protocols, primary data from laboratory instruments, and procedures of reduction and analysis of primary data, are the essential components of scientific progress. Scientific integrity is inseparable from meticulous attention to the acquisition and maintenance of these research data.

It is expected that the results of research will be carefully recorded in a form that will allow continuous access for analysis and review. Attention should be given to annotation and indexing of notebooks to facilitate detailed review of data. All data, even from observations and experiments not directly leading to publication, should be treated comparably. Research data should always be immediately available to scientific collaborators and supervisors for review. In collaborative projects involving different units, all investigators should know the status of all contributing data and have direct access to them.

Research data, including the primary experimental results, should be retained for a sufficient period to allow analysis and repetition by others of published material from those data. In some fields, five or seven years are specified as the minimum period of retention but this may vary under different circumstances.

Research data and supporting materials, such as unique reagents, belong to the National Institutes of Health, and should be maintained in the Laboratory in which they were developed. Departing investigators may take copies of notebooks or other material for further work. If the recognized senior or principal investigator departs that Laboratory, it is the responsibility of that investigator and that Institute, Center, or Division to insure that the data and unique reagents will be appropriately maintained and be accessible.

Data management, including the decision to publish, is the responsibility of the principal investigator. After publication, the research data and any unique reagents that form the basis of that communication should be made available promptly and completely to all responsible scientists seeking further information. Certain restrictions related to privacy may obtain for clinical research data.

Publication practices

Publication of experimental results is an integral and essential component of research. Other than presentation at scientific meetings, publication in a scientific journal should normally be the mechanism for the first public disclosure of new findings. Although appropriately considered the end point of a particular research project, publication is also the beginning of a process in which the scientific community at large can substantiate, correct and further develop any particular set of results.

Timely publication of new and significant results is important for the progress of science, but fragmentary publication of the results of a scientific investigation or multiple publications of the same or similar data are inappropriate. Each publication should make a unique and substantial contribution to its field. As a corollary to this principle, tenure appointments and promotions should be based on the importance of the scientific accomplishments and not on the number of publications in which those accomplishments were reported.

Each paper should contain sufficient information for the informed reader to assess its validity. The principal method of scientific verification, however, is not review of submitted or published papers, but the ability of others to replicate the results. Therefore, each paper should contain all the information that would be necessary for the scientific peers of the authors to repeat the experiments. This principle requires that any unique materials (e.g. monoclonal antibodies, bacterial strains, mutant cell lines), analytical amounts of scarce reagents and unpublished data (e.g. protein or nucleic acid sequences) that are essential for repetition of the published experiments be made available to other qualified scientists. It is not necessary to provide materials (such as proteins) that others can prepare by published procedures, or large quantities of materials (such as polyclonal antisera) that may be in limited supply, although it is desirable to do so.

Authorship

Authorship refers to the listing of names of participants in all communications, oral and written, of experimental results and their interpretation to scientific colleagues. Authorship is the fulfillment of the responsibility to communicate research results to the scientific community for external evaluation.

Authorship is also the primary mechanism for determining the allocation of credit for scientific advances and thus the primary basis for assessing a scientist's contributions to developing new knowledge. As such, it potentially conveys great benefit, as well as responsibility. For each individual the privilege of authorship should be based on a significant contribution to the conceptualization, design, execution, and/or interpretation of the research study, as well as a willingness to take responsibility for the defense of the study should the need arise. In contrast, other individuals who participate in part of a study may more appropriately be acknowledged as having contributed certain advice, reagents, analyses, patient material, space, support, etc., but not be listed as authors. It is expected that such distinctions will become increasingly important in the future and should be explicitly considered more frequently now.

In recent years, there has been a rapid increase of the average number of authors per communication. In part, this increase is due to the needs of modern research projects for contributions from many individuals, frequently those with different specialized skills. While multi-authorship is not a problem in itself, it raises many issues such as criteria for inclusion as an author, ability of each author to evaluate and defend all aspects of a study, sequence of listing of authors, and separation of various experimental results to increase numbers of communications and authorship citations. To clarify some of these concerns, consideration should be given in interdisciplinary studies to preparing brief statements of the exact contribution of each author to the work described in each communication.

Because of the variation in detailed practices among disciplines, no universal set of standards can be easily formulated. It is expected, however, that each research group and Laboratory or Branch will freely discuss and resolve questions of authorship before and during the course of a study. Further, each author should review fully material that is to be presented in public forums or submitted (originally or in revision) for publication. Each author should be willing to support the general conclusions of the study and be willing to defend the study.

The submitting author should be considered the primary author with the additional responsibility of coordinating the completion and submission of the work, satisfying pertinent rules of submission, and coordinating responses of the group to inquiries or challenges. The submitting author should assure that the contributions of all collaborators are appropriately recognized and must be able to certify that each author has reviewed and authorized the submission of the manuscript. The recent practice of some journals in requiring approval signatures from each author before publication is felt to be a useful step in regard to fulfilling the above.

Peer review and privileged information

Peer review can be defined as expert critique of either a scientific treatise, such as an article prepared or submitted for publication, a research grant proposal, a clinical research protocol, or of an investigator's research program, as in a site visit. Peer review is an essential component of the conduct of science. Decisions on the funding of research proposals and on the publication of experimental results must be based on thorough, fair and objective evaluations by recognized experts. Therefore, although it is often difficult and time-consuming, scientists have an obligation to participate in the peer review process and, in doing so, they make an important contribution to science.

Peer review requires that the reviewer be expert in the subject under review. The reviewer, however, should avoid any real or perceived conflict of interest that might arise because of a direct competitive, collaborative or other close relationship with one or more of the authors of the material under review. Normally, such a conflict of interest would require a decision not to participate in the review process and to return any material unread.

The review must be objective. It should be based solely on scientific evaluation of the material under review within the context of published information and should not be influenced by scientific information not publicly available.

All material under review is privileged information. It should not be used to the benefit of the reviewer unless it previously has been made public. It should not be shared with anyone unless necessary to the review process, in which case the names of those with whom the information is shared should be made known to those managing the review process. Material under review should not be copied and retained or used in any manner by the reviewer unless specifically permitted by the journal or reviewing organization and the author.

Clinical research

Clinical research, for the purposes of these Guidelines, is defined as research performed on human subjects or on material or information obtained from human subjects as a part of human experimentation. All of the topics covered in the Guidelines also apply to the conduct of clinical research; clinical research, however, entails further responsibilities for investigators.

The preparation of a written research protocol ("Clinical Research Protocol") according to existing guidelines prior to commencing studies is almost always required. By virtue of its various sections governing background; patient eligibility and confidentiality; data to be collected; mechanism of data storage, retrieval, statistical analysis and reporting; and identification of the principal and associate investigators, the Clinical Research Protocol provides a highly codified mechanism covering most of the topics covered elsewhere in the Guidelines. The Clinical Research Protocol is generally widely circulated for comment, review and approval. It should be scrupulously adhered to in the conduct of the research. The ideas of the investigators who prepared the protocol should be protected by all who review the document.

Clinical investigators are responsible for assuring that the proposed clinical research will be conducted only if the Clinical Center, or other clinical facilities, has the appropriate capability and support structure to insure that the research can be done safely and efficiently. The principal investigator should be familiar with the functioning of the clinical unit and should allow the investigation to continue only if the unit can provide adequate clinical care.

Investigators who are neither clinicians nor trained in clinical research may perform laboratory research on material derived from humans. To conform to the requirement of working under approved human experimentation guidelines, they should ordinarily be advised by or collaborate with trained clinical investigators.

The supervision of trainees in the conduct of clinical investigation is complex. Often the trainees are in fellowship training programs leading to specialty or sub-specialty certifications as well as in research training programs. Thus, they should be educated in general and specific medical management issues as well in the conduct of research. The process of data gathering, storage, and retention can also be complex in clinical research and sometimes not easily subject to repetition. The principal investigator is responsible for the quality and maintenance of the records and for the training and oversight of all personnel involved in data collection.

Concluding statement

These Guidelines are not intended to address issues of misconduct, i.e. fabrication, falsification, plagiarism or other practices motivated by intent to deceive. Rather, their purpose is to provide a framework for the fair and open conduct of research without inhibiting scientific freedom and creativity.

25

Reminder and update: Requirement for programs on the responsible conduct of research in National Research Service Award institutional training programs

National Institutes of Health
Alcohol, Drug Abuse, and Mental Health Administration

As stated in the NIH Guide for Grants and Contracts, Vol. 18, No. 45, December 22, 1989, administrative guidelines for the National Research Service Award (NRSA) institutional training grant applications submitted to the National Institutes of Health (NIH) and Alcohol, Drug Abuse, and Mental Health Administration (ADAMHA) have been revised "to require that a program in the principles of scientific integrity be an integral part of the proposed research training effort." This requirement applies to all competing training grant applications received after July 1, 1990. The principal goal of the NRSA grant mechanisms is to train scientists for future careers in biomedical and behavioral research. An important factor in biomedical and behavioral research is the need to maintain the highest levels of integrity in the conduct of research. The research training environment in the university setting provides a powerful context in which to promote responsible research practices.

NIH and ADAMHA recognize that the scientific community is at an early stage of developing information and methods that pertain specifically to training in research ethics for trainees. Not all methods will work in all training situations given the heterogeneity among disciplines and professions. There are no single models or paradigms. Appreciation of the heterogeneity among the biomedical and behavioral research components within the institutions calls for flexibility in approaches to effective education and training models.

Institutions must accept primary responsibility and be allowed to develop their own ways of promoting responsible conduct of research in conjunction with their training programs. Scientific and administrative leaders of the university or from outside (as consultants or speakers) could be a visible part of this effort. Applicants are urged to discuss the development of methods on this important topic with their colleagues and also look to the professional associations for guidance as well as discussions with NIH and ADAMHA staff.

An array of methods might be used at various training levels. It was stated in the NIH Guide for Grants and Contracts, December 22, 1989 notice:

"Most universities and academic institutions have practices and procedures to ensure the responsible conduct of research. These may include informal seminars and presentations on conflict of interest, data recording and retention, professional standards and codes of conduct, responsible authorship, institutional policies and procedures for handling allegations of misconduct, policies regarding the use of human and animal subjects, etc. or formal courses on bioethics, research conduct, the ideals of science, etc."

For the first 18 months of implementation of this requirement, it is expected that

From *NIH Guide*, 1990, 19 (30); (August 17), p. 1. [P. T. 44; K. W. 1014004, 1014006.]

institutions will be given considerable flexibility in order to encourage innovation in the development of methods for providing training in scientific integrity. However, descriptions of formal or informal activities related to incorporation of efforts relevant to the responsible conduct of research (i.e., ''the plan'') should be as explicit as possible (e.g., topics to be covered; faculty that may be involved; format; schedule, etc.). No application will be awarded until a description of the institution's plan to provide instruction on ethics in research training is furnished.

26
Enlarging the perspective

Ernest L. Boyer

Since colonial times, the American professoriate has responded to mandates both from within the academy and beyond. First came teaching, then service, and finally, the challenge of research. In more recent years, faculty have been asked to blend these three traditions, but despite this idealized expectation, a wide gap now exists between the myth and the reality of academic life. Almost all colleges pay lip service to the trilogy of teaching, research, and service, but when it comes to making judgments about professional performance, the three rarely are assigned equal merit.

Today, when we speak of being "scholarly," it usually means having academic rank in a college or university and being engaged in research and publication. But we should remind ourselves just how recently the word "research" actually entered the vocabulary of higher education. The term was first used in England in the 1870s by reformers who wished to make Cambridge and Oxford "not only a place of teaching, but a place of learning," and it was later introduced to American higher education in 1906 by Daniel Coit Gilman.[1] But scholarship in earlier times referred to a variety of creative work carried on in a variety of places, and its integrity was measured by the ability to think, communicate, and learn.

What we now have is a more restricted view of scholarship, one that limits it to a hierarchy of functions. Basic research has come to be viewed as the first and most essential form of scholarly activity, with other functions flowing from it. Scholars are academics who conduct research, publish, and then perhaps convey their knowledge to students or apply what they have learned. The latter functions grow *out of* scholarship, they are not to be considered a part of it. But knowledge is not necessarily developed in such a linear manner. The arrow of causality can, and frequently does, point in *both* directions. Theory surely leads to practice. But practice also leads to theory. And teaching, at its best, shapes both research and practice. Viewed from this perspective, a more comprehensive, more dynamic understanding of scholarship can be considered, one in which the rigid categories of teaching, research, and service are broadened and more flexibly defined.

There is a readiness, we believe, to rethink what it means to be a scholar. Richard I. Miller, professor of higher education at Ohio University, recently surveyed academic vice presidents and deans at more than eight hundred colleges and universities to get their opinion about faculty functions. These administrators were asked if they thought it would be a good idea to view scholarship as more than research. The responses were over-

From Ernest L. Boyer, *Scholarship Reconsidered: Priorities of the Professorate* (Princeton, NJ: Carnegie Foundation, 1990), pp. 15–25. © The Carnegie Foundation for the Advancement of Teaching. Reprinted with permission.

whelmingly supportive of this proposition.[2] The need to reconsider scholarship surely goes beyond opinion polls, but campus debates, news stories, and the themes of national conventions suggest that administrative leaders are rethinking the definitions of academic life. Moreover, faculty, themselves, appear to be increasingly dissatisfied with conflicting priorities on the campus.

How then should we proceed? Is it possible to define the work of faculty in ways that reflect more realistically the full range of academic and civic mandates? We believe the time has come to move beyond the tired old "teaching versus research" debate and give the familiar and honorable term "scholarship" a broader, more capacious meaning, one that brings legitimacy to the full scope of academic work. Surely, scholarship means engaging in original research. But the work of the scholar also means stepping back from one's investigation, looking for connections, building bridges between theory and practice, and communicating one's knowledge effectively to students. Specifically, we conclude that the work of the professoriate might be thought of as having four separate, yet overlapping, functions. These are: the scholarship of *discovery;* the scholarship of *integration;* the scholarship of *application;* and the scholarship of *teaching.*

The first and most familiar element in our model, the *scholarship of discovery,* comes closest to what is meant when academics speak of "research." No tenets in the academy are held in higher regard than the commitment to knowledge for its own sake, to freedom of inquiry and to following, in a disciplined fashion, an investigation wherever it may lead. Research is central to the work of higher learning, but our study here, which inquires into the meaning of scholarship, is rooted in the conviction that disciplined, investigative efforts within the academy should be strengthened, not diminished.

The *scholarship of discovery,* at its best, contributes not only to the stock of human knowledge but also to the intellectual climate of a college or university. Not just the outcomes, but the process, and especially the passion, give meaning to the effort. The advancement of knowledge can generate an almost palpable excitement in the life of an educational institution. As William Bowen, former president of Princeton University, said, scholarly research "reflects our pressing, irrepressible need as human beings to confront the unknown and to seek understanding for its own sake. It is tied inextricably to the freedom to think freshly, to see propositions of every kind in ever-changing light. And it celebrates the special exhilaration that comes from a new idea."[3]

The list of distinguished researchers who have added luster to the nation's intellectual life would surely include heroic figures of earlier days – Yale chemist Benjamin Silliman; Harvard naturalist Louis Agassiz; astronomer William Cranch Bond; and Columbia anthropologist Franz Boas. It would also include giants of our time – James Watson, who helped unlock the genetic code; political philosopher Hannah Arendt; anthropologist Ruth Benedict; historian John Hope Franklin; geneticist Barbara McClintock; and Noam Chomsky, who transformed the field of linguistics; among others.

When the research records of higher learning are compared, the United States is the pacesetter. If we take as our measure of accomplishment the number of Nobel Prizes awarded since 1945, United States scientists received 56 percent of the awards in physics, 42 percent in chemistry, and 60 percent in medicine. Prior to the outbreak of the Second World War, American scientists, including those who fled Hitler's Europe, had received only 18 of the 129 prizes in these three areas.[4] With regard to physics, for example, a recent report by the National Research Council states: "Before World War II, physics was essentially a European activity, but by the war's end, the center of physics had moved to the United States."[5] The Council goes on to review the advances in fields ranging from elementary particle physics to cosmology.

The research contribution of universities is particularly evident in medicine. Investigations in the late nineteenth century on bacteria and viruses paid off in the 1930s with the development of immunizations for diphtheria, tetanus, lobar pneumonia, and other bacterial infections. On the basis of painstaking research, a taxonomy of infectious diseases has emerged, making possible streptomycin and other antibiotics. In commenting on these breakthroughs, physician and medical writer Lewis Thomas observes: "It was basic science of a very high order, storing up a great mass of interesting knowledge for its own sake, creating, so to speak, a bank of information, ready for drawing on when the time for intelligent use arrived."[6]

Thus, the probing mind of the researcher is an incalculably vital asset to the academy and the world. Scholarly investigation, in all the disciplines, is at the very heart of academic life, and the pursuit of knowledge must be assiduously cultivated and defended. The intellectual excitement fueled by this quest enlivens faculty and invigorates higher learning institutions, and in our complicated, vulnerable world, the discovery of new knowledge is absolutely crucial.

The scholarship of integration

In proposing the *scholarship of integration,* we underscore the need for scholars who give meaning to isolated facts, putting them in perspective. By integration, we mean making connections across the disciplines, placing the specialties in larger context, illuminating data in a revealing way, often educating nonspecialists, too. In calling for a scholarship of integration, we do not suggest returning to the "gentleman scholar" of an earlier time, nor do we have in mind the dilettante. Rather, what we mean is serious, disciplined work that seeks to interpret, draw together, and bring new insight to bear on original research.

This more integrated view of knowledge was expressed eloquently by Mark Van Doren nearly thirty years ago when he wrote: "The connectedness of things is what the educator contemplates to the limit of his capacity. No human capacity is great enough to permit a vision of the world as simple, but if the educator does not aim at the vision no one else will, and the consequences are dire when no one does."[7] It is through "connectedness" that research ultimately is made authentic.

The scholarship of integration is, of course, closely related to discovery. It involves, first, doing research at the boundaries where fields converge, and it reveals itself in what philosopher-physicist Michael Polanyi calls "overlapping [academic] neighborhoods."[8] Such work is, in fact, increasingly important as traditional disciplinary categories prove confining, forcing new topologies of knowledge. Many of today's professors understand this. When we asked faculty to respond to the statement, "Multidisciplinary work is soft and should not be considered scholarship," only 8 percent agreed, 17 percent were neutral, while a striking 75 percent disagreed (see table). This pattern of opinion, with only slight variation, was true for professors in all disciplines and across all types of institutions.

The scholarship of integration also means interpretation, fitting one's own research – or the research of others – into larger intellectual patterns. Such efforts are increasingly essential since specialization, without broader perspective, risks pedantry. The distinction

Multidisciplinary work is soft and should not be considered scholarship

	Agree	Neutral	Disagree
All Respondents	8%	17%	75%
Research	7	9	84
Doctorate-granting	6	13	80
Comprehensive	8	14	78
Liberal Arts	8	16	77
Two-Year	9	27	63

Source: The Carnegie Foundation for the Advancement of Teaching, 1989 National Survey of Faculty.

we are drawing here between "discovery" and "integration" can be best understood, perhaps, by the questions posed. Those engaged in discovery ask, "What is to be known, what is yet to be found?" Those engaged in integration ask, "What do the findings *mean?* Is it possible to interpret what's been discovered in ways that provide a larger, more comprehensive understanding?" Questions such as these call for the power of critical analysis and interpretation. They have a legitimacy of their own and if carefully pursued can lead the scholar from information to knowledge and even, perhaps, to wisdom.

Today, more than at any time in recent memory, researchers feel the need to move beyond traditional disciplinary boundaries, communicate with colleagues in other fields, and discover patterns that connect. Anthropologist Clifford Geertz, of the Institute for Advanced Study in Princeton, has gone so far as to describe these shifts as a fundamental "refiguration, . . . a phenomenon general enough and distinctive enough to suggest that what we are seeing is not just another redrawing of the cultural map – the moving of a few disputed borders, the marking of some more picturesque mountain lakes – but an alteration of the principles of mapping. Something is happening," Geertz says, "to the way we think about the way we think."[9]

This is reflected, he observes, in:

. . . philosophical inquiries looking like literary criticism (think of Stanley Cavell on Beckett or Thoreau, Sartre on Flaubert), scientific discussions looking like belles lettres *morceaux* (Lewis Thomas, Loren Eiseley), baroque fantasies presented as deadpan empirical observations (Borges, Barthelme), histories that consist of equations and tables or law court testimony (Fogel and En-german, Le Roi Ladurie), documentaries that read like true confessions (Mailer), parables posing as ethnographies (Castañeda), theoretical treatises set out as travelogues (Lévi-Strauss), ideological arguments cast as historiographical inquiries (Edward Said), epistemological studies constructed like political tracts (Paul Feyerabend), methodological polemics got up as personal memoirs (James Watson).[10]

These examples illustrate a variety of scholarly trends – *interdisciplinary, interpretive, integrative*. But we present them here as evidence that an intellectual sea change may be occurring, one that is perhaps as momentous as the nineteenth-century shift in the hierarchy of knowledge, when philosophy gave way more firmly to science. Today, interdisciplinary *and* integrative studies, long on the edges of academic life, are moving toward the center, responding both to new intellectual questions and to pressing human problems. As the boundaries of human knowledge are being dramatically reshaped, the academy surely must give increased attention to the *scholarship of integration.*

The scholarship of application

The first two kinds of scholarship – discovery and integration of knowledge – reflect the investigative and synthesizing traditions of academic life. The third element, the *application* of knowledge, moves toward engagement as the scholar asks, "How can knowledge be responsibly applied to consequential problems? How can it be helpful to individuals as well as institutions?" And further, "Can social problems *themselves* define an agenda for scholarly investigation?"

Reflecting the *Zeitgeist* of the nineteenth and early twentieth centuries, not only the land-grant colleges, but also institutions such as Rensselaer Polytechnic Institute and the University of Chicago were founded on the principle that higher education must serve the interests of the larger community. In 1906, an editor celebrating the leadership of William Rainey Harper at the new University of Chicago defined what he believed to be the essential character of the American scholar. Scholarship, he observed, was regarded by the British as "a means and measure of self-development," by the Germans as "an end in itself," but by Americans as "equipment for service."[11] Self-serving though it may have been, this analysis had more than a grain of truth.

Given this tradition, one is struck by the gap between values in the academy and the needs of the larger world. Service is routinely praised, but accorded little attention – even in programs where it is most appropriate. Christopher Jencks and David Riesman, for example, have pointed out that when free-standing professional schools affiliated with universities, they lessened their commitment to applied work even though the original purpose of such schools was to connect theory and practice. Professional schools, they concluded, have oddly enough fostered "a more academic and less practical view of what their students need to know."[12]

Colleges and universities have recently rejected service as serious scholarship, partly because its meaning is so vague and often disconnected from serious intellectual work. As used today, service in the academy covers an almost endless number of campus activities – sitting on committees, advising student clubs, or performing departmental chores. The definition blurs still more as activities beyond the campus are included – participation in town councils, youth clubs, and the like. It is not unusual for almost any worthy project to be dumped into the amorphous category called "service."

Clearly, a sharp distinction must be drawn between *citizenship* activities and projects that relate to scholarship itself. To be sure, there are meritorious social and civic functions to be performed, and faculty should be appropriately recognized for such work. But all too frequently, service means not doing scholarship but doing good. To be considered *scholarship,* service activities must be tied directly to one's special field of knowledge and relate to, and flow directly out of, this professional activity. Such service is serious, demanding work, requiring the rigor – and the accountability – traditionally associated with research activities.

The *scholarship of application,* as we define it here, is not a one-way street. Indeed, the term itself may be misleading if it suggests that knowledge is first "discovered" and then "applied." The process we have in mind is far more dynamic. New intellectual understandings can arise out of the very act of application – whether in medical diagnosis, serving clients in psychotherapy, shaping public policy, creating an architectural design, or working with the public schools. In activities such as these, theory and practice vitally interact, and one renews the other.

Such a view of scholarly service – one that both applies and contributes to human knowledge – is particularly needed in a world in which huge, almost intractable problems call for the skills and insights only the academy can provide. As Oscar Handlin observed, our troubled planet "can no longer afford the luxury of pursuits confined to an ivory tower. . . . [S]cholarship has to prove its worth not on its own terms but by service to the nation and the world."[13]

The scholarship of teaching

Finally, we come to the *scholarship of teaching*. The work of the professor becomes consequential only as it is understood by others. Yet, today, teaching is often viewed as a routine function, tacked on, something almost anyone can do. When defined as *scholarship,* however, teaching both educates and entices future scholars. Indeed, as Aristotle said, "Teaching is the highest form of understanding."

As a *scholarly* enterprise, teaching begins with what the teacher knows. Those who teach must, above all, be well informed, and steeped in the knowledge of their fields. Teaching can be well regarded only as professors are widely read and intellectually engaged. One reason legislators, trustees, and the general public often fail to understand why ten or twelve hours in the classroom each week can be a heavy load is their lack of awareness of the hard work and the serious study that undergirds good teaching.

Teaching is also a dynamic endeavor involving all the analogies, metaphors, and images that build bridges between the teacher's understanding and the student's learning. Pedagogical procedures must be carefully planned, continuously examined, and relate directly to the subject taught. Educator Parker Palmer strikes precisely the right note when he says knowing and learning are communal acts.[14] With this vision, great teachers create a common ground of intellectual commitment. They stimulate active, not passive, learning and encourage students to be critical, creative thinkers, with the capacity to go on learning after their college days are over.

Further, good teaching means that faculty, as scholars, are also learners. All too often, teachers transmit information that students are expected to memorize and then, perhaps, recall. While well-prepared lectures surely have a place, teaching, at its best, means not only transmitting knowledge, but *transforming* and *extending* it as well. Through reading, through classroom discussion, and surely through comments and questions posed by students, professors themselves will be pushed in creative new directions.

In the end, inspired teaching keeps the flame of scholarship alive. Almost all successful academics give credit to creative teachers – those mentors who defined their work so compellingly that it became, for them, a lifetime challenge. Without the teaching function, the continuity of knowledge will be broken and the store of human knowledge dangerously diminished.

Physicist Robert Oppenheimer, in a lecture at the 200th anniversary of Columbia University in 1954, spoke elegantly of the teacher as mentor and placed teaching at the very heart of the scholarly endeavor: "The specialization of science is an inevitable accompaniment of progress; yet it is full of dangers, and it is cruelly wasteful, since so much that is beautiful and enlightening is cut off from most of the world. Thus it is proper to the role of the scientist that he not merely find the truth and communicate it to his fellows, but that he teach, that he try to bring the most honest and most intelligible account of new knowledge to all who will try to learn.''[15]

Here, then, is our conclusion. What we urgently need today is a more inclusive view of what it means to be a scholar – a recognition that knowledge is acquired through research, through synthesis, through practice, and through teaching.[16] We acknowledge that these four categories – the scholarship of discovery, of integration, of application, and of teaching – divide intellectual functions that are tied inseparably to each other. Still, there is value, we believe, in analyzing the various kinds of academic work, while also acknowledging that they dynamically interact, forming an interdependent whole. Such a vision of scholarship, one that recognizes the great diversity of talent within the professoriate, also may prove especially useful to faculty as they reflect on the meaning and direction of their professional lives.

Notes

1. Charles Wegener, *Liberal Education and the Modern University* (Chicago: The University of Chicago Press, 1978), 9–12; citing Daniel C. Gilman, *The Launching of a University and Other Papers* (New York: Dodd Mead & Co., 1906), 238–39 and 242–43.
2. Richard I. Miller, Hongyu Chen, Jerome B. Hart, and Clyde B. Killian, "New Approaches to Faculty Evaluation – A Survey, Initial Report" (Athens, Ohio; submitted to The Carnegie Foundation for the Advancement of Teaching by Richard I. Miller, Professor of Higher Education, Ohio University, 4 September 1990.)
3. William G. Bowen, *Ever the Teacher: William G. Bowen's Writings as President of Princeton* (Princeton, N.J.: Princeton University Press, 1987), 269.
4. Harriet Zuckerman, *Scientific Elite: Nobel Laureates in the United States* (New York: The Free Press, A Division of Macmillan, 1977), 282–88; citing *The World Book Encyclopedia*, vol. 14, 1975.
5. National Research Council, *Physics Through the 1990s* (Washington, D.C.: National Academy Press, 1986), 8.
6. Lewis Thomas, "Biomedical Science and Human Health: The Long-Range Prospect," *Daedalus* (Spring 1977), 164–69; in Bowen, *Ever the Teacher*, 241–42.
7. Mark Van Doren, *Liberal Education* (Boston: Beacon Press, 1959), 115.
8. Michael Polanyi, *The Tacit Dimension* (Garden City, N.Y.: Doubleday, 1967), 72; in Ernest L. Boyer, *College: The Undergraduate Experience in America* (New York: Harper & Row, 1987), 91.
9. Clifford Geertz, "Blurred Genres: The Refiguration of Social Thought," *The American Scholar* (Spring 1980), 165–66.
10. Ibid.
11. Lyman Abbott, "William Rainey Harper," *Outlook*, no. 82 (20 January 1906), 110–111; in Frederick Rudolph, *The American College and University: A History* (New York: Alfred A. Knopf, 1962), 356.
12. Christopher Jencks and David Riesman, *The Academic Revolution* (Garden City, N.Y.: Doubleday, 1968), 252.
13. Oscar Handlin, "Epilogue – Continuities," in Bernard Bailyn, Donald Fleming, Oscar Handlin, and Stephan Thernstrom, *Glimpses of the Harvard Past* (Cambridge, Mass.: Harvard University Press, 1986), 131; in Derek Bok, *Universities and the Future of America* (Durham, N.C., and London: Duke University Press, 1990), 103.

14. Parker J. Palmer, *To Know As We Are Known* (New York: Harper & Row, 1983).
15. *The New York Times,* 27 December 1954, D27.
16. Parker J. Palmer to Russell Edgerton, president of the American Association for Higher Education, 2 April 1990.

QUESTIONS FOR DISCUSSION

1. How do the multiple roles of the academic researcher create and affect collegial relationships among faculty and students?
2. How do your institution's policies on promotion and tenure reflect its commitments to teaching, research, and service to the community?
3. What are effective ways to teach good laboratory practice?

RECOMMENDED SUPPLEMENTAL READING

"The Report of a Study Group of the International Council on the Future of the University," Edward Shils, in *The Academic Ethics,* Chicago, IL: University of Chicago Press, 1983.

Higher Learning, Derek Bok, Cambridge, MA: Harvard University Press, 1986.

"The Need for an Ethical Code for Teachers of Basic Biomedical Sciences," R. E. Bulger, *Journal of Medical Education,* 1988, 63, pp. 131–133.

"PHS Workshop: Education and Training of Scientists in the Responsible Conduct of Research," Department of Health and Human Services, Washington, DC: Public Health Service, March 8–9, 1990.

PART IX

The Scientist and Industry: Conflicts of Interest and Conflicts of Commitment

INTRODUCTION

World War II marked a significant turning point in the size and productivity of scientific research, largely because governments assumed many of the costs of doing science. The achievements in engineering, physics, and medicine of that era demonstrated that science offers tremendous benefits to society that warrant taxpayer support. Governmental grants today typically fund basic rather than applied research, ideally to generate new ideas as well as useful data. Sharing of such data is fundamental to government-sponsored research, for, as Loren Lomasky argues, the findings of such work ultimately belong to the public.

Since the 1970s, however, governmental budgets for research have been unable to keep pace with the growth of scientific opportunity, and academic scientists have had to look for other sources of funding. In biotechnology in particular, the development of patentable applications offers a source of income. However, the ethical and legal uncertainties of patenting biotechnologies, especially new or modified life forms, have created tension among governments, researchers, their institutions, and financial sponsors. The policy statement "Patenting Life" from the U.S. Congressional Office of Technology Assessment recognizes that patenting biological processes has a long history, but that a number of questions remain about the future development of living organisms that might be subject to patenting.

The funding of academic research by for-profit organizations has been a feature of science since the beginning of the century, and has provided some significant developments; however, the growth of science in industry, especially in biotechnology, has heightened the potential for conflict of interest and conflict of commitment for academic scientists. Industry's desire to create products means that commercially sponsored research more likely will be in applied rather than basic science, potentially limiting its educational benefits. The importance of trade secrets in industry makes it difficult to maintain the tradition of sharing data. Researchers' desire to renew their grants from commercial sources, and in some cases the promise of personal gain, may subtly compromise their objectivity in favor of a sponsor's product.

The forces of commercialization pose challenges to the ethics of academic science that, as the Association of Academic Health Centers' report describes, may be difficult to recognize without concerted professional review. By developing their own formal policies on industry-sponsored research, individual academic institutions, laboratories, and faculties can identify and avoid many of the common pitfalls, and prepare themselves for new problems to come.

27
Sharing research data

Duncan Neuhauser

The National Research Council of the National Academy of Sciences has issued a report, *Sharing Research Data*[1] which has as its first recommendation, ''Sharing data should be a regular practice.'' Other recommendations state that investigators should share their data by the time of publication of initial major results of analysis, except in compelling circumstances. Plans for data sharing should be an integral part of a research plan whenever data sharing is feasible. Investigators should keep data available for a reasonable period after publication of results. Subsequent analyses of data by others should explicitly acknowledge the contribution of the original investigators. These are exacting standards for medical care researchers to aspire to.

This report has four recommendations for editors of scientific journals:

1) Journal editors should require authors to provide access to data during the peer review process. Although such a request would be extremely rare during the review process for *Medical Care* manuscripts, we believe that authors should, in principle, be willing to do so.

It is the expectation of the editors that the authors of papers published in *Medical Care* will allow access to their data. Keeping secret key parts of research reports in order to cash in on consulting and follow-up opportunities is inconsistent with full peer review. We have no objection to medical care researchers parleying their proprietary work into riches. In fact, if this happened, it might be good for the field. However, we are troubled by the thought that someone might exploit the peer review process, in spite of refusing to make their work available to peers, and thereby misrepresent their work as peer reviewed in the process of marketing it.

In the words of Donald Kennedy, President of Stanford:

Science relies very heavily on the capacity to replicate experiments; it is the only way at all to correct fraud. Although we referee journal articles, evaluate the logic of propositions, and check arithmetic, we cannot decide, merely from reading a report, that a result is right – only that it is not wrong in some obvious way. Accordingly, we require that scientific communications include enough detail about the way an experiment was done so that a competent investigator in the field can do it in exactly the same way. This is an exacting requirement; it compels the release of all relevant information about methods and techniques. Secret ingredients, magic sauces, and your own special glassware are fine in cookery or in product development, but in fundamental science they are out.[2]

From *Medical Care*, 1986, 24 (10), pp. 879–880.

A full description of most of the studies reported in this journal would take hundreds of pages to describe. Because this is not possible, we assume that detailed descriptions of method are available from the author on request.

2) "Journals should give more emphasis to reports of secondary analyses and to replications." We invite such submissions.

3) "Journals should require full credit and appropriate citations to original data collections in reports based on secondary analysis." We agree.

4) "Journals should strongly encourage authors to make detailed data accessible to other researchers." We assume that *Medical Care* authors accept this as a condition of submitting a paper to peer review and for publication.

The questions often raised about data sharing such as patient confidentiality, costs of re-analysis, requests by unqualified people, copyright laws, etc. are discussed in this National Research Council report, and those interested in these issues are urged to seek it out. In spite of potential problems with data sharing, the benefits of doing so greatly outweigh the risks and costs.

References

1. Committee on National Statistics, Commission on Behavioral and Social Sciences and Education, National Research Council. Sharing Research Data. Washington, DC: National Academy Press, 1985.
2. Kennedy D. The social sponsorship of innovation. In: Perpich J, ed. Biotechnology in Society. New York: Pergamon Press, 1986;26–27.

28

University-industry research relationships in biotechnology: Implications for the university

David Blumenthal, Michael Gluck, Karen Seashore Louis, Michael A. Stoto, David Wise

University-industry research relationships (UIRR's) in biotechnology have grown increasingly important for both industries and universities in the United States. Recent research indicates that nearly half the firms conducting or supporting research in biotechnology are involved in UIRR's. Their funds may account for 16 to 24% of all external support for university research in biotechnology (*1*).

The growth of UIRR's in biotechnology and other fields, however, has raised critical questions concerning their effects on institutions of higher education. Do such relationships affect the scholarly or commercial productivity of university faculty? Do UIRR's influence the commitment of faculty members to teaching or their participation in the time-consuming, sometimes tedious administrative activities so essential to the health of universities or a field of science? Do industrial research relationships encourage secrecy among scientists, disrupt relationships among scientific colleagues, or lead faculty to shift the direction of their research toward applied or commercially oriented projects?

From a survey of over 1200 faculty members in 40 of the most research-intensive U.S. universities, we report on the effect of UIRR's on faculty whose work involves the "new biotechnologies"(*2*). These fields include recombinant DNA technology, monoclonal antibody techniques, gene synthesis, gene sequencing, cell and tissue culture techniques, large-scale fermentation, and enzymology. The expansion of UIRR's in these scientific fields has been especially dramatic in recent years. UIRR's in the new biotechnologies, therefore, provide an intriguing case study for exploring both the potential risks and the potential benefits of UIRR's generally for academic institutions.

Study design

The analysis presented here is based on a survey of university faculty conducted in the winter of 1985. A sample of 1997 faculty was selected in a two-step process. First, we selected 40 universities from among the 50 schools that receive the largest amounts of federal research funds in the United States (*3*).

Second, for those 40 universities, we developed a list of 3180 life science faculty members (instructors, lecturers, assistant professors, associate professors, and full professors) included in published catalogs as members of the departments of biochemistry, molecular biology, genetics, microbiology, biology, cellular biology, or botany (*4*). We selected these departments because we judged them to be most likely to contain faculty conducting research involving the new biotechnologies. From this list, we randomly

From *Science*, 1986, 232, pp. 1361–1366. Copyright 1986 by the AAAS.

Table 1. *Characteristics of the sample. Because of question nonresponse, numbers of faculty may not add to 1238 for certain characteristics.*

Characteristic	Number	Proportion
Male	1117	0.90
Female	119	0.10
Professor	720	0.58
Associate professor	328	0.27
Assistant professor	166	0.13
Other	23	0.02
Years since completing highest degree		
0–5	45	0.04
6–10	173	0.14
11–20	485	0.39
21–30	320	0.26
31–40	161	0.13
>40	54	0.04
Total	1238	

selected 1594 individuals. A comparison group of 403 nonlife scientists was drawn from a list of 1211 faculty in departments of chemistry and engineering from the same institutions. We sought such a comparison group in order to assess the relative prevalence of UIRR's in biotechnology and in other fields known to have a long history of involvement with industry.

Each of the 1997 faculty in our sample was mailed an eight-page questionnaire dealing primarily with his or her research activities and involvement with industry. If the questionnaire was not returned within 3 weeks, a second mailing was sent. One hundred fifty-six respondents were ineligible (deceased, retired, no longer associated with the university, or incorrectly reported as a faculty member in the catalog). Of eligible respondents, 69% (993) in the life sciences and 65% (245) in chemistry and engineering returned completed questionnaires. Table 1 summarizes pertinent characteristics of respondents.

Among life science respondents, 800 of 993 (81%) did research involving the new biotechnologies. In the body of the article, we refer to these respondents as ''biotechnology'' faculty and to the remaining 193 life science respondents as ''other life science'' faculty. Unless otherwise indicated, our analyses concern respondents in our biotechnology group. In comparing groups within our sample, we used two-tailed z tests to assess differences of means or proportions. Multivariate analyses employed regressions with ordinary least-squares methodology.

We conducted a telephone survey of nonrespondents (from all disciplines) to collect minimal data regarding their research activities and involvements with industry. Of 104 nonrespondents reached, 63 provided limited information. The remainder refused, usually because they were ''too busy,'' or ''never answer questionnaires.'' Nonrespondents did not differ significantly from respondents in academic rank, the proportion receiving industrial research support, or the magnitude of industry support (as measured by the proportion of the faculty member's total direct research budget supplied by industry).

Despite our thoroughness, the data are subject to certain limitations. First, the faculty

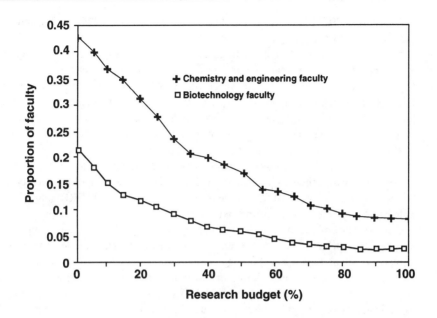

Figure 1. Extent of industry support for faculty research. Proportion of biotechnology faculty and chemistry and engineering faculty receiving at least x% of their research budget from industry sources, as x varies from 0 to 100%. For $x = 0$, the proportion of faculty with any industry funding is shown.

and universities surveyed are not representative of all faculty and academic institutions in the United States currently involved in UIRR's in biotechnology. Our faculty sample is drawn from departments that may be more involved in basic research than some other parts of universities (such as schools of agriculture) and from institutions that are more research intensive than the average American university. However, even though the population sampled is not typical of all scientists in all academic centers, it still constitutes an important and interesting group whose behavior is worthy of study.

Second, despite a high response rate for a mailed questionnaire, the fact that approximately 30% of faculty did not respond to our survey could introduce nonresponse biases into our data. Although limited information does not suggest any problems, we have no way of determining the full extent or directions of any biases created by the failure of some faculty to respond.

Third, faculty may have underreported certain behaviors or activities that they considered sensitive or embarrassing (for example, equity holding in companies) or overstated certain behaviors or activities that they considered desirable (such as publication rates and teaching time). Again, the extent of such possible biases cannot be ascertained.

Prevalence and extent of involvement in UIRR's

To ascertain the prevalence of UIRR's among faculty members, we asked respondents whether they were principal investigators (PI's) on any grants or contracts from industrial sources. Among biotechnology faculty, 23% responded affirmatively (5). These faculty were somewhat more likely to receive industry support than other life science faculty

(17%, $P = 0.007$) but considerably less likely than faculty in chemistry and engineering (43%, $P < 0.001$).

Industry supplied 7.4% of all research funds (excluding overhead) received by biotechnology faculty in our sample, and 32% of funds received by chemistry and engineering faculty. Figure 1 shows the distribution of industrial support among faculty involved in UIRR's and compares biotechnology faculty with physical scientists in the sample. Although most faculty doing work in biotechnology received a relatively small proportion of their funds from industry, 6 received at least 50% of their research support from UIRR's, and 3% received at least 75% of their funds from this source.

For the 23% of biotechnology faculty who receive some industry funds, that support constitutes 34% of their total research budget. Among biotechnology faculty involved in UIRR's, 28% received least 50% of their research support from UIRR's, and 15% received at least 75% of their funds from this source.

Our estimate of the proportion of biotechnology faculty's research support provided by industry differs considerably from our previous estimates of the proportion of university research in biotechnology supported by industry [7.4% compared to 16 to 24 (*1*)]. It should be noted, however, that this study was not designed to provide an accurate estimate of the proportion of university research in biotechnology that is funded by industry. Our sample underrepresents faculty in schools of medicine and did not include faculty from schools of agriculture, groups that might be expected to receive larger proportions of their research support from industry than do faculty in the departments surveyed (*6*).

Effects of UIRR's in biotechnology

Publication, teaching, and other traditional university activities. A major concern among critics of UIRR's in biotechnology and other fields is that faculty receiving industrial support may be less interested in and committed to traditional university activities, such as scholarship, teaching, and participation in other activities vital to the health of universities and scientific disciplines. Critics argue either that faculty will become more interested in commercializing research findings, thus pursuing subjects of less scholarly value, or else that their involvement with industry will require or encourage them to participate in time-consuming chores, such as consulting, that will compete with university activities.

To assess whether such shifts in behavior are occurring among biotechnology faculty who are involved in UIRR's, we asked respondents to tell us how many articles they had published in refereed journals during the last 3 years, how many hours of contact they had weekly (including laboratory supervision) with students or postdoctoral fellows, and whether they had served in any of several professional roles within or outside the university in the last 3 years (*7*).

Compared with colleagues doing biotechnology research, faculty receiving industry support in biotechnology reported significantly more publications and involvements with other professional activities but no statistically significant differences in teaching time (Table 2). However, such simple comparisons of faculty with and without industry support could be misleading. In order to be classified as receiving industry support, faculty in our sample had to be principal investigators on at least one industrial grant or contract. In contrast, the group without industry support includes some faculty who are not PI's

Table 2. *Selected measures of behavior among biotechnology faculty. Publications refers to publications in refereed journals during the previous 3 years. Teaching time refers to the average number of hours of contact per week with graduate students or postdoctoral fellows. Activities refers to the number of activities in universities or professional roles (university administration, professional journals, and officer in professional associations). Publication trends refers to the difference between the number of refereed publications during last 3 years and number of publications for an average 3-year period during a faculty member's career.*

Status	Publications	Teaching time	Activities	Publication trends
No industry support	11.3*	20.3	1.1*	2.2
Industry support	14.6*	22.2	1.4*	3.3

*Differences were statistically significant ($P < 0.05$).

on projects of any sort and may be less senior than or differ in other ways from principal investigators on industry projects.

To correct for such confounding effects, we performed multivariate analyses that examined the association between key faculty behaviors and industry support while controlling for the faculty member's academic rank, the number of years since completing his or her highest degree, the faculty member's total research budget from all sources, his or her involvement in consulting or other relationships with industry, and a variety of other characteristics of faculty and the universities in which they work. In taking account of sample faculties' research budgets from all sources, we effectively controlled for whether they were PI's on at least one externally funded grant or contract. Because of the way our questionnaire was constructed, faculty could report receiving research funds only for projects on which they were PI's. These multivariate analyses confirmed the significance and direction of the associations reported in Table 2.

It is possible that faculty with industry funds are publishing less than they did before they began receiving industry support, even though they still compare favorably along this dimension with faculty not participating in UIRR's. To examine this possibility, we asked faculty how many papers they had published in refereed journals during their professional careers and then compared their publication rates for an average 3-year period with their reported rates during the last 3 years (8). As Table 2 shows, biotechnology faculty with and without industry support reported publishing more in the last 3 years than they did during an average 3-year period. Faculty with industry support reported a greater increment in their publications than did other faculty. However, the difference was not statistically significant ($P = 0.14$), a finding confirmed in multivariate analysis.

Faculty who receive a large proportion of their research support from industry, or combine such heavy support with other types of industrial relationships, may be more affected by industrial support of university research than faculty with lesser levels of involvement with industry. To see whether this might be the case, we examined the reported behavior of several subgroups of biotechnology respondents: faculty who received more than 50% of their biotechnology research support from industry; faculty who received more than 50% of their research support from industry and also added at least 20% to their base salary from consulting to a for-profit company; faculty with more than 50%

of their support from UIRR's who also consulted exclusively for one biotechnology company; faculty who received more than 80% of their research support from industry; and a series of other combinations of characteristics that might signal heavy involvement with industry. Controlling for other factors, these heavily involved groups reported publication rates, hours of student or postdoctoral contact, and involvements in other professional activities that did not differ significantly from (and in some cases exceeded) those of other faculty.

The measures used here to assess the relation between faculty behavior and industrial support of their research have obvious limitations. Simple figures on publication rates and teaching time could have missed differences in the quality or nature of publications or teaching among biotechnology faculty with and without industrial support. By lumping classroom teaching together with laboratory supervision, we could have missed differences in the way faculty with and without industry funds distribute their time among these very different types of educational activities. Nevertheless, the findings should on balance prove reassuring to the university community. Certainly, our data on selected indicators provided no evidence that industrial support of faculty research in biotechnology is associated with decreased faculty productivity. If anything, the opposite seems the case.

Commercial productivity among faculty. One of the possible benefits of UIRR's in biotechnology and other fields is that they may encourage faculty to commercialize their research findings more readily than faculty without industrial research support. Such a tendency could result in greater income for the university and benefits to society through increasing the rate at which research results are transferred into practical application.

To examine this hypothesis, we asked biotechnology faculty in our sample whether their university research had resulted in any patent applications, patents, or trade secrets. Faculty with industry support were more than twice as likely (37 versus 17%, $P < 0.001$) as faculty without such support to answer affirmatively.

These data do not establish that industrial support actually increased the commercial productivity of faculty. It may be that industry successfully seeks out faculty whose work seems likely to have commercial application. However, faculty seem to feel that industrial support is helpful in producing commercially useful results from their research. Among biotechnology faculty participating in UIRR's who reported patent applications, patents, or trade secrets, 48% said that industry support had contributed significantly to the work that led to these commercialization efforts. When asked about the benefits of industrial support of university research, a majority of faculty with and without industry research funds agreed that UIRR's increase the rate of applications from basic research to some extent or a great extent (Table 3).

Involvement in UIRR's may also offer faculty opportunities to increase their personal income through royalties from licensed patents, consulting to industry, and other means. Such additional earnings may reduce pressures on universities to increase faculty salaries during periods of financial hardship and may, therefore, be counted among the benefits of UIRR's in biotechnology and other fields. In fact, involved biotechnology faculty in our sample did report that, measured as a percentage of their base salary, they earned more in additional compensation (14 versus 12% of their base salaries) each year than did faculty without industrial support for their research. Multivariate analysis controlling for faculty and university characteristics confirmed the significance ($P < 0.05$) of this association between increased faculty earnings and receipt of industry research support.

Perceived benefits of UIRR's. To capture other positive effects of UIRR's we asked biotechnology faculty about the extent to which industrial support of university research

Table 3. *Benefits reported by biotechnology faculty.*

	"To some extent or to great extent" (%)	
Question	Industry support	No industry support
To what extent does industry research support		
Involve less red tape than federal funding	76	51*
Increase the rate of applications from basic research	67	52*
Provide resources not obtainable elsewhere	63	36*
Enhance career opportunities for students	60	43*
Enhance scholarly productivity	41	20*
Produce patents that increase university revenues	41	33

*Significantly different from faculty with industry support ($P < 0.01$).

offered several possible benefits. As Table 3 shows, a majority of biotechnology respondents with industry funds reported that four of the six potential benefits occurred to some extent or a great extent. Biotechnology faculty without industrial support were consistently less enthusiastic about the consequences of UIRR's, but a majority agreed that to some extent or a great extent, UIRR's involved less red tape than federal funding and increased the rate of practical applications from basic research.

Secrecy in the university. Critics of UIRR's have argued that these arrangements may create incentives for faculty to keep their research secret and that industry is more likely to restrict publication of research findings than are other sources of support. Either effect could impede the free, rapid, and unbiased dissemination of research results. Certain of our findings lend support to these concerns.

Biotechnology faculty with industry support were four times as likely as other biotechnology faculty (12 versus 3%, $P < 0.001$) to report that trade secrets had resulted from their university research. Trade secrets were defined as "information kept secret to protect its proprietary value" (9).

To assess whether industry sponsors placed more restrictions on publications than other sources of research support, we asked biotechnology faculty the following question: "Have you personally conducted any research at your university the results of which are the property of the sponsor and cannot be published without their consent?" Respondents were then asked to identify the sponsors of this research (federal government, industry, or other).

Among biotechnology faculty involved in UIRR's, 24% (including researchers at 22 of the 40 universities in our sample) responded affirmatively to the question above and identified industry as the sponsor for which the research was conducted. Among faculty with support from sources other than industry, only 5% indicated that they had performed research under the stated conditions for such nonindustrial sponsors.

These findings should be a matter of concern for universities. Even small numbers of faculty who withhold information that they would normally share with colleagues (or make available through publication) may have a corrosive effect on the university environment. When biotechnology faculty who do not receive industry support were asked whether UIRR's pose the risk of undermining intellectual exchange and cooperation within departments, 68% said they did so to some or to a great extent. Among their colleagues with industry support, 44% agreed (Table 4) (10).

Table 4. *Risks reported by biotechnology faculty.*

	To some extent or to great extent (%)	
Question	Industry support	No industry support
To what extent does industry research support pose the risk of		
Shifting too much emphasis to applied research	70	78*
Creating pressures for faculty to spend too much time on commercial activities	68	82†
Undermining intellectual exchange and cooperative activities within departments	44	68†
Creating conflict between faculty who support and oppose such activities	43	61†
Creating unreasonable delays in the publication of new findings	40	53†
Reducing the supply of talented university teachers	40	51*
Altering standards for promotion or tenure	27	41†

*Significantly different from faculty with industry support ($P < 0.05$).
†Significantly different from faculty with industry support ($P < 0.01$).

Redirection of research. We asked biotechnology faculty the extent to which their choice of research topics had been affected by the likelihood that the results would have commercial applications. Faculty members with industry support were more than four times as likely as faculty without industry funds (30 versus 7%, $P < 0.001$) to report that such considerations had influenced their choices to some extent or to a great extent.

Although some may see such attention to commercial applications as a positive development among university faculty, others may worry that it will lead to excessive emphasis on applied investigation at the expense of more fundamental research. To a surprising degree, biotechnology faculty share this concern. Among biotechnology faculty without industrial support, 78% said that, to some extent or a great extent, UIRR's pose the risk of shifting too much emphasis to applied research. Among their colleagues participating in UIRR's, 70% agreed (Table 4).

Equity holding in biotechnology companies. Biotechnology faculty face a serious potential conflict of interest when they receive funds for their university research from companies in which they hold equity and whose products or services are based upon the faculty member's university work. In particular, such investigators may encounter especially strong economic incentives to use their university time and university facilities to do company work.

Eight percent of all biotechnology faculty in our sample (62 of 800) reported holding equity in a company whose products or services are based on their research. However, only 0.5% (4 of 800) reported that they simultaneously held equity in such a company and received funds from it for their university research. Faculty may have underreported such situations because of their sensitivity. Nevertheless, on balance our data seem to indicate that this particular form of potential conflict of interest is uncommon among biotechnology faculty in our sample.

Discussion

Data from this survey provide important insights into the consequences of UIRR's in biotechnology for university life. Some of our most significant findings speak to potential benefits of such arrangements for higher education.

Industry support of biotechnology research in universities, constituting roughly one-fifth of all available funds, is undoubtedly a welcome addition to federal funding for this dynamic area of investigation. As Table 3 shows, faculty perceive UIRR's in biotechnology to have a number of other benefits as well. Perhaps most intriguing, however, is the suggestion that UIRR's may be associated with heightened faculty productivity along a number of dimensions. Controlling for other factors, faculty in our sample who were receiving industry support tended to publish more, patent more, earn more, serve in more administrative roles, and teach just as much as faculty without industry funds.

The most obvious explanation for this observed relation between faculty accomplishments and industry support is that companies selectively support talented and energetic faculty who were already highly productive before they received industry funds. If accurate, this explanation would suggest at a minimum that industries are supporting faculty who are very important to their parent institutions.

In this respect, it is interesting to note that faculty involved in UIRR's seem capable of commercial as well as academic productivity. This lends support to the anecdotal observation that individuals who are highly successful in one dimension, such as scholarship, seem also to be capable of success in rather different dimensions, such as the production of intellectual property with potential commercial value. It should prove reassuring to universities that the commercial accomplishments of faculty involved in UIRR's do not seem to diminish their commitments to publication, teaching, or other forms of service to the university or scientific community, at least by the measures employed in our survey. This finding is consistent with other research showing that faculty who consult to outside agencies do not show diminished productivity in their university roles (*11*).

Another possible explanation for the observed productivity of faculty involved in UIRR's is that industrial support enhances their performance along some or all of the dimensions we examined. It would seem perfectly plausible that contact with industrial sponsors, even through agreements that support basic research, would increase the commercial productivity and the earnings of university faculty. Less obvious, but equally plausible, is the possibility that UIRR's could increase the scholarly productivity of faculty, either through adding to their research support, or through exposing them to new perspectives on their work. A considerable body of scholarly work suggests that interaction between scientists doing applied and basic research may enhance the work of both groups (*12, 13*).

A critical question, of course, is whether these apparent benefits of UIRR's in biotechnology for universities and their faculties are associated with any risks to traditional university values or practices. Our data strongly suggest that such risks exist.

One of the most important is an apparent tendency toward increased secrecy among faculty supported by industries. Other risks include an apparent tendency, worrisome to the great majority of respondents, for UIRR's to shift university research in more applied directions and the frequency with which industries seem to place restrictions on publication beyond requiring simply that they be allowed to review papers prior to submission. In previous work, we also reported that students and fellows supported by industry funds often face obligations to work on projects identified by industry, or to work for industries when their training is completed – conditions not imposed by governmental sponsors (*1*).

In some respects, however, even our findings concerning the risks of UIRR's in biotechnology are reassuring. Only a tiny minority of biotechnology faculty in our sample report that they hold equity in companies supporting their university research. Some observers may even find reassuring the frequency with which faculty report that they are concerned about the risks posed by industrial support of biotechnology research. These figures offer some evidence that, at least at current levels of involvement with industry, faculty remain sensitive and committed to traditional university values and practices. Although not a guarantee against erosion of these values, such faculty attitudes may indicate that they retain a capacity to police their own relationships with industrial sponsors. Those whose major interest is the field of biotechnology may also find it reassuring that biotechnology faculty are still much less likely than chemists and engineers to have connections with industry, though this, of course, may change over time.

In assessing the risks of UIRR's, however, the limits of our study should be kept in mind. Because faculty may have been unwilling to report certain behavior, we may have underestimated the prevalence of certain worrisome situations. Our quantitative measures of faculty productivity could have missed important qualitative effects of industrial support on their work. A survey of faculty inevitably fails to explore adequately the full effects of UIRR's on students. Such effects remain to be explored more thoroughly.

In addition, even the small probability of certain devastating occurrences is sufficient to engender caution. Of greatest concern may be Krimsky's (*14*) suggestion that UIRR's, precisely because they involve very talented and productive faculty, could threaten the collective judgment or ethics of scientists in a field of research. The worry here is that researchers with industrial support or other types of involvement in commercial enterprises may be influenced by their personal financial interests in judging the merits of proposals submitted for peer review to funding agencies or in commenting on public policy problems. Another related concern is that junior faculty without commercial involvements may be reluctant to speak out on certain policy issues because they fear displeasing senior faculty whose financial interests might be adversely affected.

Another difficulty in comparing the benefits and risks of UIRR's in biotechnology or other fields is that the long-run implications of current findings are hard to estimate. Furthermore, the trade-off depends on how society values the various consequences of UIRR's. Any losses to science or to university values that result from marginal increases in the level of secrecy in universities may be more than offset by net additions to knowledge that result from the infusion of industry funds into the labs of talented faculty. Marginal shifts in the direction of university work toward more applied and commercially relevant projects may have benefits for human health and economic growth that far outweigh the risks to scientific progress. In the long run, the continued well-being of universities and university science depends importantly on the health of our economy and on public perception that supporting university research contributes directly to practical results.

Though much remains to be learned, our data at least suggest some ways in which universities and government can reduce any risks that industrial support poses for involved academic institutions. First, universities should carefully monitor their relationship with biotechnology companies. Universities may want to make clear to faculty and companies that they are opposed to the protection of trade secrets resulting from industrially supported research and that the right to publish research results (with modest delays for companies to file patents) must be protected. Past research has also revealed that UIRR's with small companies (non–Fortune 500) are more likely to involve certain potentially risky arrangements than relationships with large companies (*1*).

Second, universities should be able to negotiate UIRR's that avoid objectionable restrictions on faculty behavior. Most universities are in a strong bargaining situation with respect to potential industrial sponsors (*15*). Companies are realizing substantial returns from UIRR's in biotechnology (*1*) and tend to fund strong faculty who can probably find support elsewhere if companies withdraw.

Third, government can assist universities in controlling the risks associated with UIRR's in biotechnology by continuing its support of university research. The availability of public funding will strengthen the resolve of universities and faculty in bargaining with potential industrial sponsors.

Fourth, government can further reduce the risks of UIRR's to universities by making certain that the patent system continues to provide adequate protection for the commercial value of intellectual property in the field of biotechnology. The best deterrent to secrecy in universities may be the perfection of methods that allow parties involved in UIRR's to disclose their research results while also protecting their proprietary interest in that information. Some industry observers (*16*) fear that patents may not provide adequate safeguards in the field of biotechnology and that secrecy may increase in the university and in industry as a result. In this context, much depends on how the judicial system interprets current law as biotechnology companies and universities bring suit to protect patents against what they regard as infringement (*17*).

The benefits of UIRR's in biotechnology to universities and industries make it clear that these relationships are likely to be an enduring phenomenon in American science. The associated risks for universities, and the difficulty in measuring them precisely, make it equally clear that UIRR's will continue to be controversial for some time to come. A major goal at this time should be finding ways to manage these relationships so as to preserve their benefits while minimizing any problems they create. To accomplish this, we must first increase our understanding of the impact of UIRR's on industrial productivity, university values, and the advance of science.

References and notes

1. D. Blumenthal, M. Gluck, K. S. Louis, D. Wise, *Science* **231**, 242 (1986).
2. Office of Technology Assessment. *Commercial Biotechnology: An International Analysis* (Government Printing Office, Washington, DC, 1984).
3. Among the 50 most research-intensive universities, we decided to sample faculty from only the 40 that had responded to a separate survey we conducted of university research administrators in 100 universities and medical schools. This approach allowed us to control for university characteristics in analyzing the effect of UIRR's on faculty behavior. We chose to focus on research-intensive universities because they seemed likely to have large numbers of faculty who use the new biotechnologies and because these universities play a particularly vital role in the conduct of basic research.
4. Lists of faculty members were obtained from *Peterson's Guides to Graduate Programs in the Biological, Agricultural and Health Sciences 1984* (Peterson's Guides, Princeton, NJ, 1984) and *Peterson's Guides to Graduate Programs in Engineering and Applied Sciences, 1985* (Peterson's Guides, Princeton, NJ, 1985).

5. Measuring the prevalence of industrial support in this way has the advantage that respondents can state accurately the source of their research funds. It also avoids double counting in calculating for faculty with industry support, the amounts and proportions of their research funds provided by industry. However, it may lead us to underestimate the proportion of all faculty who receive some support from industry, since non-PI's working on multi-investigator grants would not be counted. In estimating amounts of nonindustrial research support, we similarly asked faculty to tell us how much money they received as PI's from sources other than industry. This enabled us to avoid double counting funds from nonindustrial sources and is relevant to our multivariate analyses.

6. Corroboration for our original estimate of the proportion of all university research in biotechnology supported by industry can be found in a separate but as yet unpublished survey that we conducted of university administrators in nearly 100 universities and medical schools. On average, these officials estimated that industry provided 20% of external support for biotechnology research received by their institutions. However, it is still possible that our original estimate and that provided by these officials are too high. The first estimate could be excessive if the National Science Foundation's estimate of total federal support of biotechnology research in 1983, upon which our original calculations were based (*1*), was too low. Estimates by university administrators could be too high if they were including in their calculations industrial funds for research that did not meet our narrow definition of biotechnology (such as clinical research involving drug testing and new diagnostic equipment).

7. Respondents were asked whether in the last 3 years they had been chair or associate chair of the university department, head or associate head of a research institute, a university-wide administrator, a member of a review panel or study section for a federal agency, an elected officer of a professional association, or editor of a professional journal.

8. Specifically, we divided total lifetime publications by the number of 3-year intervals since the faculty member completed his or her highest earned degree. This provided an estimate of the number of refereed publications produced during an average 3-year period in that faculty member's career. We then subtracted this figure from the number of publications in the most recent 3-year period, and compared differences for faculty with and without industrial support.

9. Here again, it is possible that this relationship between trade secrecy and industry support may be explained in part by a tendency of companies to support researchers whose work has already resulted in trade secrets.

10. It should be noted that these figures report faculty perceptions of risk, rather than statements as to events or situations that have actually occurred.

11. D. C. Bok, *Harvard Magazine* (May–June 1981).

12. D. C. Pelz and F. M. Andrews, *Scientists in Organizations: Productive Climates for Research and Development* (Wiley, New York, 1966).

13. C. J. Ping, "Industry and the universities: Developing cooperative research relationships in the national interest" (National Commission on Research, Washington, DC, August 1980).

14. S. Krimsky, *geneWATCH* **1**, 5 (September–December 1984), p. 3.

15. H. Etzkowitz, *Minerva* **21**, 232 (1983).

16. A. Lemin, personal communication; H. J. P. Shoemaker, personal communication.

17. B. Cunningham, personal communication.

18. Supported by DHHS grant 100A–83, the Andrew W. Mellon Foundation, and the Alfred P. Sloan Foundation. The authors wish to acknowledge the contributions of S. Epstein, M. Kiely, and J. Durch.

29
Public money, private gain, profit for all

Loren E. Lomasky

The principle that public investment is not to be appropriated for private gain may appear self-evident. It is also thoroughly inapplicable in contemporary American economic life. Everywhere the private and public are inextricably intertwined.

I am the product of twelve years of primary and secondary education, all in public schools. My university experience was primarily in state institutions. Were it not for that prior investment in my "human capital," I would be unable to earn a living, as I now do, as a teacher of philosophy. I confess that I appropriate these earnings with great gusto. I do not regard myself as thereby raiding the public fisc. Perhaps this displays a certain lack of moral refinement on my part. If so, I am hardly alone. The vast majority of readers of the *Hastings Center Report* are in similar circumstances. We are, on average, the repositories of much public investment from which we derive our current income.

Two questions should be asked: (1) Should individuals derive private profit from public expenditures? (2) Should the state make large investments from which such profits can be derived? These are separate questions; yet they are clearly interrelated. For if the second is answered, "no," then the first becomes moot.

I am strongly inclined to believe that a negative answer *should* be given to the second. I subscribe to a classically liberal position within which the realm of permissible state action is severely circumscribed. This is not the place, however, to tilt at those particular windmills. Municipal, state, and federal instrumentalities will not any time soon undertake a weight reduction regimen. Hundreds of billions of tax dollars will be appropriated each year for what are essentially private ends. Are individuals morally obliged to forgo all prospects of gain from these appropriations?

To answer "yes" is to endorse a radically restructured economic system. Farmers are the beneficiaries of crop price supports; truckers and their customers use publicly constructed and maintained highways; broadcasters are granted rights to the electromagnetic spectrum; baseball teams play their games in municipal stadiums for which they pay negligible rent. Every corporation in America employs workers who are trained at public expense. If private gain from public expenditure is illegitimate, none of these can stand. The mixed economy gives way to one in which there is only one economic agent, the state.

I believe this to be a terrible alternative. Thoroughgoing socialism is a prescription for rigidity, irrational allocation of productive resources, and general inefficiency. Through its centralization of economic power it also places political liberties in jeopardy. But this is an old story, not worth retelling here. To uphold vintage socialism is to oppose all

From *Hastings Center Report*, 1987, 17·(June), pp. 5–7. © The Hastings Center.

private enterprise, not merely that which feeds on overflow from the public trough. The position against which I direct my criticism maintains the general legitimacy, even desirability, of private enterprise, but only when it scrupulously refrains from capitalizing on public expenditure. This position is incoherent. Its qualified endorsement of private profit-making activity is incompatible with the proposed constraint. When the public sphere is so much with us, its embrace cannot be totally avoided.

It should be clear why invocation of classical private property theory, such as that set out by Locke, is thoroughly misleading in this context. The Lockean heuristic applies in the first instance to appropriation of previously unowned items by individuals within the state of nature. The reference to the state of nature is not merely an antiquarian indulgence. It is an essential component of Locke's theory, signifying that individuals are not without prior consent to be implicated in each other's designs, let alone in an overarching social enterprise. And when a state does emerge, it functions almost entirely as the protector of the rights that individuals were alleged to enjoy in the state of nature. Classical political philosophy does not endorse the largesse-dispensing state, and it certainly does not suppose that state activity should be permitted to preempt private appropriation and exploitation of property.

I have argued that there exists no general moral presumption against deriving private income from public activities. That is not inconsistent with condemning particular instances of cashing in. A mayor may not award construction contracts to the bidder who most profusely lines his pocket with cash. I may not open up a boutique in the office that the University of Minnesota provides me. These, however, are impermissible because each involves the violation of a specific trust. Is there a corresponding violation when an individual who enjoyed the use of federal research funds attempts to profit by building an artificial heart or splicing genes? No convincing argument for that conclusion comes to mind. Quite a few specious ones do.

The profit motive and scientific knowledge

It could be claimed that medical and scientific personnel, because of the special nature of their calling, are obliged to eschew such private enrichment. They have committed themselves to the disinterested pursuit of knowledge. Discovery and application of knowledge are to be for the general welfare. It is an instance of bad faith to make these subsidiary to the end of money making.[1]

This argument is vulnerable at several points. First, this represents a contestable view of the priority of purposes that should characterize professionals. It is, definitionally, the scientist's goal to seek knowledge. Similarly, it is the barber's goal to cut hair, the accountant's to balance books, the rancher's to raise steers. Presumably, no one would require of the latter three that they set aside as a primary motivation the making of profit. The barber cuts hair because he aims thereby to gain. No moral injunction is violated. Setting knowledge above profit is one way in which the scientist can elect to structure his ends. But why should it be supposed that the reverse ordering is illicit?

Second, the argument assumes that the aim of generating knowledge is subverted by the pursuit of profit. That assumption is suspect. Discovery and application of knowledge, let us agree, can pay off in the coin of the realm. If that is the coin that jingles in my dreams, then I have a strong incentive to succeed in my scientific endeavors. This is but a particular instance of the economist's insistence that individuals are predictably and reliably motivated by self-interested concern, and that this circumstance tends to be socially beneficial: "He is. . . . led by an invisible hand to promote an end which was no part of his intention. Nor is it always the worse for society that it was not part of it. By pursuing his own interest he frequently promotes that of the society more effectually than when he really intends to promote it."[2] The hand may, on occasion, be palsied and require the assistance of a suitable prosthetic, but no evidence has yet been given that pecuniary motivation is inimical to good science.

Third, in somewhat *ad hominem* fashion, I note that a constraint against money making by scientific and medical personnel is elsewhere conspicuous by its absence. Salary schedules indicate that scientists do well, and physicians do very well indeed. If one considers also nonmonetary returns such as prestige, stimulating challenges, social opportunities, and the like, the payoff is even greater. Nor is there much evidence that this is a windfall that has fallen unbidden into checking accounts. If science-for-profit is truly illegitimate, artificial hearts are a trivial component of the malaise.

Another objection is that these profits are incommensurate with effort. A physician is entitled to income from the exercise of his profession, because he provides value-added services. But the builder of an artificial heart is merely appropriating already existing knowledge while supplying nothing of his own (or at least nothing that was not previously paid for by governmental research grants).

This represents a provincial understanding of what constitutes productive knowledge. The entrepreneur just as surely as the scientist generates useful knowledge. It is the knowledge of how scarce resources can more efficiently be applied to the satisfaction of human wants. Scientific knowledge may be good in itself, but it does not contribute to social well-being until transmuted into goods and services.

The process is not automatic; experiments are as much an aspect of the marketplace as they are of the laboratory. Some succeed while others fail. The much-discussed case of the Jarvik–7 is to the point. It may eventually return a profit to investors, but that is a distant prospect. At present, the artificial heart's ink is as red as the blood it pumps. Among the kinds of socially valuable knowledge is knowledge of which deployments of resources are productive and which are not. If the scientist-turned-entrepreneur succeeds in enriching himself, it is almost certainly because he has contributed such useful knowledge.

No investigator does more than push back ignorance a bit at the margin. Whether scientist or entrepreneur, he is the beneficiary of the entire history of human experience. The labor of previous generations and contemporaries alike provides the foundations on which each of us is able to build. No one can claim that a productive innovation stems entirely from his own effort. That should not, however, be taken as warrant for denying that individuals do generate products that are recognizably *theirs,* from which they are entitled to profit. Sociality and individual enterprise are complements, not contraries. Innovation builds on the contributions of others but in turn renders possible still further advance. The process is one on which civilization is built. It is counterproductive to allow envy or suspect ideology to subvert it.

It can be argued in response that profit from publicly funded research is legitimate, but that it should be public profit. Taxpayers have funded the research that makes the Jarvik–7 possible; therefore it is they rather than Jarvik himself who should reap the profits. The point is one of elemental fairness. People should not unduly reap benefits that derive from the contributions of others.

The argument deserves to be taken seriously. That the taxpayer is a much-abused species is a claim I have no wish to contest! Indeed, my quarrel is with its far too limited application. It is nothing short of scandalous that our political institutions routinely redistribute wealth from the less wealthy to the wealthier. That occurs, for example, when taxpayers subsidize farmers and also have to pay higher food prices. It also occurs, and in particularly blatant form, when taxpayers are required to subsidize attendance in business, law, and medical school. Those destined to be among the highest earning of our citizens are boosted into that enviable status on the backs of those distinctly less well off. Should someone wish to launch a campaign against regressive transfer payments, I would be delighted to enlist in the ranks. But, again, I am not here addressing general issues of political philosophy. Rather, I wish to consider whether there may be any special reasons why the government ought to be in the business of investing in the creation and dissemination of knowledge.

Two reasons come to mind. First, it can be claimed that knowledge is in itself a good thing. We ought to have more of it, indeed, more than individuals in their private capacity will provide. Through subsidizing the knowledge business, government causes there to be more of it.

Second, knowledge is, in the parlance of the economist, a *public good*. A public good has two defining traits: (1) if it is consumed by one person, it is difficult or impossible to prevent others from consuming it; (2) if one person consumes the good, the stock of it available to other persons is not thereby diminished. National defense is a good example. If Jones is defended from foreign aggression, it will be impossible to withhold defense from Smith, Jones's neighbor. And defense for Jones does not entail that there is less defense for Smith. Knowledge is, in the relevant respects, similar to defense. Knowledge is not diminished by being shared, nor can it easily be fenced off from appropriation by others.

Public goods will be undersupplied on the market. That is because individuals will be unable to appropriate the full product of their investment. If the good is supplied by one, all reap the benefit. Therefore, each does better when the good is produced by someone else rather than by himself. This argument may appear to reflect a somewhat jaded view of human beings as egoistic creatures who care only for themselves. That surmise is incorrect. Public goods will be undersupplied by individuals who genuinely value the welfare of others, but who value their own welfare just a little bit more. Indeed, even perfect altruists may underinvest in public goods, allocating their resources instead to bequests privately appropriable by the beneficiaries. Public goods problems are not dissolved by moral education.

The dilemma is obvious. So too is the solution. Public goods will be adequately supplied if contributions can be secured from all prospective beneficiaries. Within small groups this sometimes can be accomplished through moral suasion, but in a large collectivity institutional means for securing compliance are required. The state becomes the primary provider of public goods. All political theorists, except some extreme libertarians, agree that this is a legitimate role for government.

If knowledge is valuable in itself, that may be adequate reason to promote through governmental auspices its *discovery*. But that consideration is neutral with respect to how knowledge is to be *applied*. It is the public goods consideration that is relevant to issues of application. And here the balance is decisively on the side of encouraging the widest possible appropriation of knowledge generated through governmental programs. We cannot know in advance who will be best able to distill from the products of pure research those goods and services that most effectively satisfy the preferences of individuals. Competitive deployment of entrepreneurial energies is the surest means we know of to spread the benefits of knowledge to potential consumers, and it is the profit motive that predictably fuels the competition. It is an excess of diffidence to prohibit scientific researchers from joining the fray.

The alternatives to competitive exploitation of knowledge are either allowing knowledge to lie fallow or restricting the exploitation of publicly subsidized knowledge to public enterprises. The former is obviously self-abnegatory, the latter only slightly less so. Whatever public goods argument supports governmental production of knowledge entirely disappears when we turn to consider its application. Individuals can indeed appropriate the fruits of investment in knowledge application, and they will bend their energies to do so unless barred by edict. The market is not without flaws, but even its harshest critics concede that it is remarkably responsive to opportunities for allocative gains. The same cannot be said for state enterprises, as anyone who has walked into a post office can attest. Public monopolies are no more to be welcomed than private ones. Health care is simply too important to be left to the indifferent attention of some public corporation within the hydra that is the Department of Health and Human Services.

Yes, let us attempt to prevent private interests from illegitimately intercepting dollars that belong in the hands of taxpayers. But at the same time, we should beware of seduction by envy or abstract principles of dubious applicability. State intrusions are ubiquitous within ostensibly private enterprises. I believe that to be unfortunate. It would, though, be making a bad thing worse to use that circumstance as a pretext for diminishing further the realm within which individuals who seek profit for themselves simultaneously enrich the lives of us all.

Notes

1. For an analogous argument and objection, see Plato, *The Republic,* Book I, 342c–343b.
2. Adam Smith, *An Inquiry into the Nature and Causes of the Wealth of Nations,* IV.ii.9.

30
Patenting life: Summary, policy issues, and options for congressional action

U.S. Office of Technology Assessment

Intellectual property

Rooted in the Constitution, intellectual property law provides a personal property interest in the work of the mind. Modern intellectual property law consists of several areas of law: patent, copyright, trademark, trade secret, and breeders' rights.

Patents

A patent is a grant issued by the U.S. Government giving the patent owner the right to exclude all others from making, using, or selling the invention within the United States, and its territories and possessions, during the term of the patent (35 U.S.C. 154). A patent may be granted to whoever invents or discovers any new, useful, and nonobvious process, machine, manufacture, composition of matter, or any new and useful improvement of these items (35 U.S.C. 101). A patent may also be granted on any distinct and new variety of asexually reproduced plant (35 U.S.C. 161) or on any new, original, and ornamental design for an article of manufacture (35 U.S.C. 171).

The first patent act was enacted by Congress in 1790, providing protection for "any new and useful art, machine, manufacture, or composition of matter, or any new and useful improvement [thereof]." Subsequent patent statutes were enacted in 1793, 1836, 1870, and 1874, which employed the same broad language as the 1790 Act. The Patent Act of 1952 replaced "art" with "process" as patentable subject matter (35 U.S.C. 101). The Committee Reports accompanying the 1952 Act demonstrate that Congress intended patentable subject matter to include "anything under the sun that is made by man." However, the Supreme Court has held that laws of nature, physical phenomena, and abstract ideas are not patentable.

Patents have many of the attributes of personal property (35 U.S.C. 261). Property is generally viewed as a bundle of legally protected interests, including the right to possess and to use, to transfer by sale and gift, and to exclude others from possession. Patents are designed to encourage inventiveness by granting to inventors and assignees a limited property right – the right to exclude others from practicing the invention for a period of 17 years. In return for this limited property right, the inventor is required to file a written patent application describing the invention in full, clear, concise, and exact terms, setting

From U.S. Congressional Office of Technology Assessment, *New Developments in Biotechnology: Patenting Life* (Washington, DC: U.S. Government Printing Office, 1988), pp. 4–5, 7–9, 12–18.

forth the best mode contemplated by the inventor, so as to enable any person skilled in the art of the invention to make and use it. **Although a patent excludes others from making, using, or selling the invention, it does not give the patent owner any affirmative rights to do likewise. As with other forms of property, the right to make, use, or sell a patented invention may be regulated by Federal, State, or local law.**

Patents are more difficult to obtain than other forms of intellectual property protection. All applications are examined by the Patent and Trademark Office (PTO), which is responsible for issuing patents if all legal requirements are met. Once obtained, the enforceability of a utility patent is maintained by the payment of periodic maintenance fees.

. . .

Patenting of micro-organisms and cells

Patents on biotechnological processes date from the early days of the United States. Louis Pasteur received a patent for a process of fermenting beer. Acetic acid fermentation and other food patents date from the early 1800s, while therapeutic patents in biotechnology were issued as early as 1895.

The development of recombinant DNA technology (rDNA) – the controlled joining of DNA from different organisms – has resulted in greatly increased understanding of the genetic and molecular basis of life. Following the first successful directed insertion of recombinant DNA into a host micro-organism in 1973, scientific researchers began to recognize the potential for directing the cellular machinery to develop new and improved products and processes in a wide variety of industrial sectors. Many of these products were micro-organisms (microscopic living entities) or cells (the smallest component of life capable of carrying on all essential life processes). With the development of recombinant DNA technology, the potential of patenting the living organism resulting from the technology arose.

Prior to 1980, PTO would not grant patents for such inventions, deeming them to be ''products of nature'' and not statutory subject matter as defined by 35 U.S.C. 101. Although patent applications were rejected if directed to living organisms per se, patent protection was granted for many compositions containing living things (e.g., sterility test devices containing living microbial spores, food yeast compositions, vaccines containing attenuated bacteria, milky spore insecticides, and various dairy products). In the absence of congressional action, it took a catalytic court decision to clarify the issue of patentability of living subject matter.

The Chakrabarty case

The Supreme Court's single foray into biotechnology occurred in 1980 with its ruling in the patent law case of *Diamond v. Chakrabarty*. Chakrabarty had developed a genetically modified bacterium capable of breaking down multiple components of crude oil. Because this property was not possessed by any naturally occurring bacteria, Chakrabarty's invention was thought to have significant value for cleaning up oil spills.

Chakrabarty's claims to the bacteria were rejected by PTO on two grounds:

- micro-organisms are ''products of nature;'' and

• as living things, micro-organisms are not patentable subject matter under 35 U.S.C. 101.*

Following two levels of appeals, the case was heard by the U.S. Supreme Court, which in a 5–4 ruling, held that **a live, human-made micro-organism is patentable subject matter under Section 101 as a "manufacture" or "composition of matter."** The court reached several conclusions in analyzing whether the bacteria could be considered patentable subject matter within the meaning of the statute:

• The plain meaning of the statutory language indicated Congress' intent that the patent laws be given wide scope. The terms "manufacture" and "composition of matter" are broad terms, modified by the expansive term "any."
• The legislative history of the patent statute supported a broad construction that Congress intended patent protection to include "anything under the sun made by man."
• Although laws of nature, physical phenomena, and abstract ideas are not patentable, Chakrabarty's micro-organism was a product of human ingenuity having a distinct name, character, and use.
• The passage of the 1930 Plant Patent Act (affording patent protection for certain asexually reproduced plants) and the 1970 Plant Variety Protection Act (providing protection for certain sexually reproduced plants) does not evidence congressional understanding that the terms "manufacture" or "composition of matter" do not include living things.
• The fact that genetic technology was unforeseen when Congress enacted Section 101 does not require the conclusion that micro-organisms cannot qualify as patentable subject matter until Congress expressly authorizes such protection.
• Arguments against patentability based on potential hazards that may be generated by genetic research should be addressed to Congress and the executive branch for regulation or control, not to the judiciary.

Post-Chakrabarty events and trends

The *Chakrabarty* decision and subsequent actions by Congress and the executive branch provided great economic stimulus to patenting of micro-organisms and cells, which in turn provided stimulus to the growth of the biotechnology industry in the 1980s. In addition to the *Chakrabarty* decision, revisions in Federal patent policy promoted increased patenting of inventions in general, including living organisms and related processes. The Patent and Trademark Amendments of 1980 (Public Law 96–517) as amended in 1984 (Public Law 98–620) encourage the patenting and commercialization of government-funded inventions by permitting small businesses and non-profit organizations to retain ownership of inventions developed in the course of federally funded research.

These policies, which gave statutory preference to small businesses and nonprofit organizations, were extended to larger businesses by Executive order in 1983. The Technology Transfer Act of 1986 (Public Law 99–502) granted Federal authority to form

---

* Section 101. Inventions Patentable. Whoever invents or discovers any new and useful process, machine, manufacture, or composition of matter, or any new and useful improvement thereof, may obtain a patent therefor, subject to the conditions and requirements of this title.

consortia with private concerns. An Executive order issued in 1987 further encouraged technology transfer programs, including the transfer of patent rights to government grantees.

Increased patenting of biotechnology inventions has led to litigation, primarily related to patent infringement issues. Already, patent battles are being fought over interleukin–2, tissue plasminogen activator, human growth hormone, alpha interferon, factor VIII, and use of dual monoclonal antibody sandwich immunoassays in diagnostic test kits. It is likely that patent litigation relating to biotechnology will increase given the complex web of partially overlapping patent claims, the high value of products, the problem of prior publication, and the fact that many companies are pursuing the same products.

One negative trend arising from the increase in patent applications is the inability of PTO to process biotechnology applications in a timely manner. The number of these applications has severely challenged the process and examination capabilities of PTO. In March 1988, PTO reorganized its biotechnology effort into a separate patent examining group. As of July 1988, 5,850 biotechnology applications had not yet been acted on. **Currently, approximately 15 months lapse, on average, before examination of a biotechnology application initiates, and an average of 27 months passes before the examination process is completed by grant of the patent or abandonment of the application.** Turnover among patent examiners, lured to the private sector by higher pay, is cited as a significant reason for the delay in reviewing patents.

.   .   .

Patenting of animals

In April 1987, the Board of Patent Appeals and Interferences ruled that polyploid oysters were patentable subject matter. Subsequently, PTO announced that it would henceforth consider nonnaturally occurring nonhuman multicellular living organisms, including animals, to be patentable subject matter under general patent law. This statement initiated broad debate and the introduction of legislation concerning the patenting of animals.

The first animal patent was issued in April 1988 to Harvard University for mammals genetically engineered to contain a cancer-causing gene (U.S. 4,736,866). Exclusive license to practice the patent went to E.I. du Pont de Nemours & Co., which was the major sponsor of the research. The patented mouse was genetically engineered to be unusually susceptible to cancer, thus facilitating the testing of carcinogens and of cancer therapies. Specifically, the patent covers "a transgenic nonhuman eukaryotic animal (preferably a rodent such as a mouse) whose germ cells and somatic cells contain an activated oncogene sequence introduced into the animal ... which increases the probability of the development of neoplasms (particularly malignant tumors) in the animal." In November 1988, du Pont announced its intention to begin sales of the patented "oncomouse" in early 1989. The 1987 PTO policy and the 1988 issuance of the first patent on a transgenic animal spurred public debate on scientific, regulatory, economic, and ethical issues.

Producing transgenic animals

Most potentially patentable animals are likely to be transgenic animals produced via recombinant DNA techniques or genetic engineering. Transgenic animals are those whose

DNA, or hereditary material, has been augmented by adding DNA from a source other than parental germplasm, usually from different animals or from humans.

Laboratories around the world are conducting research that involves inserting genes from vertebrates (including humans, mammals, or other higher organisms) into bacteria, yeast, insect viruses, or mammalian cells in culture. A variety of techniques, most developed from early bacterial research, can now be used to insert genes from one animal into another. These techniques are known by a number of exotic names: microinjection, cell fusion, electroporation, retroviral transformation, and others. **Of the currently available scientific techniques, microinjection is the method most commonly used and most likely to lead to practical applications in mammals in the near future. Other methods of gene insertion may become more widely used in the future as techniques are refined and improved.** If protocols for human gene therapy, now being developed in animal models, or laboratory cultures of mammalian cells prove successful and broadly adaptable to other mammals, other gene insertion techniques could supplant microinjection.

Although the number of laboratories working with transgenic animals remains small (no more than a few hundred, worldwide), and researchers with the required skill and experience are not common, the number of research programs using these techniques has grown steadily in recent years. For reasons of convenience, much research involving transgenic mammals continues to be done using mice, although programs using several larger mammals have made significant progress. **It is anticipated that some animals of research utility or substantial economic importance will become more common as subjects of transgenic modifications in the near future (within 5 to 10 years). Beyond mice, the major research efforts involving transgenic modifications focus on cattle, swine, goats, sheep, poultry, and fish.**

Producing transgenic animals by microinjection, although tedious, labor intensive, and inefficient (only a small fraction of injected eggs develop into transgenic animals), compares favorably in at least three respects with traditional breeding techniques:

- The rapidity with which a specific gene can be inserted into a desired host means that **the time it takes to establish a line of animals carrying the desired trait is much reduced.**
- The specific gene of interest can be transferred with great confidence, if not efficiency, and if proper purification protocols are followed, **without any accompanying, unwanted genetic material.**
- With proper preparation, **genes from almost any organism can be inserted into the desired host,** whether it is a mouse or some other animal. Historically, genetic material exchanged by classical hybridization (crossbreeding) could only be transferred between closely related species or different strains within a species.

If there is a fundamental difference arising from the new techniques, it is that breeders have greatly augmented ability to move genes between organisms that are not close genetic relatives (e.g., human and mouse, or human and bacterium). Most transgenic animal research in the near future will likely focus on traits involving a single gene. Manipulation of complex traits influenced by more than one gene, however, such as the amount of growth possible on a limited food regimen, or behavioral characteristics, will develop more slowly (perhaps within 10 to 30 years) because of greater technical difficulty and the current lack of understanding of how such traits are controlled by genes.

Species barriers and species integrity

Some concern has been raised over negative impacts transgenic animals might have on their own species, based on the assertion that transferring genes between species transgresses natural barriers between species, and thus violates their "integrity" or identity.

Modern biologists generally think of species as reproductive communities or populations. They are distinguished by their collective manifestation of ranges of variation with respect to many different characteristics or qualities simultaneously. The parameters that limit these ranges of variation are fluid and variable themselves: different species may have substantially different genetic population structures, and a given species may look significantly different in one part of its range than it does in another while still demonstrably belonging to the same gene pool or reproductive community. Although research into the nature of species continues to be vigorous, marked by much discussion and disagreement among specialists, general agreement among biologists exists on at least one point: **nature makes it clear that there is no universal or absolute rule that all species are discretely bounded in any generally consistent manner.**

The issue of species integrity is more complex and subtle than that of species barriers. If a species can be thought of as having integrity as a biological unit, that integrity must, because of the nature of species, be rooted in the identity of the genetic material carried by the species. Precisely how a species might be defined genetically is not yet apparent.

Any genetic definition of species, grounded in the perception of a species as a dynamic population, rather than a unit, cannot be simple; it must be statistical and complex. Therefore, **to violate the "integrity" of a species it is not sufficient to find a particular gene, once widespread throughout the species, now entirely replaced by a different gene.** Such changes occur repeatedly throughout the evolutionary history of a lineage and are described as microevolutionary. These changes are usually insufficient to alter a species in any fundamental way or to threaten any perceived genetic integrity.

If it is possible to challenge the integrity of a species, it would have to be by changing or disrupting something fundamental in its genetic architecture, organization, or function. Mammals like mice, cattle, or humans may contain from 50,000 to 100,000 or more genes. Whatever it is in the organization and coordination of activity between these genes that is fundamental to their identity as species, it is not likely to be disrupted by the simple insertion or manipulation of the small number of genes (fewer than 20) that transgenic animal research will involve for the foreseeable future.

The right of a species to exist as a separate, identifiable creature has no known foundation in biology. Species exist in nature as reproductive communities, not as separate creatures. The history of systematics and taxonomy (the disciplines of naming and describing species) demonstrates that species' existence has often been independent of scientists' shifting understanding or abilities to discern this existence. Furthermore, most of the domestic animals that are now the subjects of transgenic research (with the possible exception of some fish), and are likely to be for the foreseeable future, are already the products of centuries, and in many cases millennia, of human manipulation.

Federal regulation and animal patents

To gain an understanding of the potential use and regulation of genetically altered animals that might be patented, OTA asked selected Federal agencies the following questions:

* How are genetically altered animals currently used in research, product development, and mission-oriented activities conducted or funded by your agency?
* What are the potential uses of such animals during the next 5 years?
* How does (or would) your agency regulate such animal use? What statutes, regulations, guidelines, or policy statements are relevant?

Several agencies currently use transgenic animals. The National Institutes of Health is currently the largest user of such animals for biomedical research projects. USDA has conducted research on the genetics of animals for many years. USDA's Agricultural Research Service reported projects involving the use of growth hormone in sheep and swine, and chickens engineered by recombinant DNA technology to be resistant to avian leukosis virus. USDA's Cooperative Research Service is in the early stages of supporting extramural research projects involving genetically engineered animals. The National Science Foundation (NSF) currently funds research involving transgenic animals in a range of experiments, all involving laboratory animals. With the use of transgenic animals becoming central to whole lines of investigation, NSF expects that work with such animals will increase. The Agency for International Development (AID) funds research involving conventional and transgenic animals at international research centers that are only partially funded by the United States. Accordingly, AID has minimal control over such research activities.

Several Federal agencies regulate experimental use or commercial development of genetically altered animals. Because current statutes regulate various uses and protections for animals, no single Federal policy governs all uses of genetically altered animals. In the absence of a single policy, Federal agencies will rely on existing statutes, regulations, and guidelines to regulate transgenic animal research and product development. **Current federally funded research efforts could lead to patents on animals. The patentability of an animal, however, does not affect the manner in which the animal would be regulated by any Federal agency.**

Economic considerations

Economic considerations will influence the order in which different transgenic animals are produced for commerce. Transgenic animals used for biomedical research are likely to be developed first, primarily due to extensive research in this area. Transgenic agricultural animals are also likely to be produced, although large-scale commercial production of such livestock and poultry is unlikely in the near future (5 to 10 years). **The largest economic sectors likely to be influenced by animal patents are the different markets for agricultural livestock and some sectors of the pharmaceutical**

industry. The principal agricultural markets involve poultry, dairy, and red meat. These markets are organized quite differently, and are subject to different degrees of economic concentration. Poultry is most concentrated (though still diffuse by the standards of other industries, such as automobiles) and the dairy and red meat sectors much more diffuse. Different economic forces are important in markets as well: Federal price supports are of major importance in the dairy market, while the market for poultry is more open and competitive.

It is difficult to predict the manifold consequences of any particular approach to protecting intellectual property, especially across so wide a range of economic activity as that spanned by patentable animals. This range embraces diverse sectors of the agricultural livestock markets, pharmaceutical and other chemical production, as well as academic research or industrial testing. The economics of patenting and the effect on inventors and consumers will be determined by the potential use of the animal, its market, its reproduction rate, and its relative value.

The existence of animal patents and the degree to which they are employed in the different markets may introduce some new economic relationships. It is not now clear that these are likely to have any substantially adverse effects on the major markets or existing market forces. **The same types of pressures that have driven economic choices in the past are likely to continue to dictate them in the future. If an innovation increases costs (e.g., if a patented animal costs more than the unpatented alternative) it is unlikely to be adopted unless it commensurately increases outputs or product values.** It therefore seems that although cost savings can be anticipated to follow from animal patenting in some areas (e.g., pharmaceutical production or drug testing), innovations attributable to patented animals are likely to advance more slowly in low margin operations such as raising beef cattle.

In some cases, efficient alternatives to protection of intellectual property via patents are feasible. Trade secrets or contractual arrangements might serve well where the animals involved have a high intrinsic value and are limited in number (e.g., animals used for pharmaceutical production). When faced with the complexity of the markets for pork or beef production, however, such alternatives are clearly less practical, although the same complexity complicates any scheme for enforcement or royalty collection associated with patenting animals per se.

Ethical considerations

A number of ethical issues have been raised in regards to patenting animals. Many of these arguments focus on the consequences that could occur subsequent to the patenting of animals. Other arguments focus on religious, philosophical, spiritual, or metaphysical grounds. These arguments have been used to support and oppose the concept of animal patenting.

Many arguments relating to the consequences of animal patenting are difficult to evaluate since they are speculative, relying on factual assertions that have yet to occur or be proven. Arguments based largely on theological, philosophical, spiritual, or metaphysical considerations are likewise difficult to resolve, since they usually require the assumption of certain presuppositions that may not be shared by other persons. Thus, such arguments are not likely to be reconciled with those persons holding opposing and often strongly held beliefs.

Most arguments that have been raised both for and against the patenting of animals concern issues that would be materially unchanged whether patents are permitted or not. Most arguments center on issues that existed prior to the current patenting debate (e.g., animal rights, the effect of high technology on American agriculture, the distribution of wealth, international competitiveness, the release of novel organisms into the environment). It is unclear that patenting per se would substantially redirect the way society uses or relates to animals.

Many concerns about the consequences of patenting can be addressed by appropriate regulations or statutes, rather than by amendments to patent law. Other arguments, particularly those of theological, philosophical, spiritual, or metaphysical origin, need to be debated more fully and articulated more clearly.

31
New opportunities create new problems

Association of Academic Health Centers

In recent years, cooperative endeavors between academic institutions and industry have raised new public concerns about potential conflicts of interest. The increased commercial possibilities that have accompanied the expansion of the biomedical research field have led to perceptions in academe, government and industry that such situations threaten to compromise not only the objectivity and obligations of researchers, but also the missions of academic institutions. Concerns also focus on the inherent differences in outlook and philosophy of universities and industry, which pose ethical dilemmas for both institutions and scholars.

The existence of conflicts of interest has long been recognized by universities, which have attempted to develop institutional policies to manage these conflicts. Conflicts of interest are neither unique to academic health centers nor confined to the biomedical research field. However, the special value placed on health, and the special trust placed in universities, make academic health centers particularly vulnerable to public scrutiny and accountability. Moreover, the three-fold, interrelated missions of academic health centers – the education of health professionals, the conduct of biomedical research, and the delivery of patient care services – combined with the basic values of the universities of which they are a part, create a unique institutional environment and raise special problems. These missions can be a source of unavoidable conflict in themselves. They can produce ambiguities and conflicts as individuals are faced with competing goals and obligations – many of which affect the well-being of the public.

The mission of patient care can generate an additional set of conflicts of interest. They arise in the management of faculty practice plans, clinics, and proprietary ventures of the university faculty to which certain academic health center patients may be referred. These issues in clinical care are profound and complex. They are affected by the larger social debate – not focused on academic health centers – about the propriety of a whole range of financial arrangements among hospitals, physicians, suppliers, and companies in the health field. Legislation and regulations have emerged from this debate, and it seems likely that more is on the way.[1] However, these issues in clinical care are not the main focus of this report. Instead, we address principally conflicts more uniquely related

From Association of Academic Health Centers, *Conflicts of Interest in Academic Health Centers* (Washington, DC: AAHC, 1990), 1–16. This report is a product of the Task Force on Science Policy. The Board of Directors of the Association of Academic Health Centers (AHC) has approved its release as an AHC document. The views expressed in this report are those of the task force and do not necessarily represent the views of the Board or the membership at large. The preparation of this paper was supported in part by the Josiah Macy, Jr. Foundation. Copyright 1990 by the Association of Academic Health Centers.

to the university's primary missions of research, and teaching, and endeavors that derive from them.

This report analyzes how potential conflicts of interest may arise in the context of research or related activities of faculty, staff and students in academic health centers. While some of the sources of conflict and principles that are suggested to guide action are more widely applicable, this report focuses specifically on what *academic health centers* can do to identify, avoid and manage conflicts of interest within the university culture. It is not intended as a blueprint for regulation by state or federal governments.

Many groups are concerned about conflict of interest issues. For example, at the 1982 Pajaro Dunes, California conference, presidents of major research universities and corporate chief executive officers analyzed corporate-research relationships. "The premise of the conference was that collaboration between universities and industry will benefit all parties if the university's ideals are in no way distorted by industry's millions." Although the discussion was useful, no consensus was achieved on most issues. Nevertheless, the conference reached agreement on the controversial issue of university investments in proprietary companies. The group concluded that these investments are ill advised "unless . . . there are sufficient safeguards to avoid adverse effects on the morale of the institution."[2]

While most universities have developed policies and procedures to manage conflicts of interest, academic health centers conduct some kinds of research that may generate unique concerns. Principal among these is research (either basic or clinical) to develop or evaluate products intended for clinical application which may have great commercial value.[3] Another problem results from the fact that in contemporary biomedical research, the boundary is increasingly blurred between the foundational work conducted in academic health center laboratories and the immediately derivative product development work which is often done in the commercial sector.

These issues are complex, and some of them are of concern to many audiences. But they are principally matters that concern the university and the academic health center, and the AHC believes accordingly that the primary responsibility for managing these conflicts and for establishing appropriate guidelines for faculty behavior must rest with the academic institutions. For their part, research sponsors, and especially the federal government, have only a limited, albeit sharply defined, area of interest in these matters, namely to ensure that the research they support is conducted and reported with integrity. Similarly, the Food and Drug Administration, in approving drugs, medical devices and diagnostic products, and the Health Care Financing Administration, in deciding whether to pay for them, have interests in assuring that the data on which they form their conclusions are trustworthy.

Academic institutions vary greatly in their approaches to faculty governance, administration, culture, history and research portfolios. Nonetheless, they share a need to develop clear policies and comprehensive procedures regarding conflicts of interest that will satisfy the requirements of the individual institutions while being implemented more broadly in a generally consistent fashion. Some degree of consistency of policy is especially important to provide reasonable assurances to research sponsors and the public and to accommodate an era in which collaboration of investigators from many different institutions is increasingly common.

A. Defining conflicts of interest

Like many important concepts, "conflict of interest" is susceptible to many meanings. It is often used in debate as if merely affixing it to an opponent proves misconduct. This view is mistaken for several reasons. First, "conflict of interest" has meaning only with reference to *an explicit body of norms that the actor and others would agree constrain their behavior*. Only those subject to some professional code, or some generally accepted standards of practice or performance, are expected to avoid "conflicts of interest." Second, some conflicts of interest are unavoidable and acceptable. The mere existence of a conflict does not imply wrongful behavior; more specifically, it does not connote professional or scientific misconduct.

In an abstract sense, conflicts of interest are ubiquitous. One might say that a person has a conflict of interest whenever the person's own interests are different from those of others, or when the person has two conflicting desires or goals. But such a definition would make the concept so universal as to be meaningless. A physician would therefore always have a "conflict" between his or her interests in treating patients effectively, limiting health costs, making money, avoiding malpractice, being reasonably available, and having some time for family and personal activities. Similarly, a researcher may wish to gain fame and obtain additional funds, but also wish to report the truth. If one views these as "conflicts of interest," the concept has no limit.

Therefore, a useful discussion of conflicts of interest must begin with a definition that excludes conflicts that are trivial or unavoidable. The definition also must be more than a projection of individual values; more than merely that a conflict "is in the eye of the beholder." Conflicts of interest can be discussed concretely only if it is widely agreed that a given person *is supposed to obey a particular set of norms*.

Fortunately, in the case of professions it is possible to be more specific. The essence of a profession is that its members commit themselves to a set of standards and behavioral norms higher than or different from merely the morals of the marketplace. Sometimes, state licensing rules even incorporate a professional code of ethics. In the health professions, one can refer to the Principles of Medical Ethics, the Code of Ethics of the American Academy of Ophthalmology, the Principles of Psychologists, the Principles of Ethics of the American Dental Association, the Code for Nurses of the American Nurses' Association, and similar codes.[4] These embodiments of professional norms – although not exhaustive of the informal standards that guide professionals – nevertheless provide tangible points of reference.

As one moves from clinical care to teaching, research, and university administration, however, it is not so easy to identify a "code of professional ethics" that addresses the problems or that provides guidance for their resolution. Conduct in an academic health center implicates a variety of professional codes (*e.g.*, for physicians or psychologists); federal regulations (*e.g.*, on human subjects); state laws (*e.g.*, on pharmacy licensure); university rules (*e.g.*, on approval of research protocols); and contractual requirements (*e.g.*, on teaching commitment). Proper conduct often requires considering some or all of these obligations – as well as old-fashioned common sense, honesty, and fairness. But sorting these out – especially when they conflict – is far from a simple task.

In addition, it is important to distinguish between *conflict of interest* and *conflict of commitment:*

Conflict of interest has two distinct components – conflict of interest which most often involves money, and conflict of commitment, which most often involves time. Conflict of interest exists whenever an individual's personal ties could unduly influence a professional judgment. Conflict of commitment exists when an individual's primary loyalties are in doubt. Both types of conflict are part of the territory when a University invites the spirit of entrepreneurialism into its midst. Universities are institutions that purport to serve the public good, while entrepreneurs . . . are interested in private gain.[5]

This distinction is incorporated, for example, in the University of Illinois "Interim Guidelines and Procedures on Conflicts of Interests Policies" (1988):

1. A 'conflict of commitment' exists when the external or other activities and undertakings of an academic staff member are so substantial or demanding of the staff member's time and attention as to interfere, or appear to interfere, with the individual's responsibilities to the unit to which the individual is assigned, or to students, or to the University.
2. A 'conflict of interest' may take various forms, but arises when an academic staff member is or may be in a position to influence the University business, research, or other decisions in ways that could lead to any form of personal gain for the academic staff member or the staff member's family, or give improper advantage to others to the University's detriment.

Based on our own experiences and the analysis above, we believe that a serviceable definition is that:

A potential or actual conflict of interest exists when legal obligations or widely recognized professional norms are likely to be compromised by a person's other interests, particularly if those interests are not disclosed.

This definition underlies our analysis in the remainder of the Report.

B. History of research collaboration between industry and academe

The collaboration of academic researchers with government and industry has a long tradition in this country, particularly in the fields of chemistry, engineering, and agriculture.[6] For example, Alexander Graham Bell collaborated for years with MIT physics professor Charles Cross, who already had a device for electronic transmission of sound when Bell arrived in our country. Cross became a consultant to the Bell Telephone Company and later, to AT&T.[7] In the ensuing decades, it became widely recognized that the American system, in which there are many interchanges between researchers, teachers, and industry, has tremendous advantages both for the progress of scholarship and for the expansion of commerce. Within the last decade, industrial sponsorship of research has accelerated with the active encouragement of the federal government, as biotechnology, information technology, and related fields have become burgeoning areas of our economic life. Under President Carter, the White House staff expressed concern about delays in the flow of knowledge and technology from universities to industry and then to the public.[8] Congress responded by providing tax credits for industrial research, and by creating incentives through the presumption that the university – rather than the government – owns inventions resulting from federally supported research.[9]

Congress also enacted the Stevenson-Wydler Technology Innovation Act in 1980 (Pub.

L. 96–480), which established a national policy of encouraging cooperative arrangements among industry, government and academic institutions. This was followed in 1986 by the Federal Technology Transfer Act (Pub. L. 99–502) which was viewed as virtually mandating collaboration between government scientists and private industry.[10] Executive Order 12591, signed by President Reagan in 1987, required federal agencies to designate officials responsible for facilitating technology transfer, in order to encourage further collaboration.

There are good reasons for universities and industry to work together, and these federal policies have encouraged and strengthened such relationships. Cooperative Research and Development Agreements ("CRADAs"), authorized by the Technology Transfer Act, have been implemented in a number of federal agencies. The Veterans Administration, for example, supplemented its $210 million appropriation for research this year with over $300 million from industry, private donations, health service fees, and other sources.[11] Similarly, the National Institute of Science and Technology (NIST) (formerly, the National Bureau of Standards) receives roughly half of its research funds from private sources. In addition, hundreds of scientists from industry conduct their own research in NIST laboratories, and there are many joint ventures and collaborative agreements supporting other research relationships between NIST and industry.[12] Similarly, employees of the National Institutes of Health (NIH) are encouraged to collaborate with industry. NIH has occasionally called for proposals that require industry and academic institutions to submit joint applications for grants and contracts in particular areas of research and development.

Individual states have followed the example of the federal government by establishing regional economic development programs and research centers to encourage collaboration between universities and industry – in part to revive aging local industries and to promote economic growth.

Universities themselves have encouraged closer collaboration with industry, because of the potential benefits to both the academic institutions and the community at large that flow from such relationships. These benefits include: (1) invigoration of teaching and research training, (2) providing additional financial support for socially useful research, (3) stimulating cross-fertilization of research ideas and early identification of commercial potential by bringing university faculty and staff into closer contact with industry, (4) expediting the pace of technology transfer, and (5) helping universities to retain outstanding personnel by enabling them to work on "cutting edge" projects with adequate resources.

As Paul Gray, president of MIT and Vice-Chairman of the President's Council on Competitiveness has said: "I have become convinced that America has a unique advantage in its research universities, where exploration of the frontiers of science is supported by governmental and private funds, and where the channels between academia and commerce are well marked to permit the application of new discoveries to create products and processes of economic benefit to society. No other country has that capacity or linkage."[13] Likewise, former Duke University President Terry Sanford has said that "universities should do all that is reasonably possible to earn returns on inventions, and should not be timid in making prudent arrangements to assure the target fair return."[14]

While the new opportunities for university-industry relationships have created great benefits, they have also been seen as creating potential problems. With increasing frequency and urgency, some charge that these relationships can create "conflicts of interest" that may distort research practices, taint academic objectivity, erect barriers to collegiality, and in other ways compromise the core values of academic institutions. Gilbert Omenn, Professor and Chairman of Environmental Health at the University of Washington, has summarized well the balance of risks and benefits in university/industry relationships:

For the university and faculty members, their potential advantages are enhanced income, resources for program expansion, broadened opportunities for students, access to special equipment or research tools, and longer-term support for high-risk projects, possibly with fewer strings attached. On the other hand, ... such relationships carry the potential risk of creating imbalances of faculty, students, and space; of using up the "seed corn" of basic knowledge while seducing students and faculty into more targeted, narrower training and research; of inhibiting communication, publication, peer review, and sharing of strains and reagents; and of losing public confidence and jeopardizing government funding.[15]

We begin by asking why concerns over conflicts of interest in biomedical research have recently become so prominent.

C. Sources of concern

1. *Outside Sponsors.* The potential for conflicts of interest has increased with the recent growth in industrially sponsored research and in entrepreneurial activities on the part of faculty. During the early part of the century, university research was supported almost exclusively by student fees, tuition, endowments and other university funds (including state funding in the case of state institutions), and by some private foundations. After World War II, the federal government (through DoD, NSF, and NIH) became the major source of external funds. Although government support in the physical sciences and engineering is predominantly through contracts that are highly regulated through the Federal Acquisition Regulations, support in the biomedical sciences has been largely through investigator-initiated grants, which traditionally have had very little regulation or oversight. Thus, the relation in the biomedical sciences has been primarily based on trust with few requirements for formal accountability.

In the 1970s, government support did not keep pace with the rapidly rising cost of teaching and research, particularly in fields such as biomedical research, microelectronics, optics and nuclear engineering. As a result, universities increasingly turned to industry for additional support. "Industry funds going to universities to support R & D have increased about five-fold in the last decade."[16] Although the amount of industrial support for research in health sciences has risen dramatically since the 1970s, most of that money has been spent "in-house"; consequently, industry supports only a small fraction of the total biomedical research conducted at academic institutions.[17] While proportionately small, industrial support in biomedical research often involves the kinds of products intended for clinical application that capture public interest.

2. *Medical Service Fees.* The proportion of medical school funding derived from earned service fees – faculty practice plans and hospital fees – has tripled, from about 12% in 1970 to more than 30% in 1980 and nearly 40% in 1988.[18] One study concluded in 1983 that income from the private practice of medicine was already the largest single source of funding for the nation's medical schools.[19] This emphasis on the provision of medical services and increasing dependence on the need to generate clinical fees has had a profound impact on the internal dynamics of academic health centers, and on the way the public views them.

3. *International Competition.* Another cause for public concern has been the loss of confidence in America's intellectual standing and commercial competitiveness, and the apparent ability of some other nations (the Japanese and occasionally Europeans) to transfer basic research breakthroughs more quickly into new products. There is increasing pressure on universities to produce commercial payoffs in return for the tax and funding subsidies they receive.

4. *Entrepreneurial Activities.* Still another reason for increased concern over conflicts of interest is that researchers and clinicians have become more entrepreneurial. Such activities on the part of physicians generally have caused the public and legislators to wonder about the altruism of those in the health field. The lag time between basic research findings and their clinical and commercial applications has shortened significantly in recent years. As a result, the basic biological sciences have become potentially more profitable, and entrepreneurial opportunities for research scientists have markedly increased.

5. *Public Policy and Ethical Issues.* Major healthcare centers are unavoidably involved in some of the society's most sensitive ethical issues. These include the availability or "rationing" of scarce medical resources, care of the terminally ill, abortions and AIDS. Moreover, the public no longer waits passively to receive the latest medical advances. Instead, associations concerned with specific diseases – AIDS, arthritis, cancer – press to keep their concerns at the top of funding agendas, while other groups, concerned with specialized issues such as genetic engineering and use of animals in research, challenge whether and how certain research should be conducted. There is pressure to accelerate reporting of scientific breakthroughs, FDA approval of new products, and the development of new medical technologies. When the stakes – and emotions – are high, it is inevitable that the ethics and motivations of participants will be scrutinized.

6. *Mistrust of Professionals and Institutions.* The rise of consumerism in the 1960s and 1970s provided the impetus for greater accountability to the public of all kinds of public and private entities. Surveys repeatedly show a declining public respect for most professions. The public appears to be increasingly unwilling to cede independence and authority to teachers, doctors, lawyers, accountants, or government officials. This is not entirely surprising, since professionals receive large benefits from society in the form of a license granting them a monopoly over certain services. In return, professionals owe certain obligations to the society that grants this benefit. The public has particularly strong concerns about integrity in matters concerning health and biomedical research. Because of the long tradition of trust in the doctor-patient relationship, there is a great sense of betrayal when that trust is violated.

Because universities and hospitals receive public benefits in the form of research grants, tax exemptions, training support, and other fees, government regulation and public accountability are to be expected. Congress has been examining with new vigor the taxability of ancillary ventures of tax-exempt entities which may not be "substantially related" to their tax-exempt purposes. In this environment, any suggestion of a private pecuniary motive or conflict of interest receives sharp scrutiny.

The result of the trends outlined above is that society is now less willing to leave the academic world entirely to its own devices. Instead there are efforts – through legislation, regulation, political pressure, and targeted funding – to influence research agendas and activities, particularly at academic health centers. There are parallel efforts to monitor and regulate those activities. Preserving trust and retaining public confidence will be essential for maintaining the vigor and intellectual independence of academic research in the health sciences.

D. Federal oversight

Until academic institutions themselves demonstrate the ability to deal with conflicts of interest in a way that satisfies legislators and the public, there will be pressures to attempt to manage such conflicts through statute and regulations, some of which may be ill-advised. The government has both the authority and the responsibility to ensure that public monies are properly spent and that regulatory decisions (such as determining the safety and efficacy of drugs and devices) are based upon reliable data and independent analyses. Federal activity in the latter half of the 1980s illustrates the willingness of government to step in and regulate the conduct of biomedical research. For example:

- The 1985 amendments to the Public Health Service Act, 42 U.S.C. § 289(b), require recipients of PHS funding to have in place procedures for investigating and responding to allegations of scientific misconduct. PHS has recently issued final implementing regulations. 54 *Fed. Reg.* 32446–51 (1989).
- NIH recently proposed guidelines on conflicts of interest, although they were later withdrawn after being subject to widespread criticism. *NIH Guide to Grants and Contracts,* Vol. 18, No. 32 (Sept. 15, 1989).
- Recent amendments to the Animal Welfare Act imposed additional requirements for review of animal research, and the care and use of laboratory animals. 7 U.S.C. § 2145.

There is little doubt that these legislative and regulatory actions have been prompted by skepticism about how health professionals, faculties and research institutions balance objectivity and entrepreneurship, how well they transfer results to the public and how effective they are in maintaining high ethical standards. How much farther Congress moves toward regulation depends in part on how willing and effective the private sector and academia are in conforming their conduct to credible standards, and in communicating accurately and effectively to the public and the government what is being done.

Notes

1. *See, e.g.,* Omnibus Budget Reconciliation Act of 1989 § 6204 (Physician Ownership of and Referral to Health Care Entities); Medicare and Medicaid Anti-Kickback Law, 42 U.S.C. § 1320a–7(b); "Medicaid and Medicare Program: Fraud and Abuse OIG Anti-Kickback Provisions," 54 *Fed. Reg.* 3088 (Jan. 23, 1989).
2. B. Culliton, "Pajaro Dunes: The Search for Consensus," 216 *Science* 155, 156 (Apr. 9, 1982). See full statement in 9 *J. Coll. & Univ. L.* 533 (1983).
3. B. Healy, *et al.,* "Conflict of Interest Guidelines for a Multicenter Clinical Trial of Treatment After Coronary-Artery Bypass Graft Surgery," 320(14) *New Eng. J. Med.* 949 (Apr. 6, 1989).
4. *See also,* R. Chalk, *et al. Professional Ethics Activities in the Scientific and Engineering Societies,* American Association for the Advancement of Science (1980).
5. C. K. Gunsalus and J. Rowan, "You and the Big U: Protecting Your Interests and Your Name – Conflict of Interest Considerations in Spin-off Licensing," presented at the 2nd Conference

on the University Spin-Off Corporation, Virginia Polytechnic Institute, Blacksburg, VA (May 16–17, 1989).

6. Institute of Medicine, *Government and Industry Collaboration in Biomedical Research and Education* (1989) at 4 and 33–34; D. Nelkin, R. Nelson and C. Kiernan, "Commentary: University Industry Alliances," 12(1) *Science, Technology, and Human Values* 65–68 (Winter, 1987).

7. P. Gray, testimony at a Hearing on *Is Science for Sale? Conflicts of Interest vs. the Public Interest,* Committee on Government Operations, Subcommittee on Human Resources and Intergovernmental Operations, 101st Cong. 1st Sess. (June 13, 1989) (hereinafter *"Weiss Hearing"*).

8. E. L. MacCordy, "The Impact of Proprietary Arrangements on Universities," in *Biotechnology-Professional Issues and Social Concerns,* American Association for Advancement of Science (1988) at 13.

9. Ibid.

10. Ibid. at 5, citing NIH Deputy Director William Raub.

11. Ibid. at 7.

12. Ibid. at 9–10.

13. P. Gray, Testimony in *Weiss Hearing* (June 13, 1989), *supra,* note 7.

14. Quoted in B. Reams, University-Industry Research Partnerships 8 (1986). *See also,* "Pajaro Dunes Conference Draft Statement," 9 *J. College & Univ. Law* 533 (1983); A. Bearn, "The Pharmaceutical Industry and Academe: Partners in Progress," 71 *Am. J. Med.* 81–88 (1981); G. Keyworth, "Federal R & D and Industrial Policy," 220 *Science* 1122 (June 10, 1983); Testimony of Victor J. Marder, M.D., of University of Rochester Medical Center at Hearing on *Federal Response to Misconduct in Science: Are Conflicts of Interests Hazardous to Our Health?,* before the Committee on Government Operations, Subcommittee on Human Resources and Intergovernmental Relations, 100th Cong., 2d Sess. (Sept. 29, 1988) ("Combining the strengths of the pharmaceutical industry, the academic environment, and hospital network and research, tangibly expands our resources and potential for breakthroughs in medical knowledge and care").

15. G. S. Omenn, "University/Industry Research Linkages; Arrangements Between Faculty Members and their Universities," presented at AAAS Symposium on *Impacts of Commercial Genetic Engineering on Universities and Non-Profit Institutions* (Washington, D.C., Jan. 6, 1982).

16. D. Nelkin, R. Nelson and C. Kiernan, "Commentary: University-Industry Alliances," 12(1) *Science, Technology and Human Values,* 65 (Winter, 1987).

17. *NIH Data Book* (1988) Tables 3 and 3.1, at 4. *See also,* ibid., Fig. 2.1, at 3.

18. L. Taksel, P. Jolly, and R. Beran, "US Medical School Finances," 262(8) *J.A.M.A.* 1020, 1023 (Aug. 25, 1989).

19. R. H. Ebert and S. S. Brown, "Academic Health Centers," 303(20) *New Eng. J. Med.* 1200 (May 19, 1983).

QUESTIONS FOR DISCUSSION

1. Do the responsibilities and commitments of academic scientists working under a grant from a commercial enterprise differ from those of scientists employed in that company's laboratories? If so, how? If not, why not?
2. Is the patenting of living organisms ethically problematic? If a genetically altered mouse can be patented, could a dog, a primate, or a human being likewise be patented if created with similar techniques?
3. Should researchers whose work results in commercial products be held personally responsible in the event that the products are later found to cause harm?

RECOMMENDED SUPPLEMENTAL READING

Science as Intellectual Property: Who Controls Scientific Research, Dorothy Nelkin, New York: Macmillan, 1984.

Research Funding as an Investment: Can We Measure the Returns? Office of Technology Assessment (OTA), OTA-TM-SET–36, Washington, DC: U.S. Government Printing Office, 1986.

"Responsibility, Risk, and Informed Consent," Peter F. Carpenter, in Karen B. Eckelman (ed.), *New Medical Devices: Invention, Development, and Use,* Washington, DC: National Academy Press, 1988, pp. 138–145.

"Collaborative Research in Biomedicine: Resolving Conflicts," K. E. Hanna, Background paper, Institute of Medicine (IOM) Committee on Government-Industry Collaboration in Biomedical Research and Education, Washington, DC: Institute of Medicine, 1989.

"Policy on Conflicts of Interest and Commitment," Harvard University Faculty of Medicine, Cambridge, MA: Harvard University, March 22, 1990.

PART X

The Scientist in Society: Interactions, Expectations, and Obligations

INTRODUCTION

Are scientists morally responsible for the application of their findings? Physicists have long debated their role in the development and control of nuclear weapons, but this question is applicable to biological scientists as well. For example, the availability of the birth control pill has been linked to social phenomena ranging from the economic empowerment of women to the disintegration of the family and an epidemic of infertility. Could the researchers whose work led to oral contraceptives have anticipated their effects and tried to shape them? If so, should they have done so?

In 1975, in an unprecedented act of professional self-governance, leading researchers in recombinant DNA called for a moratorium on certain aspects of their work until its appropriate goals and limits could be established. In a related area, the explosion of information from the Human Genome Project is anticipated to have vast consequences, and a portion of the project's funding is designated for studying its ethical and social ramifications.

The public's view of scientists is marked by tension: people are eager for scientific miracles, but many also mistrust the power of science and motives of researchers with highly technical expertise. To serve the social goals of science, researchers must educate the public about their work and ensure that their self-regulation merits public confidence.

However, Frank von Hippel and Rosemary Chalk note that even in science "whistle-blowers" are often punished by colleagues who resent public scrutiny of their work. Dorothy Nelkin further illustrates how awe of science complicates true public understanding, and makes appropriate science policy inherently difficult. Even if scientists cannot dictate the ways in which their findings will be used, they have a responsibility as professionals and citizens to make their knowledge accessible and meaningful to governmental decision makers and the public at large so that its benefits, risks, and limits are adequately recognized.

32
Summary statement of the Asilomar Conference on Recombinant DNA Molecules

Paul Berg, David Baltimore, Sydney Brenner, Richard O. Roblin III, and Maxine F. Singer

I. Introduction and general conclusions

This meeting was organized to review scientific progress in research on recombinant DNA molecules and to discuss appropriate ways to deal with the potential biohazards of this work. Impressive scientific achievements have already been made in this field and these techniques have a remarkable potential for furthering our understanding of fundamental biochemical processes in pro- and eukaryotic cells. The use of recombinant DNA methodology promises to revolutionize the practice of molecular biology. Although there has as yet been no practical application of the new techniques, there is every reason to believe that they will have significant practical utility in the future.

Of particular concern to the participants at the meeting was the issue of whether the pause in certain aspects of research in this area, called for by the Committee on Recombinant DNA Molecules of the National Academy of Sciences, U.S.A. in the letter published in July, 1974* should end; and, if so, how the scientific work could be undertaken with minimal risks to workers in laboratories, to the public at large, and to the animal and plant species sharing our ecosystems.

The new techniques, which permit combination of genetic information from very different organisms, place us in an area of biology with many unknowns. Even in the present, more limited conduct of research in this field, the evaluation of potential biohazards has proved to be extremely difficult. It is this ignorance that has compelled us to conclude that it would be wise to exercise considerable caution in performing this research. Nevertheless, the participants at the Conference agreed that most of the work on construction of recombinant DNA molecules should proceed provided that appropriate safeguards, principally biological and physical barriers adequate to contain the newly created organisms, are employed. Moreover, the standards of protection should be greater at the beginning and modified as improvements in the methodology occur and assessments of the risks change. Furthermore, it was agreed that there are certain experiments in which the potential risks are of such a serious nature that they ought not to be done with presently available containment facilities. In the longer term, serious problems may arise in the large scale application of this methodology in industry,

---

*Report of Committee on Recombinant DNA Molecules: "Potential Biohazards of Recombinant DNA Molecules," *Proc. Nat. Acad. Sci. USA* **71**, 2593–2594, 1974.

From *Proceedings of the National Academy of Science,* 1975, 72, 1981–1984. Summary statement of the report submitted to the Assembly of Life Sciences of the National Academy of Sciences and approved by its Executive Committee on 20 May 1975.

medicine, and agriculture. But it was also recognized that future research and experience may show that many of the potential biohazards are less serious and/or less probable than we now suspect.

II. Principles guiding the recommendations and conclusions

Although our assessments of the risks involved with each of the various lines of research on recombinant DNA molecules may differ, few, if any, believe that this methodology is free from any risk. Reasonable principles for dealing with these potential risks are: (*i*) that containment be made an essential consideration in the experimental design and, (*ii*) that the effectiveness of the containment should match, as closely as possible, the estimated risk. Consequently, whatever scale of risks is agreed upon, there should be a commensurate scale of containment. Estimating the risks will be difficult and intuitive at first but this will improve as we acquire additional knowledge; at each stage we shall have to match the potential risk with an appropriate level of containment. Experiments requiring large scale operations would seem to be riskier than equivalent experiments done on a small scale and, therefore, require more stringent containment procedures. The use of cloning vehicles or vectors (plasmids, phages) and bacterial hosts with a restricted capacity to multiply outside of the laboratory would reduce the potential biohazard of a particular experiment. Thus, the ways in which potential biohazards and different levels of containment are matched may vary from time to time, particularly as the containment technology is improved. The means for assessing and balancing risks with appropriate levels of containment will need to be reexamined from time to time. Hopefully, through both formal and informal channels of information within and between the nations of the world, the way in which potential biohazards and levels of containment are matched would be consistent.

Containment of potentially biohazardous agents can be achieved in several ways. The most significant contribution to limiting the spread of the recombinant DNAs is the use of biological barriers. These barriers are of two types: (*i*) fastidious bacterial hosts unable to survive in natural environments, and (*ii*) nontransmissible and equally fastidious vectors (plasmids, bacteriophages, or other viruses) able to grow only in specified hosts. Physical containment, exemplified by the use of suitable hoods, or where applicable, limited access or negative pressure laboratories, provides an additional factor of safety. Particularly important is strict adherence to good microbiological practices, which to a large measure can limit the escape of organisms from the experimental situation, and thereby increase the safety of the operation. Consequently, education and training of all personnel involved in the experiments is essential to the effectiveness of all containment measures. In practice, these different means of containment will complement one another and documented substantial improvements in the ability to restrict the growth of bacterial hosts and vectors could permit modifications of the complementary physical containment requirements.

Stringent physical containment and rigorous laboratory procedures can reduce but not eliminate the possibility of spreading potentially hazardous agents. Therefore, investigators relying upon ''disarmed'' hosts and vectors for additional safety must rigorously test the effectiveness of these agents before accepting their validity as biological barriers.

III. Recommendations for matching types of containment with types of experiments

No classification of experiments as to risk and no set of containment procedures can anticipate all situations. Given our present uncertainties about the hazards, the parameters proposed here are broadly conceived and meant to provide provisional guidelines for investigators and agencies concerned with research on recombinant DNAs. However, each investigator bears a responsibility for determining whether, in his particular case, special circumstances warrant a higher level of containment than is suggested here.

A. *Types of containment*

1. Minimal Risk. This type of containment is intended for experiments in which the biohazards may be accurately assessed and are expected to be minimal. Such containment can be achieved by following the operating procedures recommended for clinical micro-biological laboratories. Essential features of such facilities are no drinking, eating, or smoking in the laboratory, wearing laboratory coats in the work area, the use of cotton-plugged pipettes or preferably mechanical pipetting devices, and prompt disinfection of contaminated materials.

2. Low Risk. This level of containment is appropriate for experiments which generate novel biotypes but where the available information indicates that the recombinant DNA cannot alter appreciably the ecological behavior of the recipient species, increase significantly its pathogenicity, or prevent effective treatment of any resulting infections. The key features of this containment (in addition to the minimal procedures mentioned above) are a prohibition on mouth pipetting, access limited to laboratory personnel, and the use of biological safety cabinets for procedures likely to produce aerosols (e.g., blending and sonication). Though existing vectors may be used in conjunction with low risk procedures, safer vectors and hosts should be adopted as they become available.

3. Moderate Risk. Such containment facilities are intended for experiments in which there is a probability of generating an agent with a significant potential for pathogenicity or ecological disruption. The principal features of this level of containment, in addition to those of the two preceding classes, are that transfer operations should be carried out in biological safety cabinets (e.g., laminar flow hoods), gloves should be worn during the handling of infectious materials, vacuum lines must be protected by filters, and negative pressure should be maintained in the limited access laboratories. Moreover, experiments posing a moderate risk must be done only with vectors and hosts that have an appreciably impaired capacity to multiply outside of the laboratory.

4. High Risk. This level of containment is intended for experiments in which the potential for ecological disruption or pathogenicity of the modified organism could be severe and thereby pose a serious biohazard to laboratory personnel or the public. The main features of this type of facility, which was designed to contain highly infectious microbiological agents, are its isolation from other areas by air locks, a negative pressure environment, a requirement for clothing changes and showers for entering personnel, and laboratories fitted with treatment systems to inactivate or remove biological agents that may be contaminants in exhaust air and liquid and solid wastes. All persons occupying these areas should wear protective laboratory clothing and shower at each exit from the containment facility. The handling of agents should be confined to biological safety cabinets in which the exhaust air is incinerated or passed through Hepa filters. High risk containment includes, in addition to the physical and procedural features described above, the use of rigorously tested vectors and hosts whose growth can be confined to the laboratory.

B. Types of experiments

Accurate estimates of the risks associated with different types of experiments are difficult to obtain because of our ignorance of the probability that the anticipated dangers will manifest themselves. Nevertheless, experiments involving the construction and propagation of recombinant DNA molecules using DNAs from (*i*) prokaryotes, bacteriophages, and other plasmids, (*ii*) animal viruses, and (*iii*) eukaryotes have been characterized as minimal, low, moderate, and high risks to guide investigators in their choice of the appropriate containment. These designations should be viewed as interim assignments which will need to be revised upward or downward in the light of future experience.

The recombinant DNA molecules themselves, as distinct from cells carrying them, may be infectious to bacteria or higher organisms. DNA preparations from these experiments, particularly in large quantities, should be chemically inactivated before disposal.

1. Prokaryotes, Bacteriophages, and Bacterial Plasmids. Where the construction of recombinant DNA molecules and their propagation involves prokaryotic agents that are known to exchange genetic information naturally, the experiments can be performed in minimal risk containment facilities. Where such experiments pose a potential hazard, more stringent containment may be warranted.

Experiments involving the creation and propagation of recombinant DNA molecules from DNAs of species that ordinarily do not exchange genetic information, generate novel biotypes. Because such experiments may pose biohazards greater than those associated with the original organisms, they should be performed, at least, in low risk containment facilities. If the experiments involve either pathogenic organisms or genetic determinants that may increase the pathogenicity of the recipient species, or if the transferred DNA can confer upon the recipient organisms new metabolic activities not native to these species and thereby modify its relationship with the environment, then moderate or high risk containment should be used.

Experiments extending the range of resistance of established human pathogens to therapeutically useful antibiotics or disinfectants should be undertaken only under moderate or high risk containment, depending upon the virulence of the organism involved.

2. Animal Viruses. Experiments involving linkage of viral genomes or genome segments to prokaryotic vectors and their propagation in prokaryotic cells should be performed only with vector–host systems having demonstrably restricted growth capabilities outside the laboratory and with moderate risk containment facilities. Rigorously purified and characterized segments of non-oncogenic viral genomes or of the demonstrably non-transforming regions of oncogenic viral DNAs can be attached to presently existing vectors and propagated in moderate risk containment facilities; as safer vector–host systems become available such experiments may be performed in low risk facilities.

Experiments designed to introduce or propagate DNA from non-viral or other low risk agents in animal cells should use only low risk animal DNAs as vectors (e.g., viral, mitochondrial) and manipulations should be confined to moderate risk containment facilities.

3. Eukaryotes. The risks associated with joining random fragments of eukaryote DNA to prokaryotic DNA vectors and the propagation of these recombinant DNAs in prokaryotic hosts are the most difficult to assess.

A priori, the DNA from warm-blooded vertebrates is more likely to contain cryptic viral genomes potentially pathogenic for man than is the DNA from other eukaryotes. Consequently, attempts to clone segments of DNA from such animal and particularly primate genomes should be performed only with vector–host systems having demonstrably restricted growth capabilities outside the laboratory and in a moderate risk containment facility. Until cloned segments of warm-blooded vertebrate DNA are completely characterized, they should continue to be maintained in the most restricted vector–host system in moderate risk containment laboratories; when such cloned segments are characterized, they may be propagated as suggested above for purified segments of virus genomes.

Unless the organism makes a product known to be dangerous (e.g., toxin, virus), recombinant DNAs from cold-blooded vertebrates and all other lower eukaryotes can be constructed and propagated with the safest vector–host system available in low risk containment facilities.

Purified DNA from any source that performs known functions and can be judged to be non-toxic, may be cloned with currently available vectors in low risk containment facilities. (Toxic here includes potentially oncogenic products or substances that might perturb normal metabolism if produced in an animal or plant by a resident microorganism.)

4. Experiments to Be Deferred. There are feasible experiments which present such serious dangers that their performance should not be undertaken at this time with the currently available vector–host systems and the presently available containment capability. These include the cloning of recombinant DNAs derived from highly pathogenic organisms (i.e., Class III, IV, and V etiologic agents as classified by the United States Department of Health, Education and Welfare), DNA containing toxin genes, and large scale experiments (more than 10 liters of culture) using recombinant DNAs that are able to make products potentially harmful to man, animals, or plants.

IV. Implementation

In many countries steps are already being taken by national bodies to formulate codes of practice for the conduct of experiments with known or potential biohazard.*[†] Until these are established, we urge individual scientists to use the proposals in this document as a guide. In addition, there are some recommendations which could be immediately and directly implemented by the scientific community.

A. Development of safer vectors and hosts

An important and encouraging accomplishment of the meeting was the realization that special bacteria and vectors which have a restricted capacity to multiply outside the

---

*Advisory Board for the Research Councils, "Report of the Working Party on the Experimental Manipulation of the Genetic Composition of Micro-Organisms. Presented to Parliament by the Secretary of State for Education and Science by Command of Her Majesty, January 1975." London: Her Majesty's Stationery Office, 1975, 23pp.

[†]National Institutes of Health Recombinant DNA Molecule Program Advisory Committee.

laboratory can be constructed genetically, and that the use of these organisms could enhance the safety of recombinant DNA experiments by many orders of magnitude. Experiments along these lines are presently in progress and in the near future, variants of λ bacteriophage, non-transmissible plasmids, and special strains of *Escherichia coli* will become available. All of these vectors could reduce the potential biohazards by very large factors and improve the methodology as well. Other vector–host systems, particularly modified strains of *Bacillus subtilis* and their relevant bacteriophages and plasmids, may also be useful for particular purposes. Quite possibly safe and suitable vectors may be found for eukaryotic hosts such as yeast and readily cultured plant and animal cells. There is likely to be a continuous development in this area and the participants at the meeting agreed that improved vector–host systems which reduce the biohazards of recombinant DNA research will be made freely available to all interested investigators.

B. Laboratory procedures

It is the clear responsibility of the principal investigator to inform the staff of the laboratory of the potential hazards of such experiments before they are initiated. Free and open discussion is necessary so that each individual participating in the experiment fully understands the nature of the experiment and any risk that might be involved. All workers must be properly trained in the containment procedures that are designed to control the hazard, including emergency actions in the event of a hazard. It is also recommended that appropriate health surveillance of all personnel, including serological monitoring, be conducted periodically.

C. Education and reassessment

Research in this area will develop very quickly and the methods will be applied to many different biological problems. At any given time it is impossible to foresee the entire range of all potential experiments and make judgments on them. Therefore, it is essential to undertake a continuing reassessment of the problems in the light of new scientific knowledge. This could be achieved by a series of annual workshops and meetings, some of which should be at the international level. There should also be courses to train individuals in the relevant methods since it is likely that the work will be taken up by laboratories which may not have had extensive experience in this area. High priority should also be given to research that could improve and evaluate the containment effectiveness of new and existing vector–host systems.

V. New knowledge

This document represents our first assessment of the potential biohazards in the light of current knowledge. However, little is known about the survival of laboratory strains of bacteria and bacteriophages in different ecological niches in the outside world. Even less is known about whether recombinant DNA molecules will enhance or depress the survival of their vectors and hosts in nature. These questions are fundamental to the testing of any new organism that may be constructed. Research in this area needs to be undertaken and should be given high priority. In general, however, molecular biologists who may construct DNA recombinant molecules do not undertake these experiments and it will be necessary to facilitate collaborative research between them and groups skilled in the study of bacterial infection or ecological microbiology. Work should also be undertaken which would enable us to monitor the escape or dissemination of cloning vehicles and their hosts.

Nothing is known about the potential infectivity in higher organisms of phages or bacteria containing segments of eukaryotic DNA and very little about the infectivity of the DNA molecules themselves. Genetic transformation of bacteria does occur in animals, suggesting that recombinant DNA molecules can retain their biological potency in this environment. There are many questions in this area, the answers to which are essential for our assessment of the biohazards of experiments with recombinant DNA molecules. It will be necessary to ensure that this work will be planned and carried out; and it will be particularly important to have this information before large scale applications of the use of recombinant DNA molecules is attempted.

33
The high cost of hype

Dorothy Nelkin

On January 28, 1986, a long-standing and comfortable partnership between NASA and the press was shattered, when the space shuttle Challenger exploded seconds after lift-off, killing all aboard.[1] The press reaction to the explosion was one of grief, disillusionment, and rage. For many longtime space journalists the event was a personal tragedy. "Those people were me," wrote a Houston reporter. "The shining star of technology for 30 years has dimmed." The *Miami Herald* compared the "countdown to disaster" to a "Greek tragedy, peppered with portents of the doom to come." The *New York Times* wrote of its disillusionment with an agency that "has symbolized all that is best in American technology . . . computerized, at the cutting edge of technology, sophisticated in its public relations strategy, squeaky-clean in its integrity."[2]

The space program had been important to the development of science journalism as a profession. The many months at Cape Canaveral had brought together journalists interested in science and technology, and attracted new writers to the field. For 30 years they had covered the space program as an awesome and pioneering venture, a source of national prestige. The first space shuttle in 1981 assumed symbolic dimensions in the popular press as an affirmation of American faith in science and technology, a solution to problems of military security, a "sweet vindication of American know-how." In effect, the press reports of space launches incorporated all the images that are so characteristic of science and technology journalism.

Fascinated with the technology, reporters for years had simply accepted what NASA fed them, reproducing the agency's assertions, promoting the prepackaged information they received, and rarely questioning the premises of the program, the competence of the scientists, or the safety of the operation. Only three days before the accident, a *Boston Globe* reporter joked about NASA's public relations: "How does NASA spell publicity? Christa McAuliffe," referring to the school teacher who was among the astronauts. Three days later, McAuliffe was called "the victim of a PR campaign."

After the accident an angry press felt betrayed. *Newsweek* announced that "the news media and NASA, wedded by mutual interest from the earliest days of the space program, are in the midst of a messy divorce." Having suddenly lost faith in the veracity of NASA, some newspapers even engaged in electronic war games, using high-technology interception antennas and experimental laser cameras to get stories about the recovery of the shuttle that NASA wanted to conceal.[3] The press was filled with self-incrimination, as reporters accused themselves of accepting "spoon-fed news," of ignoring the safety problems of NASA by focusing only on the launches, of "treating the shuttle like a running photo opportunity," of letting readers down. More than any other event, the Challenger accident brought press and public awareness of the importance of probing and critical science journalism.

Science writers, in effect, are brokers, framing social reality for their readers and shaping the public consciousness about science-related events.[4] Through their selection of news about science and technology they set the agenda for public policy. Through their presentation of science news they lay the foundation for personal attitudes and public actions. For they are often our only source of information about the technical choices that significantly affect our lives.

Press coverage of science and technology is increasing, reflecting the pervasiveness of science and technology in business, politics, and health. Scientific and technological choices affect our work, our health, our lives. We pay for their implementation and bear their social costs. Public understanding of their social implications, their technical justifications, and their political and economic foundations is in the interest of an informed and involved citizenry. It is also critical to the health of our scientific and technological enterprise. The high cost of public naiveté regarding science and the nature of scientific evidence has been apparent in many controversies – over the value of animal experimentation, the appropriate precautions to prevent the spread of AIDS, the risks of a nuclear power plant explosion, and the teaching of evolution in the schools.

The press can play an important role in enhancing public understanding, but it frequently fails to do so. There are many examples of brilliant science reporting, written with analytic clarity, critical insight, and provocative style; but too often science in the press is more a subject for consumption than for public scrutiny, more a source of entertainment than of information.[5] Too often science is presented as an arcane activity outside and above the sphere of normal human understanding, and therefore beyond our control. Too often the coverage is promotional and uncritical, encouraging apathy, a sense of impotence, and the ubiquitous tendency to defer to expertise.

Science is practiced by an elite, but its impact extends to us all. Yet political questions of scientific responsibility and accountability are seldom considered news; nor are the ideologies or social priorities that guide science policy decisions. Focusing on individual accomplishments and dramatic or controversial events, journalists convey little about the sociology of science, the structure of scientific institutions, or the daily routines of research. We read about the results of research and the stories of success, but not about the process, the dead ends, the wrong turns. Who discovered what is more newsworthy than what was discovered or how. Thus science in the press becomes a form of sport, a "race" between scientists in different disciplines or between competitive nations.

There is little in this type of reporting to help the reader understand the nature of scientific evidence and the difference between science and unverified opinion. As a result, when new problems emerge as the focus of public concern, people are ill-prepared to deal with scientific information. The persistent fear of catching AIDS through casual contact with AIDS victims despite scientific evidence to the contrary is a case in point.

The reporting of technology, like that of science, tends to be promotional. Many writers convey a fervent conviction that new technology will create a better world. But the message is polarized – we read of either promising applications or perilous effects, of triumphant progress or tragic risks. Impending breakthroughs are reported with zeal, and technological failures are reported with alarm. But the long-term political and social consequences of technological choices are seldom explored. Thus technology in the press becomes a side show unrelated to events at center stage.

This study has suggested that many of these characteristics of science and technology reporting follow from the nature of the relationship between journalists and their sources. Many scientists today, concerned about their legitimacy in the political arena and anxious to receive support for their work, are sensitive to their image in the press. Hoping to shape that image, they are becoming adept at packaging information for journalists. Like advocates in any field, they are prone to overestimate the benefit of their work and minimize its risks. Indeed, the problems of science and technology reporting can often be traced to the influence of sources advocating their ideas.

For their part, journalists, especially those with limited experience in science reporting, are vulnerable to manipulation by their sources of information. They are concerned about balance and objectivity and accept the ideology of science as a neutral source of authority, an objective judge of truth. Some science writers are in awe of scientists; others are intimidated. But most are bewildered by the complexity of technical issues. The difficulty of evaluating a complex and uncertain subject converges with the day-to-day constraints of the journalistic profession to reinforce the tendency to rely uncritically on scientific expertise. While political writers often go well beyond press briefings to probe the stories behind the news, science reporters tend to rely on scientific authorities, press conferences, and professional journals. The result? Many journalists have adopted the mind-set or "frame" of scientists, interpreting science in terms defined by their sources, even when those sources are clearly interested in projecting a particular view.

Thus while art, theater, music, and literature are routinely subjected to criticism, science and technology are almost always spared. While political writers aim to analyze and criticize, science writers seek to elucidate and explain. Few are the outlets for journalists who would serve as critical commentators on, or probing investigators of, science and technology. Rare are the Walter Lippmanns or I. F. Stones of science who write regularly in the press.[6] Unaggressive in their reporting and relying on official sources, science journalists present a narrow range of coverage. Many journalists are, in effect, retailing science and technology more than investigating them, identifying with their sources more than challenging them.

If the reporting of science and technology is so uncritical, why is there continued tension between scientists and the press? The communities of science and journalism differ in certain fundamental and important respects. To begin with, they often differ in their judgments about what is news. In the scientific community, research results become reliable and therefore newsworthy through replication by and endorsement of professional colleagues. Prior to publication in reputable journals, scientific papers are carefully evaluated and approved through the system of peer review. This system of establishing reliability is critical to the structure of science, and especially to the process of scientific communication. For scientists, then, research findings are tentative, undigested, provisional – and therefore not newsworthy – until certified by peers to fit into the existing framework of knowledge. For journalists, on the other hand, certified and established ideas are "old news" – of far less interest than new and dramatic, though possibly tentative, research. Seeking to entertain as well as to inform, they are attracted to nonroutine, nonconventional, and even aberrant events.[7] This difference between scientists and journalists often becomes a source of contention when overzealous researchers seek press coverage of "hot" research prior to the time-consuming process of peer review.

In their search for credible perspectives on controversial issues, journalists often rely on the opinions of scientists who have become well-known public figures. Nobel Prize winners are frequently cited in fields well outside their specialized expertise, journalists having sought their opinions simply because of their general prestige in science and the familiarity of their names. Scientists suspect such use of unverified opinion. Arnold Relman, editor of the *New England Journal of Medicine,* expressed the scientists' view: "If a [politician] makes a statement of what the policy of his government is or what he thinks or what he is going to vote, that's news. . . . News of a new development in science is coupled with evidence. Opinion is not important, it's evidence. Opinion is cheap and can be misleading in science, but opinion in politics or public affairs is another matter."[8]

Certain professional practices that are part of journalism conflict with scientific expectations about appropriate styles of communication. For example, while both groups are committed to communicating truth, journalists must often omit the careful documentation and precautionary qualifications that scientists feel are necessary to accurately present their work. While scientists are socialized to qualify their findings, journalists may see qualifications as protective coloration. Furthermore, readability in the eyes of the journalist may be oversimplification to the scientist. Indeed, many accusations of inaccuracy are traceable to reporters' efforts to present complex material in a readable and appealing style.

Journalistic conventions intended to enhance audience appeal may also violate scientific norms. For example, to make abstract technical decisions more concrete, science writers often examine the personal choices of their technical informants ("Would you live at Love Canal?"), undermining the idea that technical decisions are based on depersonalized evidence. To create a human interest angle, journalists also personalize science; but the focus on individual accomplishments and the presentation of scientists as stars contradicts communal norms, which favor a collective image of science as an objective and disinterested profession. Similarly, to convince their editors about the newsworthiness of science and technology, journalists tend to emphasize the uniqueness of individual events (the "first" discovery, the "breakthrough"). Although many scientists actively contribute to the breakthrough syndrome, ideally they prefer to emphasize continuity and the cumulative nature of research.

The journalistic preoccupation with conflict and aberration, intended to attract the reader's interest, is a further source of strain. In covering disputes journalists tend to create polarities: technologies are either risky or they are safe. The quest for simplicity, drama, and brevity precludes the complex, nuanced positions that scientists prefer. But the polarized presentation of technical disputes also reflects journalists' norms of objectivity – their belief that verity can be established by balancing conflicting claims. This approach further contributes to strain, for objectivity to a scientist is based on the understanding that claims must be verified by empirical means – hardly by balancing opposing views.

Differences in the use of language add to the strain. The language of science is intended to be precise and instrumental. Scientists communicate for a purpose – to indicate regularities and aggregate patterns, and to provide technical data. In contrast, journalistic language has literary roots. Journalists will choose words for their richness of reference, their suggestiveness, their graphic appeal. They are likely to prefer a "toxic dump" to a "waste disposal facility."

In any discourse, language is organized to address the background and assumptions of the anticipated audience.[9] Scientists direct their professional communication to an audience that is trained in their discipline. They take for granted that their readers share certain assumptions and therefore will assimilate the information conveyed in predictable ways.[10] Journalists, on the other hand, write for diverse readers who will interpret the information in subjective terms, depending on their interests, objectives, and technical sophistication.[11] Thus, while scientists talk of aggregate data, reporters write of the immediate concerns of their readers: "Should I use saccharin? Will I be harmed?"[12]

Often words that have a special meaning in a scientific context will be interpreted differently by the lay reader. For example, the word "epidemic" has both technical and general connotations. Scientists use the word "epidemic" to describe a cluster of incidents greater than the normal background level of cases. If the background level is zero, then six cases are technically an epidemic. To the public or the journalist an epidemic implies thousands of cases, a rampantly spreading disease.

Confusion over the definition of "evidence" occurs among scientists as well as in the press, often confounding the discourse of risk disputes. Biostatisticians use the word "evidence" as a statistical concept. But for biomedical researchers the critical experiment may also be defined as evidence. Most lay people accept as credible evidence anecdotal information or individual cases. So, too, do journalists. Such differences frequently lead to misunderstanding. In reports about the health effects of exposure to toxic chemicals at Love Canal and Times Beach, for example, scientists and journalists held different assumptions – about the definition of credible evidence concerning the validity of animal tests, the neighborhood's habitability, and the adequacy of containment of the chemicals. Thus, when scientists described the health effects of dioxin with a cryptic "no evidence," meaning no statistically significant evidence, journalists interpreted their response as an effort to cover up the problem, since they knew of individual cases.

Similar linguistic confusion marked the dispute over the report written by the National Academy of Sciences panel on food additives, when the Academy's placement of saccharin in a "moderate risk category" was interpreted by the press to mean it was a "moderate cancer-causing agent."

Perhaps the most important source of strain between scientists and journalists lies in their differing views about the appropriate role of the press. Scientists often talk about the press as a conduit or pipeline, responsible simply for transmitting science to the public in a way that it can be easily understood. They expect to control this flow of information to the public as they do within their own domain. Confusing their special interests with general questions about the responsibility of the press, they are reluctant to tolerate independent analysis of the limits or flaws of science. They assume that the purpose of journalism is to convey a positive image that will promote science, and they see the press as a means of furthering scientific goals.

This view of journalism is reflected in scientists' complaints about the press and its effects on public attitudes. Scientists tend to attribute negative public attitudes about science and technology to problems of media communication, ultimately to journalists, who, they believe, distort the flow of information from scientists to the public. Alternatively, however, problems of scientific communication could as easily be attributed to the sources of information, to suppression of facts, to manipulation of information, or to overeager, promotional public relations.[13]

Many science journalists, of course, have a perception of their role that is not too different from that of scientists. They see their mission as one of recording "official history" – of elucidating and even eulogizing science. But there are some who are beginning to question their role as "self-appointed trumpets" for science and technology. Reacting to events such as Three Mile Island, Love Canal, or the Challenger explosion, and to the economic implications of large and costly scientific endeavors, they are beginning to suspect promotional hype about science and technology, and to raise probing questions in their interviews with scientists: Who pays? Who is responsible? What's in it for the public? What are the stakes?

While "gee whiz," "cosmic breakthrough" articles continue to dominate press coverage of science and technology, a number of journalists today want to probe scientific issues so that, as one journalist put it, "public expectations do not get out of control." "It is not enough for us to report the new discoveries or gadgetries; we must delve deeper into their effects on people and public policy." "I want to take some of the awesomeness out of science." "I want to create a better-informed citizenry able to deal with problems." These are among the goals expressed by at least some journalists today.

Efforts to improve the standards of science journalism are also apparent in the increased professionalization of the field. The professional organization of science writers is the National Association of Science Writers (NASW), founded in 1934 by a dozen veteran science writers[14] to "foster the dissemination of accurate scientific knowledge by the press of the nation in cooperation with scientific organizations and individual scientists."[15] Convinced of the public importance of science, these writers were concerned about the minimal level of press coverage. Struggling to convince their editors that science was news, the NASW founders hoped that professionalizing their specialty would enhance its visibility, recognition, and prestige. Moreover, a professional society could provide credentials to improve reporters' relations with scientists. Said David Dietz, one of the founders and Scripps Howard's science editor, "Membership in the NASW would be the kind of credential a scientist would appreciate."[16]

The NASW remained a very small organization until after World War II, when press coverage of science and technology began to expand. Reflecting this expansion, it grew from 113 members in 1950 to 413 members in 1960 and 830 in 1970. It has 1200 members today. The organization brings together prospective employers and science writers, encourages recruitment into the specialty, and facilitates contacts with reliable scientific sources of information. Its newsletter disseminates professional "gossip," information on NASW activities and members, and special articles of interest to the advancement of the profession.[17]

In 1960 NASW spawned an independent nonprofit organization, the Council for the Advancement of Science Writing (CASW), a group whose membership includes writers, editors, educators, and scientists. The council raises funds to support the development of curriculum in schools of journalism, as well as annual briefings (the "New Horizons in Science" program) in which distinguished scientists talk about current scientific advances. The CASW also supports regional science reporting workshops, a fellowship and internship program, and special courses for journalists on such topics as biostatistics.

Formal training in science is increasingly viewed as essential background for science journalists, and special courses have proliferated. There are about 43 programs in science journalism in 67 colleges and universities. Fourteen offer masters degrees in the field. These programs include science requirements, so that soon most younger reporters specializing in science writing will have some science background.

Other efforts have been initiated by scientists. In order to reduce mutual suspicion between scientists and journalists and to assure that timely and reliable information reaches the press, the Scientists' Institute for Public Information (SIPI) has organized a Media Resource Service (MRS). As a clearinghouse, MRS includes a computer file of about 20,000 scientists and engineers who have agreed to answer queries from reporters. It receives over 50 telephone calls a week from journalists who are seeking reliable sources on a very wide range of subjects that call for scientific information. When a crisis such as the Chernobyl accident or the space shuttle explosion occurs, hundreds of reporters will call. If the subject of inquiry is a disputed one, MRS routes journalists to several scientists selected to represent a spectrum of opinion. The organization also brings together scientists and journalists in round table discussions of controversial scientific issues such as animal experimentation or the disposal of toxic wastes. Their purpose is to enhance both the technical sophistication of journalists and the political sophistication of scientists involved in these disputes.[18]

The success of MRS suggests that a significant number of scientists are willing to work for better relations. But tension between science and journalism is likely to persist. For the differences between these two communities are fundamental – following, as they do, from the institutional constraints and external pressures that each profession must face. Improving the scientific knowledge of journalists and enhancing the political understanding of scientists are both important, but maintaining their differences is also essential if each community is to fulfill its unique social role.

Indeed, the tension can itself be healthy. If the popular press is to play its traditional role as a watchdog over major social and political institutions, if it is to mediate between science and the public and facilitate the public discourse about crucial policy issues, both scientists and journalists must accept and come to terms with an uneasy and often adversarial relationship. Scientists must restrain the promotional tendencies that lead to controls on information or to oversell, and they must open their doors to more probing investigation. And journalists on their part must try to convey understanding as well as information. It is not enough to merely react to scientific events, translating and elucidating them for popular consumption. To understand science and technology, readers need to know their context: the social, political, and economic implications of scientific activities, the nature of evidence underlying decisions, and the limits as well as the power of science as applied to human affairs.

Notes

1. This section on the Challenger accident was developed with the help of Susan Lindee, a Cornell University doctoral student.
2. *Houston Chronicle,* February 1, 1986; *Miami Herald,* February 23, 1986; and *New York Times,* February 5, 1986.
3. *New York Times,* March 20, 1986.
4. For a theoretical perspective on the hegemonic role of the press see Stuart Hall, "Culture, the Media and the Ideological Effect," in James Curran, M. Gurevitch, and J. Woollacott (eds.), *Mass Communication and Society* (Beverly Hills, Calif.: Sage, 1979), chap. 13.
5. See discussion in Robert Young, "Science as Culture," *Quarto,* December 1979, p. 7; and Langdon Winner, "Mythinformation," in Paul T. Durbin (ed.), *Research in Philosophy and Technology,* vol. 7 (Greenwich, Conn.: JAI Press, 1984), pp. 287–304.
6. There are, of course, notable exceptions. Daniel Greenberg, who publishes a newsletter entitled *Government and Science Report* and sometimes writes a science policy column for the *Wash-*

ington Post. The *New York Times* has hired several reporters from *Science* who have been writing some interpretive and critical articles. The news and comments section of *Science* also publishes critical commentary; however, *Science* is a specialized publication read mainly by scientists and science policy professionals.

7. L. E. Trachtman, "The Public Understanding of Science Effort," *Science, Technology and Human Values,* vol. 6, summer 1981, pp. 10–15.

8. Arnold Relman, "Special Report on Medicine and the Media," *P & S,* April 1982, p. 22.

9. See Erving Goffman, "Felicity's Condition," *American Journal of Sociology* 89, July 1983, pp. 1–53.

10. J. C. Pocock, "Ritual Language and Power," *Politics, Language and Times* (London: Methuen, 1970).

11. Richard Whitley, in Terry Shinn and Richard Whitley (eds.), *Expository Science* (Dordrecht: D. Reidel, 1985), points out that the many different nonscientific groups that constitute the audience for scientific information seek such information for specific purposes and assimilate it accordingly.

12. Quoted in Harold I. Sharlin, *EDB: A Case Study in the Communication of Health Risk,* (Washington, D.C.: Environmental Protection Agency, 1985).

13. See, for example, David Rubin, "What the President's Commission Learned about the Media," in T. Moss and D. Sills (eds.), *The Three Mile Island Accident* (New York: New York Academy of Sciences, 1981), pp. 95–106.

14. Howard Blakeslee (Associated Press), Ferry Colton (Associated Press), Watson Davis (Science Service), David Dietz (Scripps Howard), Victor Henderson *(Philadelphia Inquirer),* Thomas Henry *(Washington Star),* Waldemar Kaempffert *(New York Times),* Gobind Behari Lal (Hearst), William Laurence *(New York Times),* John O'Neill *(New York Herald Tribune),* Robert B. Potter *(American Weekly),* and Allen Shoenfield *(Detroit News).*

15. The charter is reproduced in Carolyn D. Hay, *A History of Science Writing in the United States,* master's thesis, Northwestern University, 1970.

16. Quoted in Hay, op. cit., p. 54.

17. Another professional newsletter, *Sciphers,* appeared in 1979, published by the Science Writing Educators Group at the University of Missouri.

18. A similar organization, the Center for Health Communication, has been formed at the Harvard School of Public Health to clarify and interpret health information for journalists. The communications office of the American Association for the Advancement of Science plays a similar role.

34
Due process for dissent

Frank von Hippel and Rosemary Chalk

On August 23, 1977, Glenn Greenwald, a chemist in the Public Utilities Department of the City of North Miami Beach, Florida, was called to 800 N.E. 182nd Terrace by a resident who complained that the water coming out of the tap tasted, smelled and looked peculiar. Greenwald agreed, and his tests showed that the water contained an abnormally small amount of free chlorine.

Laboratory analysis completed the next day revealed coliform bacteria in the water sample, and Greenwald decided that action was needed. Unable to find his supervisor, he asked his department head for an immediate flushing of the water distribution system in the area. Such flushings are accomplished by opening a neighborhood's fire hydrants, usually at night, but – trusting Greenwald's judgment – the department head ordered immediate action.

Greenwald's supervisor was irate when he learned of the flushing: he doubted that the action had been necessary and he feared that the residents of the affluent neighborhood where it had taken place might become unduly alarmed. He therefore told Greenwald that he should consider resigning if he could not work through channels.

But the contamination problem had not been solved by the flushing, and – in contrast to his superiors – Greenwald continued to believe that there was a potential health hazard. He wanted to continue tests and to advise residents of the house officially not to drink their tap water until further notice. His supervisors agreed to the continued testing but refused to authorize the official notice.

On the third day after Greenwald had first visited 800 N.E. 182nd Terrace, a teen-age resident asked him why the testing was still going on. Greenwald described the contamination problem, and suggested that the family not drink the water until the problem had been cleared up. Later that same day, however, when the chemist told his supervisor and department head of this conversation, he was summarily discharged for insubordination.

Greenwald promptly took his case to the city's Civil Service Board, which three months later upheld his firing. Then he took his case to the U.S. Department of Labor, appealing under the employee protection section within the Safe Drinking Water Act of 1974. The relevant part of this legislation states that "No employer may discharge any employee or otherwise discriminate against any employee . . . because the employee has . . . participated . . . in any . . . action to carry out the purposes of this title." The Labor Department's administrative law judge who heard the case agreed that Greenwald's discharge was indeed a violation of the Safe Drinking Water Act. The Judge went on to observe that

From Frank von Hippel, *Citizen Scientist* (New York: American Institute of Physics, 1991), pp. 40–42, 49–51.

"to punish or discriminate against a chemist for recommending a procedure which, at worst, would be a precautionary step, would be to demand that all subordinates at all levels remain silent if so instructed until harm has occurred or is imminent." But Greenwald's was an empty victory. Since his complaint had not been filed within a 30-day statutory limit contained in the Act, the judge had to recommend to the secretary of labor that the appeal be dismissed.

The dilemma of the employed professional

Glenn Greenwald's experience in exercising his professional responsibility highlights a serious dilemma for modern scientists and engineers. Early assessments of adverse impacts of technologies on society are often made by professionals working within large organizations, but such organizations are usually eager to avoid what they describe as "premature" disclosure of concerns which may later prove to be insubstantial. Since judgments of the importance of such concerns typically involve value judgments as well as professional judgments, there is often considerable room for disagreement.

The tension between an organization's concern to control its own affairs and the public's interest in knowing of possible hazards is mirrored in a tension of loyalties within its professional employees. Scientists and engineers are expected to be loyal to their organization's management, and they are so instructed by their professional societies. In its "Guidelines to Professional Employment for Engineers and Scientists," the Engineers Joint Council writes that:[1]

the professional employee must be loyal to the employer's objectives and contribute his creativity to these goals.

But – because of their special expertise – engineers and scientists also have special responsibilities for the protection of the public. The "Engineer's Code" of the National Society for Professional Engineers states, for example, that:

the engineer will have proper regard for the safety, health, and welfare of the public in the performance of his professional duties. If his engineering judgment is overruled by nontechnical authority, he will clearly point out the consequences. He will notify the proper authority of any observed conditions which endanger public safety and health. . . . He will regard his duty to the public welfare as paramount. . . .

Ordinarily these expectations do not conflict. Occasionally, however, as in Greenwald's case, an issue cannot be resolved within organizational channels, and an employee is moved by feelings of professional responsibility to make sure that his concerns are heard by higher levels of management or responsible outside individuals. If without authorization, an employee makes known his or her concerns to individuals outside the organization he or she is said to have "blown the whistle."

Though the public is clearly more receptive to criticism of large organizations today than formerly, such "whistle-blowing" remains an extreme and rather rare manifestation of the phenomenon of dissent. Many technical dissenters win an audience – and eventually a resolution of their concerns – within their organizations. And the vast majority of dissenters whose employers are unresponsive either do not feel strongly enough about their dissents or are too timid to blow whistles publicly. Unfortunately, most managements see dissenting employees as challenging the legitimacy of management's authority, and "whistle-blowing" is taken as a challenge to the credibility of the organization as a whole. Dissent therefore provides the ingredients for a confrontation between a technical expert and his or her management – an intimidating prospect for most employees. After finding that they are unable to obtain a full hearing for their concerns without antagonizing their supervisors, most dissenters therefore decide to "swallow the whistle" rather than blow it.

.   .   .

Protecting the public

In 1972 Ralph Nader remarked on the relatively small number of corporate employees who "go public" with their concerns about potential hazards caused by their company's activities:[2]

Corporate employees are among the first to know about industrial dumping of mercury or fluoride sludge into waterways, defectively designed automobiles, or undisclosed adverse effects of prescription drugs and pesticides. They are the first to grasp the technical capabilities to prevent existing product or pollution hazards. But they are very often the last to speak out.

Congress also noticed this anomaly and therefore started to include "employee protection sections" in federal safety and environmental laws. The sections are designed to protect from retaliation employees who bring to governmental attention hazards regulated under these laws. The protections include provision for a hearing before a Department of Labor examiner. In general, however, the Department has not been aggressive in enforcing the protections; it has even neglected to issue procedures or to notify employees of the existence of their protections. For example, Glenn Greenwald learned too late that he was required to file his complaint within 30 days after being fired.

In areas not covered by employee protection legislation, the courts have occasionally intervened on behalf of employees who were dismissed by private organizations for attempting to uphold the law. Thus, for example, the West Virginia Supreme Court ruled in favor of a bank employee who complained of retaliation for trying to bring his employer into compliance with state consumer protection laws. The Court found that "the rule that an employer has an absolute right to discharge at will an employee must be tempered by the principle that, where the employer's motivation for the discharge is to contravene some substantial public policy principle, then the employer may be liable to the employee for damages occasioned by the discharge."[3]

In the case of federal employees, Congress concluded that "whistle-blowers" need special protection. The case which was most effective in convincing Congress of this fact was that involving A. Ernest Fitzgerald, a cost analyst (civilian employee) for the Air Force.

In brief, after Fitzgerald disclosed to a congressional committee a $2 billion cost overrun on the C-5A military air transport development contract, his civil service tenure was found to have been granted by a computer error (an extremely rare discovery) and then

Secretary of the Air Force, Robert C. Seamans, abolished Fitzgerald's job as part of a "retrenchment program."[4] Fitzgerald spent years in the courts and hundreds of thousands of dollars in legal expenses before he was finally reinstated.

In response to such cases, Congress included a section in the Civil Service Reform Act of 1978 barring reprisals by federal officials against employees who disclose information "concerning the existence of any activity which the employee . . . reasonably believes constitutes . . . mismanagement . . . or a substantial and specific danger to the public health or safety." However, under the Reagan administration, the Office of Special Counsel, which was set up to protect whistle-blowers, turned down 99 percent of the cases that came to it because, in the special counsel's view, "most whistle-blowers are malcontents."[5]

Even with conscientious enforcement, no amount of due-process protection will protect dissenters who have become *persona non grata* in their organizations from subtle harassment. For such circumstances, in which work situations are made demoralizing by managements who want to be rid of employees but do not retaliate against them openly, additional remedies must be sought. One possibility suggested to us is a job placement service that would give a high priority to finding positions for conscientious dissenters whose employment situations have become untenable; such services could be operated by professional societies.

Dealing with the issues

Whatever due-process protections to dissenting professional employees are provided will have little value, however, unless they are imbedded in a process which deals effectively with the substance of the dissent. Those who would develop due-process procedures for dissenters must keep in mind the necessity for providing open and balanced reviews of the issues being raised. Too often review groups present unsubstantiated conclusions which cast doubt on the integrity of the review process and become the foci of new controversies.

Fortunately, to some extent the protection of conscientious dissent will facilitate the development of impartial reviews: if dissenters cannot be silenced, it becomes more difficult to ignore their concerns.

In summary, then, silencing dissenters as bearers of ill-tidings may seem in the short term to be the simplest way to deal with the difficult problems which they raise. But, in the longer term, enhancing the professionalism of scientists and engineers, and defending them when they follow its dictates, are vital to the welfare of our entire society.

References

1. Engineers Joint Council, *Guidelines to Professional Employment for Engineers and Scientists.* New York: E. J. C., August 1, 1978.
2. Nader, R.; Petkas, P.; and Blackwell, K. eds. *Whistle-Blowing.* New York: Grossman, 1972, p. 4.
3. For an overview of federal and state whistleblower protections, see Katz, S. M. and Kohn, M. D., *Antioch Law Journal* 4, Summer 1986: pp. 99–132.

4. *The Dismissal of A. Ernest Fitzgerald by the Department of Defense* (record of hearings on November 17 and 18, 1969). Washington, D.C.: U.S. GPO, 1969.
5. Devine, T. M. and Aplin, D. G., ''Abuse of Authority: The Office of the Special Counsel and Whistleblower Protection,'' *Antioch Law Journal* 4, Summer 1986: pp. 5–71.

35
Ethical issues in human genome research

Thomas H. Murray

Scientific research into human genetics has been a continuing source of intriguing, and at times formidable, ethical issues. The recent worldwide interest in a project to map and ultimately sequence the estimated three billion base pairs of the human genome has generated controversy over the effect such knowledge might have on us, as well as about the wisdom of investing so much research funding – an estimated $3 billion over 15 years in the United States alone – on such a targeted effort.

The latter question is largely a matter of science policy rather than ethics. As an investment of scarce resources, the genome initiative may not be the wisest at this time. Respectable arguments have been made on both sides of the question. But even if it is not the wisest way to spend research resources, that would not make it unethical. The confusion may lie in the profligate manner in which epithets such as unethical or immoral are used to tarnish a person or enterprise we do not like.

It is difficult to define ethics comprehensively. In general, the study of ethics is understood as the attempt to understand good and bad, right and wrong. Some writers distinguish between ethics and morality, drawing on the association between morality and mores – the accepted ways of a people, both stemming from the same Latin root. For these authors, ethics connotes systematic study whereas morality suggests the more common, everyday, rough-and-ready practical effort to do good and avoid evil. Many contemporary scholars use ethics and morality interchangeably, except in special circumstances where the meaning of the two diverge. They will be used as synonyms in this article.

Field of bioethics

A precise definition of ethics may be difficult to find, but there is considerable agreement on what is meant by bioethics. Bioethics is the study of ethical issues in medicine, health care, and the life sciences. As a formal field of study, bioethics is approximately 20 years old, although a few pioneering scholars were writing in the 1950s on issues that were later incorporated into bioethics. From its earliest stirrings, bioethics has paid considerable attention to human genetics, wrestling with such issues as prenatal genetic testing and abortion, genetic manipulation, and eugenics. In the past 5–10 years, the field of bioethics has grown rapidly, expanding the range of questions scholars ask, and even experiencing controversy over method (1).

From the standpoint of bioethics, research on the human genome presents no completely novel ethical questions, at least for now. That is partly because of the nature of new

From *FASEB Journal*, 1991, 5, pp. 55–60.

ethical questions, which typically are variants of ethical questions that scholars and others have wrestled with before. This embeddedness of questions in experience with analogous questions means that we do not have to invent every response totally anew, but rather can draw on the history of scholarly analysis that has come before. The acceleration of knowledge about human genetics promised by genome research assures that the ethical questions presented will be plentiful and significant. They may be grouped into three categories: *1)* the possibility of greatly increased genetic information about individuals and populations; *2)* the manipulation of human genotypes and phenotypes; and *3)* challenges to our understanding of ourselves, individually and collectively.

Uses and misuses of genetic information

Genome research will allow us to learn a great deal about the genetic makeup of individuals, especially their propensities toward diseases. In many instances, our powers to predict the likelihood (or in some cases certainty) of disease will come years or decades before any effective treatment for the disease is available. Nancy Wexler, known for her work on Huntington's disease, has dubbed this genetic prophecy (2).

Huntington's disease

Huntington's disease is inherited in an autosomal dominant manner. The first symptoms usually appear in the victims' 30s or 40s, after they have had an opportunity to have children. The disease is progressive and invariably fatal, causing uncontrolled movements and dementia. The gene has not yet been discovered, but markers close to it have been found, at a recombination frequency of as little as 1%, permitting an indirect test (linkage analysis) for the defective allele in families with adequate and informative DNA from multiple members. Presymptomatic testing has been made available for people at risk of Huntington's disease, but only a fraction of those eligible have chosen to be tested (3).

As dramatically as any disease, presymptomatic testing for Huntington's disease illustrates the psychological dynamics and ethical difficulties likely to arise with testing for genetic predisposition (4). Until recently, testing for Huntington's disease had taken place only under research protocols that included substantial counseling in advance of the actual genetic testing, as well as follow-up supportive counseling. Experience has shown that the process of explaining genetic risks is complex; understanding often comes only slowly and painfully, the psychological burdens of genetic disease can be massive, and not everyone wants to know his or her own risk. Using linkage analysis poses additional problems. It relies on DNA samples from affected and unaffected relatives of the person wishing to know. The tests may yield information about the risks of other family members who may not wish to know their own status; family members may not wish to participate, which yields conflict.

Huntington's disease is rare, with few if any new mutations. Individuals at risk are likely to know that they are. On the other hand, genetic testing for recessive diseases with high prevalence of carriers in identifiable populations is likely to affect many. Cystic fibrosis (CF)* is one such example.

***

* Abbreviations: CF, cystic fibrosis; PKU, phenylketone urea; OTA, U.S. Congress Office of Technology Assessment; TIL, tumor infiltrating lymphocytes; hGH, human growth hormone; EPO, erythropoietin.

Cystic fibrosis and carrier screening

The gene that causes CF has been identified, and the most frequent variant has been cloned (5). It appears that CF can be caused by a variety of mutant alleles for the gene that sits on the long arm of chromosome 7. The most common mutant allele is known as ΔF508. It accounts for approximately 68% of known CF-inducing chromosomes. Other alleles can also cause CF, but are not yet well-characterized.

CF occurs in approximately 1 of every 2500 live births in white populations, which implies (for an autosomal recessive disease) a carrier frequency of roughly 1 in 25. The potential market in the U.S. alone for a screening test is enormous. The prospect of such widespread screening for CF carriers provokes ethical concerns.

First there are questions of accuracy. Would the test correctly identify those who carry a CF gene as well as those who do not? For a test that would pick up 75% of individuals carrying a CF gene, one-quarter of the carriers would be missed. For those planning to have a child, only 56% of couples at risk would have both partners identified as carriers (6). A person whose test results are negative (with a test of the same sensitivity) would have his or her probability of being a carrier reduced from 1 in 25 to 1 in 99 – better odds, but still not certain.

A second set of concerns is prompted by the history of population screening for such recessive disorders as sickle cell trait and phenylketone urea (PKU). Screening programs were often adopted without careful planning, and without provision for appropriate follow-up to assure that the programs' purposes would be achieved. Carrier screening programs sometimes have resulted in misunderstanding, stigmatization of carriers, and other problems. Properly designed screening programs would avoid such outcomes.

A crucial part of any acceptable screening program would be adequate explanatory and supportive counseling. Public misinformation about genetics is substantial. Many physicians do not have a good grasp of genetics (7). One recent study estimated the counseling requirements of a population screening program for CF carriers. Using modest estimates of the counseling time needed by unaffected and affected couples, the authors concluded that 651,000 hours would be required. In light of the number of certified genetic counselors (450) and clinical geneticists (500) in the U.S., the supply appears grossly inadequate to meet the expected demand (6).

At present, CF presents a volatile mixture pushing toward increased testing – enthusiasm for scientific breakthroughs, anxious prospective parents, and commercial enterprises eager to find profitable outlets for their biotechnologic skills. Just as we may hope that the development of CF carrier screening benefits from the history of other genetic screening efforts, so we may also hope that future screening programs for genetic diseases that will be discovered in genome research will benefit from our experience with CF screening. Professional bodies are beginning to speak out in favor of responsible positions. The American Society of Human Genetics, for example, has stated recently that routine carrier screening is not appropriate (8).

Genetic testing for presymptomatic disease and carrier screening are only two of the uses to which knowledge gained in the Human Genome Initiative might be put. Prenatal screening for genetic disease is another; it stirs controversy because one of the choices upon finding that a fetus is afflicted with genetic disease is abortion. Much scholarship has been devoted to the ethics of abortion, with no resolution of the political battle (9, 10).

These three forms of screening are done, at least purportedly, for the benefit of the individual being screened. New uses of genetic tests are evoking controversy. In these proposed uses, the test is being done not for the good of the person being tested, but rather for some organization – for example, a prospective employer or insurer.

Genetic testing in the workplace

In 1938, the geneticist J. B. S. Haldane observed that not all workers exposed to a particular occupational hazard became symptomatic. He postulated that the difference in response to toxic exposures was at least in part genetically determined. If we could assure that individuals who were genetically susceptible to the disease were steered to other occupations, Haldane reasoned, we could reduce the number of people who became ill (11). Workplace genetic screening was justified by its consequences for public health. In Haldane's time, the technology to do genetic screening was not available. But his rationale for workplace genetic screening was revivified in the 1960s and 1970s with suggestions that new screening techniques might make it possible to put his idea into practice (12).

The early proponents of workplace genetic screening did not foresee the political, economic, and ethical complexities their idea would later reveal. The first publicized case of such screening was by a U.S. corporation. A plant owned by this company screened for sickle cell trait among its black workers. The company maintains that the screening was purely voluntary, initiated at the request of an organization of black employees, and that the results were not used in hiring or placement decisions. The journalist who reported the story claims otherwise (13).

Debate about the ethics of workplace genetic testing has focused on the purposes for which such tests might be used. Four purposes have been identified: diagnosis, research, information, and exclusion (14). Genetic tests, like many other procedures, can be helpful in diagnosis and research. Their use in those contexts is governed by the ethics of medical diagnosis and treatment and the ethics of research with human subjects. No novel moral dilemmas attend the use of genetic tests for those purposes.

Genetic tests may also be used before hiring or placing a particular worker to uncover a genetic susceptibility believed to put the individual at greater risk of occupational disease associated with hazards in that workplace. The crucial distinction here is between giving the tests voluntarily, with the information given to the worker who then decides whether to accept any additional risk, or compelling workers to take the tests and using the results to exclude workers who may have genetic susceptibilities.

A program of voluntary testing to inform workers of their risks is ethically defensible. In general, we believe that the individuals affected are the ones with the greatest ethical right to decide whether or not to accept risks. There are some risks that are so nearly certain to occur and cause grievous harm that we do limit choices for individuals. Except for such circumstances we usually allow competent adults to decide for themselves what risks are acceptable to them.

With presymptomatic genetic testing, a program of workplace genetic testing should include effective education and counseling to prevent misunderstanding of the results and to deal with emotional responses to learning that one has genetic risks. A carefully designed program of workplace genetic testing to inform workers, leaving the choice up to individual workers about whether to accept risks, does not confront any insurmountable ethical barriers. The same cannot be said for compelled genetic testing.

Compulsory genetic testing, leading to possible exclusion from jobs, has been controversial. Critics argue that it violates deeply held notions of individual autonomy and could be used in socially undesirable ways. For example, testing for sickle cell anemia followed by exclusion of those with the trait would effectively exclude one of every eight black job candidates in the U.S. Where workers are plentiful, employers might prefer to screen out susceptible workers rather than invest in equipment to reduce exposure to hazards. The prospect of such undesirable effects, along with our respect for individual liberty and choice, make compulsory workplace genetic testing ethically problematic.

The U.S. Congress Office of Technology Assessment (OTA) studied workplace genetic screening in the early 1980s (15). The OTA report concluded that the present state of genetic testing and knowledge about genetic contributions to workplace disease did not justify screening employees for genetic susceptibility. A survey reported in the same study shows some use of genetic tests by U.S. employers, but ambiguities in the report make it impossible to know if the tests were used for legitimate and unproblematic purposes, such as diagnosing the illness of an employee or for the controversial purpose of excluding so-called hypersusceptibles. The OTA is writing another report on genetic testing in the workplace to be released in the fall of 1990.

From reducing illness to reducing cost

The most important movement in the ethics of workplace genetic testing has been away from the original vision of a public health measure to screening as a way of reducing illness-related costs with no effect on the overall incidence of disease.

Although there is still little evidence that workplace genetic screening could identify individuals with increased risks of workplace-related disease, there is increasing reason to believe that genetic screening for common diseases such as arterial disease (including coronary disease), stroke, and cancer may soon be possible. Other disabling diseases, including mental diseases such as depression and schizophrenia, might also become the targets of genetic screening. Employers might find such tests attractive ways to save money by screening prospective employees and hiring those without evidence of genetic susceptibilities to disease.

Employee illness, at least in the U.S., costs employers money. With health insurance costs becoming an increasingly larger proportion of employers' expenses, employers are looking for ways to diminish health-related costs including health insurance, disability insurance, the cost of lost productivity from ill workers, and the cost of training replacement workers for skilled positions.

The combination of increased employer concerns about the costs of illness and the prospect of genetic tests for predisposition to common, costly diseases are fertile ground for the use of such tests to screen workers.

The ethics of genetic screening for non-workplace-related disease differ in part from genetic screening for workplace-related disease. Working in the particular workplace does not put the worker at an increased risk; the disease to which the person may be susceptible is not related to the workplace. The information to be gained from such tests is not relevant to the individual's choice of whether to work in that environment, although it might be relevant to other life choices, such as diet, exercise, and other health-related behavior. Being denied a job because of predisposition to a non-workplace-related disease is as great an affront to an individual's liberty as a denial for predisposition to a workplace-related disease. But here there is no compensating reduction in risk to the individuals denied employment nor is there any public health benefit; those who will die from heart disease or cancer will still die from it – unemployed and possibly unemployable.

Employers are not the only ones likely to be interested in people's predisposition to common disabling and killing diseases. Companies selling life, disability, or health insurance are also interested in genetic tests.

Genetic testing in insurance

Insurance works on the principle of sharing risk. When the risk is equally uncertain to all, then all can be asked to contribute equally to the insurance pool. Not all individuals have the same risk of dying, for example. The older one is (beyond early childhood), the greater the risk of death. Older people are charged more for the same amount of life insurance than younger people. Some occupations are riskier than others. Test pilots pay more for life insurance than accountants. None of this seems unfair. The ethics of discriminating according to genetic predisposition, on the other hand, seems much more ethically complex.

Insurance companies have begun to think about what to do with tests for genetic predisposition to disease (16). As the authors of an industry-sponsored report see it, two factors may force insurers to use genetic tests. First, once such tests become available in medical practice, individuals can be tested privately to learn whether they have enhanced risks of disease. People who learn they have higher risks are more likely to buy insurance and are more likely to buy larger amounts. In the insurance industry, this phenomenon is known as adverse selection – the tendency to purchase insurance when one expects to file a claim. Second, competition among insurance companies will tend to drive companies toward screening for predisposition. If one company begins using such tests, it would be able to offer lower rates to individuals who do not have genetic predisposition to disease and higher rates to those with such predispositions. Individuals offered the lower rates are more likely to purchase insurance from that company, whereas the ones with genetic predisposition to disease will seek insurance from another company that does not do genetic testing. The latter company will either have to raise its rates (to avoid bankruptcy) or it will also have to use genetic tests.

Genetic manipulation

Probably the most widely discussed and fear-inspiring use of genetic science is genetic manipulation, especially gene therapy. Other uses of genetics to manipulate human physique, physiology, or behavior may be equally significant and raise important ethical issues of their own.

Gene therapy

Many human diseases are caused by abnormal alleles. The idea that the most effective way to correct such genetic deficiencies is by replacing, correcting, or supplementing the malfunctioning gene has been discussed for almost two decades, but has only recently become technically plausible (17). The ethics of gene therapy have been discussed exhaustively. Indeed, there may be no other manifestation of modern genetics that has received such thorough ethical examination or that must pass through such extensive scientific and ethical review. In June of 1980 the general secretaries of the three largest religious bodies in the U.S. wrote to the President expressing concern about genetic manipulation. Partly in response to this concern, a U.S. Presidential Commission issued a report (18), as did an office of the U.S. Congress (19).

In the U.S., research on gene therapy funded by the National Institutes of Health must pass multiple levels of review, including a special subcommittee of the Recombinant DNA Advisory Committee. The subcommittee has issued several revisions of a "Points to Consider" document, outlining the many scientific and ethical considerations that must be satisfied before a research protocol could be approved (20).

Scholarly discussion of the ethics of human gene therapy has reached a high level of sophistication, with both ethicists (21) and scientists (22) making substantive contributions. The most important question in the debate over the ethics of gene therapy is whether gene therapy is ethically distinctive from other forms of medical therapy. There are questions about such a novel and potentially risky therapy – for example, how to obtain genuine informed consent from patients in desperate circumstances. But these kinds of questions are not decisively different for gene therapy than for other highly innovative therapies for devastating diseases. The main ethically significant difference between gene therapy and other therapies is the potential for the changes wrought in an individual by gene therapy to be passed onto offspring of the treated person. Other therapies affect directly only the life of the particular individual being treated. The prospect of intentional genetic changes being passed on indefinitely struck most commentators as distinctive and significant for at least two reasons. First, the principle of informed consent that justifies many of the risks of medical experimentation cannot apply in any simple way to the descendants of subjects of gene therapy research. These persons were not yet conceived at the time of the research, and hence cannot be said to consent to risks to their own genome. Second, whatever harm might be caused by gene therapy might be magnified manyfold if it were passed onto future generations rather than dying out with the subjects of the current research.

Considerations such as these led to a crucial distinction in the ethics of gene therapy research: germ-line vs. somatic cell line gene therapy. Only genetic alterations in germ-line cells have the potential to be passed on to future persons. Genetic changes in a person's somatic cells will die with that individual. Somatic cell gene therapy, then, to the extent that it is reliably confined to somatic cells only, is ethically analogous to other novel medical therapies. The ethically distinctive element of gene therapy is only characteristic of germ-line manipulation.

Most scholars agree that research on somatic cell gene therapy is ethically defensible with the usual safeguards for research with human beings. There is less consensus about germ-line therapy. Some argue that there is no conclusive argument against germ-line gene therapy, and that the prospect of curing genetic disease not merely for the person under treatment but for all of his or her descendants could justify research. However, scholars and public bodies agree that it is better to exercise caution and not engage in any germ-line gene therapy research at this time. Further debate over the ethics of germ-line gene therapy is likely.

The distinctiveness of germ-line gene therapy can be questioned. Of course, other medical therapies or other human interventions can have genetic consequences for future generations. Mutagenic drugs, such as those often used in cancer treatment, and radiation therapy cause genetic changes, as do many environmental or occupational exposures. Such changes, if they are incorporated stably into germ-line cells, can be passed on to future generations. Even standard, nonmutagenic therapies have genetic consequences for populations when they permit the survival and reproduction of individuals who would otherwise have perished or who did not have children. Future discussions will help to clarify the meaning and significance of the distinction between germ-line and somatic cell gene therapy.

Other uses of recombinant DNA in humans

Ironically, the first approved experiment using recombinant DNA in humans was not gene therapy per se but involved labeling patients' tumor infiltrating lymphoyctes (TIL cells) with a gene that conferred resistance to neomycin. This biochemical flag allowed researchers to track the survival and migration of cells believed to fight the advanced melanoma from which these individuals suffered (23). The first true approved gene therapy experiment is just now under way (24). Genetic engineering techniques are also being developed that might enhance the cancer-fighting properties of cells such as TILs.

Modifying people with biotechnology

Gene therapy may have attracted most of the public's attention, but other applications of new genetic knowledge that might be generated by the genome project could have more immediate and wider impact. The ability to clone a human gene, incorporate it into a microorganism or mammalian cell line, and produce and purify the gene product can have substantial ethical consequences. Human growth hormone (hGH) is now produced this way; before the introduction of biosynthetic hGH the only supply was from pituitaries of human cadavers. hGH was scarce; its only major therapeutic use was for hGH-deficient pituitary dwarfs.

Once biosynthetic hGH became available, the temptation to use it to make non-hGH-deficient children taller and to gain the competitive advantage that height gives in certain cultures (including the U.S.) became strong, and anecdotal reports of parents trying to obtain it for their normal children circulated. Thus far, misuse has been deterred by a restrictive policy that makes hGH available only through certain hospital pharmacies, even though it is not a drug whose sale is restricted by law. Recent research, however, indicating that hGH may mitigate or reverse some of the effects of aging in individuals who have low levels of endogenous hGH may presage more uses for hGH that will make the current method of control unworkable. Should hGH become widely available for indications other than short stature, we may see complex ethical problems as the knowledgeable, wealthy, and adventurous seek it for their children (25).

In a similar manner, although for a more restricted group, another fruit of genetic research is having unintended social and ethical consequences. Biosynthetic erythropoietin (EPO) may offer enormous benefit to hundreds of thousands of people suffering from chronic anemia, such as those undergoing hemodialysis for treatment of end-stage renal disease. EPO induces the production of erythrocytes and can increase the oxygen-carrying capacity of the blood. Athletes engaged in sports requiring endurance such as distance running, skating, skiing, or cycling may gain a competitive advantage from EPO comparable to that obtained from blood doping – autologous or homologous blood infusion to raise the blood's ability to carry oxygen to rapidly metabolizing tissue. Using blood doping or performance-enhancing drugs to gain a competitive advantage is ethically suspect and prohibited by many sports authorities (26). The organizations that oversee sports, such as the International Olympic Committee, have classified EPO as a performance-enhancing drug and are seeking ways to discourage its use among competitive athletes.

hGH and EPO are only among the first of the fruits of contemporary genetics that will pose difficult ethical problems as people seek to use them not to treat disease but for nontherapeutic purposes.

Challenges to our self-understanding

There is a tendency in bioethics, as in other fields, to focus on the immediate, practical dilemmas posed by new developments. It may be that the most important challenges posed by the human genome project will not be the pragmatic concerns discussed thus far, but will have to do with the way we understand ourselves, our nature and significance, and our connections with our ancestors and descendants.

One manifestation of the genome initiative will be increased understanding of our genetic similarity with other species. Scientists have tried to estimate DNA homology between humans and other primates to clarify evolutionary relationships among primate species (27). These early efforts to gauge genetic similarity seem to indicate that human DNA is strikingly similar to that of chimpanzees, at least as assessed by the relatively crude measures thus far available. Human DNA appears to be related to more distant species as well. Comparisons of synteny between mouse and human chromosomes show a substantial degree of correspondence, which suggests an evolutionary relationship, coincidentally giving researchers clues to where in the genome to search for a particular gene if its homolog has been found in mice (or humans) (28).

Evidence of our genetic relationship with other species is nothing more than additional confirmation of the theory of evolution. On the other hand, if more and more sophisticated tests of similarity continue to show how much like other species we are, genetically speaking, we may reevaluate not only our molecular but also our moral relationship with nonhuman forms of life.

Genetics as explanation/excuse?

One of the most common ethical and legal questions is whether and to what extent a person is responsible for something. We ask if the individual who committed a violent act was responsible for his behavior – morally blameworthy, legally culpable. We ask if the inventor was responsible for the new device (credit rather than blame being at stake here), the scientist for the discovery, the author for the idea, style, and specific words.

We also ask about responsibility for larger issues than discrete acts or inventions. We question whether the overweight person is responsible for his or her obesity, and by extension, for the illnesses to which obesity is a contributing factor, and perhaps for the expense of caring for those illnesses. We ask whether alcoholics are responsible for their addiction and for the consequences of acts committed while they were inebriated.

On an even broader level, we ask whether groups who do especially well (or especially poorly) in various social and economic realms experience the outcomes they do because of some intrinsic traits and abilities or because of lack of opportunity.

Genetics frequently provides an explanation or excuse for individual behaviors or traits, as well as for group differences. The genome project will enhance the tendency to give genetic explanations for individual and group differences in two ways. First, research will suggest genetic correlates for a wide range of human traits and behavior. Some may prove to be spurious, but others will withstand scrutiny. Whenever such a genetic correlate is suggested for some ethically, legally, or economically consequential outcome, there will be a temptation to explain it as fundamentally – that is exclusively or exhaustively – genetic, and hence outside the individual's responsibility or capacity to control. Researchers have recently reported a link between a dopamine receptor gene and alcoholism (29). Others have warned against attributing too much significance to this finding (30).

Second, in the initial rush of findings of genetic connections to important human traits and behavior, both scientists and the public may become too eager to embrace genetic explanations for a vast range of ethically significant phenomena. The phenomena in question may range from illness, including mental illness, addiction, occupational and environmental illness, to the educational and occupational attainments of different racial and ethnic groups.

History is rich with examples of scientific perspectives used inappropriately for political purposes. Frequently, genetic or earlier hereditarian theories have been the subject of such misuse. The first large-scale intelligence testing program in the U.S. was the Army alpha program, which was designed to screen incoming recruits according to their intellectual capacities. Certain groups did not fare well on the test, including immigrants from southern Europe. Because the results conveniently fit the beliefs of those overseeing the testing, they accepted the tests as valid measures of intrinsic ability rather than as the profoundly culture-bound instruments they were. They also overlooked the fact that many of these immigrants spoke English poorly or not at all: the test was in English.

In recent decades the debate has been over the heritability of intelligence and the reason for disparities in IQ test scores among racial and ethnic groups (31). The political consequences of such debates are clear: if educational and economic inequalities are caused by social inequities, then society has an obligation to remedy those inequities; if, on the other hand, the inequalities in outcome are a function of (which in political debate can rapidly be translated into determined by) inherited differences, then we do not have to be so troubled, or worry about our own unjust actions.

The questions raised here also have important, in some instances profoundly important, legal ramifications that must be thoroughly explored. As George Annas has written:

Although we are utterly unprepared to deal with issues of mandatory screening, confidentiality, privacy, and discrimination, we will likely tell ourselves that we have already dealt with them well . . . (p. 20) (32).

The point here is not that we should ignore the influence of genetics on human affairs. Scientists should be the last people to abandon evidence in favor of sentimental, comforting illusion. Lucidity demands that we confront the truth as it is. Rather, we must learn not to overinterpret what we find. We must learn how to communicate effectively among ourselves and with the public about the limits of our knowledge.

Last, we must acknowledge the limited ethical and political significance of our genetic knowledge. When the founders of the United States wrote that all men (all people) are created equal, they did not mean this as a statement of biological fact, but as an ethical, legal, and political proclamation: before the collectivity of the state, all persons must be regarded as equal – each due equal respect, equal liberty, and equal protection, among other fundamental rights. The sciences of inequality, with genetics at the forefront, will force us to reinterpret what equal treatment and equal regard mean in an enormous range of contexts. But they need not threaten the ethical core of that commitment.

References

1. Jonsen, A. R., and Toulmin, S. (1988) *The Abuse of Casuistry: A History of Moral Reasoning.* University of California, Berkeley
2. Wexler, N. S. (1989) The oracle of DNA. In *Molecular Genetics in Diseases of Brain, Nerve, and Muscle* (Rowland, L. P., Wood, D. S., Schon, E. S., and DiMauro, S., eds) Oxford University Press, New York
3. Jenkins, J. B., and Conneally, P. M. (1989) The paradigm of Huntington disease. *Am J. Hum. Genet.* **45,** 169–175
4. Bird, S. J. (1985) Presymptomatic testing for Huntington's disease. *JAMA* **253,** 3286–3291
5. Rommens, J. M., Ianuzzi, M. C., Kerem, B., Drumm, M. L., Melmer. G., Dean, M., Rozmahel, R., Cole, J. L., Kennedy, D., Hidaka, N., Zsiga, M., Buchwald, M., Riordan, J. R., Tsui, L.-C., and Collins, F. S. (1989) Identification of the cystic fibrosis gene: chromosome walking and jumping. *Science* **245,** 1059–1065
6. Wilfond, B. S., and Fost, N. (1990) The cystic fibrosis gene: medical and social implications for heterozygote detection. *JAMA* **263,** 2777–2783
7. Holtzman, N. A. (1978) Rare diseases, common problems: recognition and management. *Pediatrics* **62,** 1056–1060
8. Caskey, C. T., Kaback, M. M., and Beaudet, A. L. (1990) The American Society of Human Genetics statement on cystic fibrosis. *Am. J. Hum. Genet.* **46,** 393
9. Callahan, D. (1970) *Abortion: Law, Choice and Morality.* Macmillan, New York
10. Luker, K. (1984) *Abortion and the Politics of Motherhood.* University of California, Berkeley
11. Haldane, J. B. S. (1938) *Heredity and Politics.* Allen and Unwin, London
12. Stokinger, H. E., and Mountain, J. T. (1963) Tests for hypersusceptibility to hemolytic chemicals. *Arch. Environ. Hlth.* **6,** 57–64
13. Severo, R. (1980) Screening of blacks by DuPont sharpens debate on genetic tests. *New York Times.* 4 February, p. 1
14. Murray, T. H. (1983) Warning: screening workers for genetic risk. *Hastings Center Rep.* **13,** (Feb.) 5–8
15. United States Congress Office of Technology Assessment. (1983) *The role of genetic testing in the prevention of occupational disease.* U.S. Government Printing Office, Washington, D.C.
16. Genetic Testing Committee to the Medical Section of the American Council of Life Insurance (1989) *The potential role of genetic testing in risk classification.* American Council of Life Insurance, Washington, D.C.
17. Anderson, W. F. (1984) Prospects for human gene therapy *Science* **226,** 401–409
18. President's Commission for the Study of Ethical Problems in Medicine and Biomedical and Behavioral Research. (1982) *Splicing life: the social and ethical issues of genetic engineering with human beings.* U.S. Government Printing Office, Washington, D.C.
19. U.S. Congress Office of Technology Assessment. (1984) *Human gene therapy – a background paper.* Washington, D.C. OTA-BP-BA–32

20. Human gene therapy subcommittee, NIH recombinant DNA advisory committee. (1989) Points to consider in the design and submission of protocols for the transfer of recombinant DNA into human subjects. National Institutes of Health. Bethesda, Maryland

21. Walters, L. (1986) The ethics of human gene therapy. *Nature (London)* **320**, 225–227

22. Anderson, W. F. (1985) Human gene therapy: scientific and ethical considerations. *J. Med. Philos.* **10**, 275–291

23. Culliton, B. J. (1989) Gene test begins. *Science* **244**, 913

24. Marwick, C. Preliminary results may open door to gene therapy just a bit wider. *JAMA* **262**, 1909

25. Murray, T. H. (1987) The growing danger from gene-spliced hormones. *Discover* **8**, 88–92

26. Murray, T. H. (1983) The coercive power of drugs in sports. *Hastings Center Rep.* (Aug) **13**, 24–30

27. Koop, B. F., Goodman, M., Xu, P., Chan, K., and Slightom J. L. (1986) Primate n-globin DNA sequences and man's place among the great apes. *Nature (London)* **319**, 234–238

28. McKusick, V. A. (1990) *Mendelian Inheritance in Man,* 8th Ed. Johns Hopkins University Press, Baltimore

29. Blum, K., Noble, E. P., Sheridan, P. J., Montgomery, A., Ritchie, T., Jagadeeswaran, P., Nogami, H., Briggs, A. H., and Cohn, J. B. (1990) Allelic association of human dopamine D receptor gene in alcoholism. *JAMA* **263**, 2055–2060

30. Gordis, E., Tabakoff, B., Goldman, D., and Berg, K. (1990) Finding the gene(s) for alcoholism. *JAMA* **263**, 2094–2095

31. Jensen, A. R. (1973) *Educability and Group Differences.* Harper and Row, New York

32. Annas, G. (1989) Who's afraid of the human genome? *Hastings Center Rep* **19**, (July/August) 19–21

QUESTIONS FOR DISCUSSION

1. Why is the public image of the researcher so often the stark contrast between the "mad scientist" and the "brilliant, technological savior"? What effect do these stereotypes have on real scientists and their work?

2. What role do bench scientists have in setting the standards for children's education in their disciplines? What are the possible consequences of scientific illiteracy for science and society?

3. What responsibility do researchers in different fields have to ensure that the public understands their work? Why is such education useful for society and scientists alike?

RECOMMENDED SUPPLEMENTAL READING

"Scientific Societies and Public Responsibilities," Doris K. Miller, in *The Social Responsibility of Scientists, Annals of the New York Academy of Sciences,* 1971, 196, pp. 247–255.

"Whistleblowing and Leaks," Sissela Bok, in *Secrets: An Ethical Examination of Concealment and Revelation,* New York, Pantheon Books, 1984, pp. 210–229.

Science, Technology, and Society, Rosemary Chalk (ed.), Washington, DC: American Association for the Advancement of Science, 1988.

"Man-made Death: A Neglected Mortality," Richard Rhodes, *Journal of the American Medical Association,* 1988, 260, pp. 686–687.